ENOUGH

A Memoir

REBECCA BRICKER

Folio&Leaf

To beautiful Giverny,
a place I'll always love

To Bruges,
the lovely fairy-tale city that stole my heart

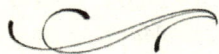

ALSO BY REBECCA BRICKER

By Chance

The Sound of His Voice

The Secret of Marie
Le Secret de Marie (French edition)

Not a True Story

Tales from Tavanti:
An American Woman's Mid-Life Adventure in Italy

Chapter 1

Our romance began slowly, as some love affairs do.

When it escalated into something amazingly wonderful, my Frenchman and I had already known each other a few years.

It was an unlikely romance, really. But then, unlikeliness often makes a love story more compelling. And when you're a main character in an unlikely love story, you tend to get swept up in the breathless drama of it and can easily ignore the warning signs that you should have paid attention to.

An early warning in this love affair came during the first hour of my maiden visit to the place that would become my new home. My Frenchman, whose name is Henri, had invited me to spend Easter week with him at his apartment in Giverny, the village in the Normandy countryside made famous by Claude Monet.

A couple of months earlier, Henri had shown me a few photos of his place and had sketched a floor plan, which turned out to be a tad inaccurate. I had ignored the clutter in the pictures and optimistically clung to high hopes.

On my arrival day, he had met me at Charles de Gaulle Airport near Paris and whisked me off to Giverny's historic Hôtel Baudy for lunch. We lingered, enjoying each other's company and the bright prospects of what was to come. We had found LOVE in our golden years. (I was then 63 and he was 74.) We couldn't believe our good fortune.

I was a happy new bride-without-a-marriage-certificate, which turned out to be a good thing, in retrospect. My Frenchman and I were clear about two things: no marriage and no co-mingling of funds, except that we would share the rent, utilities and the expense of his housekeeper at *chez nous*.

When we arrived at his apartment, a short distance from the Baudy, he parked at the front door and led me inside. I tried very hard not to dwell on the filthy towel that had been stuffed in the cat entrance at the bottom of the front door or the faded fabric that had been nailed over the door's ten windowpanes. Nailed. In the jumble of furniture that crowded a large living-dining area, I took note of the giant harmonium he said had come from a monastery. I had enjoyed playing my grandmother's old pump organ as a girl. Maybe the harmonium and I would become friends.

Beyond the windows at the far end of the room, I could see waves of corrugated plastic sheets that formed a roof where years of baked-on dirt and grime had collected. I walked over to the windows (which had no curtains, hung or nailed) and saw, below, the main hall of my Frenchman's museum – his pride and joy – which housed a vast collection of antique machinery and steam engines from around the world. Henri calls himself the museum's "curator," but as I soon learned, he is the museum's lifeblood and soul.

Henri showed me the kitchen, which seemed frozen in time with its 25-year-old fridge and a "Lady Europa" dishwasher that was about the same age. We sat down on rickety barstools at a long butcher's table that he had painstakingly refinished. His petite pharmacy of vitamins and meds sat at one end, along with a vintage chrome-plated toaster and matching teakettle. He opened the lid before switching on the kettle and removed a couple of eggs that he had hard-boiled that morning.

"You boil eggs in your kettle?" I asked.

"*Pourquois pas?*" he said. Why not, indeed.

I noticed an empty, white-china gravy boat sitting outside, on the kitchen window ledge, but decided that question could wait until another day.

We didn't linger over our tea. He was eager to show me the new bed he had purchased for us.

Actually, I knew the bed was intended for me. During our six-month courtship, we reluctantly had decided that we would need separate bedrooms because of our snoring issues. I'm a soft sporadic snorer, with occasional loud snorts that wake him up. He's a volcanic snorer who rocks the walls and my eardrums with every breath. On our "honeymoon" trip to Malta, earplugs and a pillow over my head were no help. My best friend in the middle of those nights was Goddess Ativana (I think of her, in my version of modern-day mythology, as the Sand Man's mistress).

I sat down on the edge of the new bed. "It's memory foam," I said, running my hand over the mattress. I hate memory-foam mattresses. They're hot and you can't change positions easily. I knew it had been an expensive purchase, so I said nothing more.

We got under the sheets, the color of charcoal, and we gave that memory foam something to remember.

In the afterglow of all that, as we sighed and snuggled together under those hideous charcoal sheets, the apartment's front door opened.

I pulled the charcoal sheet tight around me. "Who's that?"

My thoughts immediately went to his unmarried sister, Bernadette, who was very much on the scene. Although she lived elsewhere, she visited daily, tending to her many pots of flowers and preparing meals for family and friends in a large eat-in kitchen adjacent to the museum. I had spent an evening with Henri and Bernadette on a previous visit. If I hadn't known better, I would have thought they were husband and wife, as I watched them standing amicably at the stove together, he carving the meat and she stirring the gravy. I was sure she had many male admirers. She was blonde and chic, with a perfect figure she flaunted in form-fitting jeans and trendy T-shirts that she fashionably tucked in at her belt buckle. Despite her many romantic prospects, I wondered, even back then, if her one true love was Henri.

"It might be Bernadette," he said, confirming my guess.

"What? She walks in without knocking?" I pulled the sheet tighter.

3

"Or maybe it's Sofie," he said.

"Who's Sofie?"

"She's the housekeeper. She was here yesterday, but maybe she forgot something."

"She doesn't knock either?"

He said nothing and within a few minutes he was snoring. Henri takes naptime seriously.

I could hear the clatter of teacups and saucers in the sink as our visitor washed up. She slid the barstools back into place and then walked toward the bedroom, which is next to the kitchen. I held my breath as she passed the closed bedroom door on her way down the hall to the bathroom, where she turned on the washing machine. A few minutes later, I could hear her setting up a drying rack in the boiler room, next to the bedroom.

This went on for 45 minutes, all while Henri snoozed. Any minute I thought the bedroom door would burst open with a woman carrying laundry that she intended to fold on the bed.

I finally nudged the Frenchman awake. "What's going on? She can't be blind. Surely, she saw your car parked out front and the two teacups on the counter."

He sighed. "It's Pauline."

"Who's Pauline?"

"My first wife."

I sat up, still clutching the sheet. "What the FUCK?!"

"She comes a few days a week to help out. She does the dishes and the washing. And she brings eggs from her chickens."

"She does this out of the kindness of her heart? Your ex-wife."

"I pay her."

"I'm already seeing a way to cut our expenses here."

My Frenchman looked so quintessentially French, lying in his new big bed with his new much-younger girlfriend while listening to the bustle of his first wife emptying his Lady Europa dishwasher.

"Does she know about me?"

"Yes, I told her on Sunday you were coming today."

"You didn't ask her not to come today?"

He shrugged. "It's her regular day."

In a few minutes, the tidying up stopped. I didn't actually hear the front door close, but all went quiet. I lay back on the pillow and closed my eyes, trying to calm myself.

"I feel like I'm in a bad French movie."

Henri ignored that comment and asked if I liked the bedding. "Bernadette went with me to the shop. I let her choose everything."

"You asked your sister to choose our bedding?"

"Who else would I ask?"

"What about me, the woman who's lying here next to you."

He looked puzzled, as though the thought hadn't occurred to him. "I wanted it to be a surprise."

"It is," I said, somewhat sarcastically.

And just then, the front door opened again.

A woman called out something in French. Henri didn't answer her.

"Pauline again?"

"No, that's Bernadette."

"Maybe she wants to know if I like the bedding?"

"You don't like it?"

"Charcoal is not my favorite color."

His sister left without further intrusion. Henri sat up and smiled at me.

I should have known then that what was to come in this unlikely love story would be far more than I thought I was signing up for.

Henri padded off in the nude and came back in a red, terrycloth bathrobe that made him look like Father Christmas. Henri could easily play Father Christmas. He is short and stocky, with a gray stubbly beard, a little round belly and a twinkle in his eyes that could light a fire.

"Would you like a glass of wine?" he asked.

That seemed like a very good idea. *Une bonne idée*, as the French say.

I put on my robe and followed him into the kitchen. There on the counter was a tray set for his breakfast the next morning. For *our* breakfast, actually. Instead of one coffee mug, there were two.

A small cardboard egg carton sat next to the mugs. Henri flipped open the lid and looked at the four eggs inside. Grinning, he said, "I usually get only two."

Chapter 2

I had met Henri a few years earlier at a B&B where I stayed during my many visits to Giverny. I was doing research for a book about American Impressionist painter Theodore Robinson, who used to come to Giverny with his Parisian model, a mystery woman named Marie.

The B&B was in an 18th-century water mill (*moulin*, in French) that featured in many of Robinson's Giverny paintings. In my favorite of his paintings, Marie sits pensively with a book in her lap on a stone bridge next to the moulin. There was speculation that Robinson may have used the room where I usually stayed – with its enormous arched window and vaulted ceiling – as a makeshift studio space.

My first memory of Henri was on a fall evening. I'd had dinner at the Baudy and was feeling a bit chilled from my walk back to the moulin. I heard laughter and a fire crackling in the moulin's sitting room when I returned. I poked my head in to say good night, and the proprietors, Olivier and Maxine, invited me to join them for a nightcap, which I gladly accepted. There's nothing like a shot of calvados – Normandy's high-octane apple brandy – to warm heart, soul and toes. They were sitting at a small table with Henri, who pulled up a chair for me. He didn't introduce himself. I thought he was a neighbor who had stopped by for a drink. He was friendly and spoke English well. He told me he had traveled extensively in his work as a mechanical engineer and had spent a lot of time in the States.

Henri often stopped by the moulin in the mornings to have

coffee with Olivier and Maxine. I discovered during a later visit that Henri was Olivier's much-older brother.

I didn't know much else about Henri. He was always cordial with the B&B guests. But there was a sadness about him. He rarely smiled. I never heard him laugh. On one of my visits, I watched him from an upstairs room as he sat in the moulin's garden alone, drinking his coffee and having a smoke. He stared vacantly at nothing.

I would later learn that he had lost the love of his life – a partner of some 25 years – to early-onset dementia. She was still alive, in fact, at a nearby care facility. When he told me that story, I was at his museum, watching a film reel of the events that had been held there over the years. He pointed her out to me in one segment. "That's my wife," he said. "I don't see her anymore. She doesn't know me."

As he came to know more about me, at least the project that kept bringing me back to Giverny, he offered to help me with my research. "My family has lived here for four generations," he told me. "I know a lot about Giverny's history."

I wasn't surprised to find out that Henri's family had known Claude Monet. Henri's grandmother lived next door to Monet and knew him well. When her husband died in World War I, his body was never recovered and, without papers certifying his death, the French government withheld her widow's benefits. Monet stepped in and loaned her money. Henri still has the loan document Monet drew up in his own hand.

Henri was born in Giverny in 1943. The village was occupied by Germans then. He was a sickly newborn who couldn't digest milk. A Jewish doctor, who had been forced into German military service, was stationed in the village and saved Henri's life with his kit of medicines and food rations.

After World War II, Monet's house and gardens fell into decline. By the 1950s, the property had been abandoned, and Henri and his friends ran wild there. They skated on the lily pond in winter and fished off the iconic Japanese bridge in summer.

Henri knew every nook and alley of Giverny. I enlisted his

help on one visit as I searched for a garden where Robinson had photographed Marie for some of his paintings of her. I had read that the garden belonged to a house that had been rented in the 1890s by a Boston artist named Mariquita Gill. She herself had done paintings of the garden, which had a distinctive tree with a bent limb that looked like a flexed arm. The same tree appeared in several of Robinson's photos of Marie.

One morning as Henri and I sat together at the moulin's breakfast table, he studied the images I had on my laptop of Gill's painting and Robinson's photos of the garden. Ever the engineer, Henri drew a diagram showing that Gill had taken artistic license in the placement of the tree in her painting. Robinson's photos showed the tree was not by the garden gate, as Gill had rendered it. Even if the tree were still alive – a big IF, given that Robinson's photos were more than 120 years old – it wouldn't be in the spot where it appears in the painting.

A childhood friend of Henri's happened to be at the moulin that morning and he, too, looked at the images. He and Henri discussed possible locations in the village I should explore. Gill was not as well-known as other American painters who were part of Giverny's art colony at that time, so the house wouldn't be marked on the tourist map of the village.

The man casually mentioned to Henri that he had a painting by a prominent Giverny artist of that era, John Leslie Breck, also from Boston. Breck infamously made a play for Monet's stepdaughter, Blanche, and Monet ran him out of the village.

The painting was of a "har," the man said.

I quickly figured out he meant "hare." Paintings of dead hares, dangling by their paws with blood oozing beneath their fur are, to me, a grotesque, animal-art sub-genre, but it would be a noteworthy painting because it was done by Breck.

"Do museums know about this painting?" I asked the man.

He shrugged.

"Has it ever been exhibited?"

He said it had been shown once at a museum in Vernon, the town across the river from Giverny.

I would come to find out that any number of paintings by renowned artists are squirreled away in Giverny.

Several years after Monet moved to Giverny in 1883, his impressionistic landscapes lured young bohemian painters – many of them Americans who were studying art in Paris – to the luminous Seine River Valley. When they arrived in Giverny, in the late 1880s, Angelina and Lucien Baudy, seeing a ripe business opportunity, converted a modest cafe-grocery store they owned in the village to a *pension*, with 20 bedrooms, a dining room, three painting studios, a billiard room and a ballroom. It became known as the American Painters Hotel. A gracious hostess, Madame Baudy expanded her menu of Normandy dishes to include American favorites such as Boston baked beans, porridge and cornflakes. She imported five brands of whiskey, an exotic drink in France at the time. The Baudy dining room became a makeshift gallery where painters-in-residence displayed their work. Paintings were a form of currency – the way impoverished artists paid for room and board and other expenses. It's said that Monet, in his starving-artist days, once threatened to throw himself in the Seine when a butcher refused to accept payment in the form of a painted canvas.

Madame Baudy's dining-room gallery drew the attention of Paris art galleries and collectors. But some paintings from that era passed into private hands. Henri says he knows of at least five Monet paintings in Giverny that are privately owned – some, he thinks, are unknown to museums. The garden walls are high in Giverny for good reason.

For a couple of days, I walked on tiptoes down the village lanes, peering over walls, hoping to find an old tree with a bent limb. Henri promised to vouch for me if I got reported as a peeper to the gendarmes.

Henri enjoyed hearing my stories over coffee in the mornings as my research unfolded. He was impressed by how much I knew about the artists who had come to Giverny. I had studied art history in college and had read extensively about the Impressionist movement and its painters. It was a joy for me to see the locations where they painted in Giverny. The scenes haven't changed much. Even the railing on the bridge, where Marie posed for Robinson, is the same. The only difference is a welding mark where Henri and Olivier mended a break in the wrought iron some years ago.

Olivier mentioned to Giverny's mayor, who had stopped by the moulin for coffee one spring morning, about my search for Gill's house. The mayor, a balding older man who looked a bit like Monet, stroked his white beard as he studied the images on my laptop. I also showed him a Robinson painting of Marie in the same garden, with a glimpse of the rooftops beyond the top of the wall. He sent me up to the northwest corner of the village, which was nestled against a hill.

From the slope, I had a good view of a walled garden below. The gnarled trees there looked quite old. One was barely upright and had the stub of a broken, bent limb. I couldn't be absolutely sure it was the garden where Robinson had painted Marie. But it had a good vibe.

I looked up at the cloudy sky and said, "Theo, give me a sign." As I got into my car, I looked back at the garden, just as sunbeams lit up forsythia blooms beyond the garden wall.

I took that as a sign.

The next year, my novel *The Secret of Marie* was published. There was a little champagne celebration in Giverny, attended by the mayor and an official from the Monet Foundation. I have a nice photo of me with Henri. He has an arm affectionately around my shoulder, with a big smile on his face.

I began work on another novel set in Giverny and neighboring

Vernonnet, where painter Pierre Bonnard lived for many years. Intrigued by the stories of Giverny's secret cachet of masterworks, I concocted an art-forgery story about a painting that Bonnard had hidden away of a young model who committed suicide after he broke off their engagement. A month before her death, he had married his long-time mistress who had insisted he destroy the paintings he had done of his young, jilted fiancée. I made up the forgery story, but my account of Bonnard's tortured love life was true.

Of course, this new project meant more trips to Giverny to do research about Bonnard. Henri had introduced me to the owners of the Bonnard house, a lovely couple who had staged the rooms to look as though Bonnard still lived there, based on his paintings and photos of the place. They invited me to come for lunch one day and asked a local friend who was fluent in English to join us.

The divine woman who was my translator that day is someone I fondly call Madame Red Shoes. Her red Mary Jane-style shoes are her signature. In her mid-80s, she had the style and bounce in her step of a 17-year-old coquette. Mademoiselle Red Shoes would be just as apt.

Madame Red Shoes – whose real name is Marie Noëlle Révérend – was herself an artist. She liked doing portraits and still lifes in pastels, sculpting busts of Monet and making pottery. Ceramic bowls adorned with red-glazed cherries were her specialty. When I first met her, she wove her white hair in a flower-laced braid that circled her head like a crown. But later, she cut off the braid and let her curls unfurl. Truly, a mademoiselle at heart whose company and confidence I would enjoy in my new life to come.

~⌐

All this time, during my research trips to Giverny, I was living in Italy. A few years earlier, when my son and only child started college, I sold my house in Pasadena, California and moved to Florence. I had been a single mother for 10 years – a chapter of my life I thoroughly enjoyed – but I felt, when my son left home, it was time to turn the page. So off I went to Italy.

My first year in Florence inspired my first book, a memoir that I thought of as Under the Tuscan Sun Gone Wrong. Within the first month of my arrival, I discovered I was living next door to a Mafia princess whose Papa-from-Palermo complained to the building management that I had parked in his daughter's garage space for a week (I accidentally took her spot, but just for one night). I awoke one morning to find my apartment door wide open – a DON'T MESS WITH US message, my Italian acquaintances cautioned me. An inauspicious beginning, but great material for a book.

I lived in Italy for several years, in awe of its beauty and history, but constantly frustrated by its inefficiency and bureaucracy. Then came a change in Italy's tax laws: If I stayed on as a resident, Italy would tax my worldwide income at a rate somewhere between 35-45 percent, maybe higher. Despite a tax treaty with the U.S. that supposedly prevents double taxation, I would, in fact, be double-taxed on my book royalties. What's more, there would be a "wealth tax" on my savings and investments – not just on interest and dividends, but on the principal.

The accountant who explained this to me – a chic Italian woman with suede boots up to her thighs – said smugly, "You Americans love Italy. This is the price you have to pay."

I smiled and replied, "I don't love it that much."

I was contemplating my options during a visit to Giverny. Henri took me for a drive one morning, up to a bluff above the chalky cliffs that overlook the Seine.

"You have a big decision to make," he said after I told him about my tax situation.

"I'm not going to stay in Italy. But I need to figure out where to go next."

As I looked out over the breathtaking view on that bright September morning and thought about my love for Giverny, a move to this part of France made sense. But I didn't know what new hurdles I might face, especially if I had to go back to the U.S. and start the daunting visa-application process again. The thought of that was overwhelming.

Henri asked me to meet him for dinner that evening at the Hôtel Baudy. I told him I would be joining the artist group that was staying at the moulin for their last evening in the gardens. In those days, painters and photographers were allowed in the gardens after hours to enjoy the solace Monet had known. The American organizers of the painting program were good friends of mine and had offered me a room at the moulin, at a discount, just a week earlier when they received a late cancellation. I loved that I could hop on a plane from Florence and join them on short notice.

I promised Henri I would break away from the group in time to see the sun set from the Baudy terrace. "It's the most beautiful time of day in Giverny," he told me.

"I wouldn't miss it."

As it turned out, I almost did. A sudden shower poured down on those of us at the gardens that evening. I was standing on the Japanese bridge as the rain began. The painters frantically joined me for cover, under the dense wisteria bower, and tried to shield their canvases with plastic from their supply kits.

A short while later, sunbeams streaked through the clouds and suddenly a rainbow appeared, as if arching upward from the surface of the pond.

After the rain stopped, I hurried out of the gardens and rushed down Rue Claude Monet toward the Baudy, where I could see Henri waiting for me at the front door.

He smiled as I apologized for being late and for my rain-splattered appearance. My already curly hair had taken on an amazing life of its own.

When we sat down at our table, I couldn't wait to show Henri the photo I had taken of the rainbow.

He looked at me with such affection. "I'd say that's a very good omen."

Later that evening, I joined the artists at the moulin for a farewell round of calvados. The camaraderie at the table was so in keeping with Giverny's art-colony spirit. It's what I've always enjoyed about Giverny.

It was late when I returned to my room, a cozy attic space tucked under the roof of the moulin's half-timbered tower.

I checked my email and was surprised to see a message from Henri:

Thank you for these moments spent together. It's a great pleasure for me. We have very similar tastes and ideas. I would like to talk about them with you for a longer time.

And then he ended with "*Je t'aime.*" I love you.

I remembered the night of my first visit to the moulin many years earlier. It was late September, the end of the season, and I was the only guest. Olivier and Maxine lived elsewhere in the village then, so I was truly alone. To be sure of that, on the first night of my stay, I climbed the stairs of the tower, turning on lights and checking behind doors in the guest rooms. When I opened the last door on the top floor, I found myself at the foot of the dark stairwell leading to the attic. I felt a rush of cold air – a whoosh that felt more like a *presence*. I shut the door tight and ran back downstairs to my room.

I had told Henri the story of that night and how I had pushed a dresser against the door of my room and calmed myself by singing to the phantom of the moulin.

I couldn't have imagined then that 13 years later, I'd be sitting in the attic room where the phantom lived, reading a loving message from Henri.

There was hubbub at breakfast the next morning as the artist group gathered to say their good-byes. Luggage and easels were going out the door as Henri entered, at his usual time. He sat down next to me at the table and poured himself a cup of coffee and refilled my cup as well. I casually asked him if he'd take me to the train station that afternoon. I was leaving, too, that day.

Henri picked me up a few minutes early. We made small talk en route. He parked across from the station and turned off the engine.

He leaned toward me and smiled, then kissed me gently on the lips.

We spoke of when we'd meet again. I suggested that we find a place, new to both of us, where we could spend a few days together and get to know each other better. He liked that idea.

He walked me to the entrance of the station and kissed me again. And then he left, choosing not to wait with me for the train to arrive.

It was my first lesson about my Frenchman: He doesn't like good-byes.

Chapter 3

Henri and I chose Malta for our rendezvous. It was new to us both and alluringly exotic. I booked the B&Bs; he reserved the rental car. We coordinated our flights so that he, at his insistence, would arrive before me. "I want to be there to greet you," he said. Henri was courting me.

I felt strangely calm about this tryst. The anticipation of sex with a new lover can be both thrilling and unnerving. But the moment I saw him at the gate, as he rushed to embrace me, I wanted nothing more than to spend the next few days tangled in bedsheets.

We got horribly lost on our way from the airport in Luqa. The street signs were in Arabic, which our GPS navigator couldn't pronounce. It should have taken us 20 minutes to get to the B&B in Valletta, but we spent an hour and a half trying to find our way through the labyrinthine streets. It was early evening by the time we checked in, so we headed down to the harbor for a wonderful seafood dinner. Henri generously shares his food and fed me buttery shrimp from his fork.

There was a nip in the air that night. It was early November. I shivered a little as I pulled my jacket around me on our walk up from the harbor to our B&B. Henri slipped his arm around my waist. I don't remember what we talked about. All I could think about was that in a very short while we'd be in bed together.

Months later I would ask him if he had felt nervous that night. He said, "Not at all. Were you?"

Yes, I was nervous. But that slipped away as I gave myself to him that night.

I wondered how long it had been since he had last made love. At one point, he whispered, "I haven't felt like this since..." He didn't finish his sentence. But I realized that Henri was a man whose profound loss had left him starving for love.

~

Our time on Malta was a lot like a honeymoon.

One evening, we decided, from our tangle of sheets, we needed room service. We called a local couscous restaurant, recommended in our B&B's guide to the neighborhood. I hung out the window of our Maltese balcony, waving to the delivery driver who was a block away looking for our street number, while Henri was on the sidewalk below talking to him by phone. Henri spoke Spanish and a little Arabic and guided our dinner to the B&B's front door.

I set the table on our boxed balcony — an enclosed porch that is a traditional feature of Maltese architecture. The balconies are typically painted in bright colors. Ours, appropriately, was red. Romantic that I am, I had packed a few tea-light candles in my suitcase. I lit them just as Henri entered the room with our dinner-to-go in hand. The man who rarely smiled was grinning from ear to ear.

When we sat down to our candlelight dinner, Henri asked, "What about the violins?"

"No problem." I cued my laptop's iTunes playlist to Vivaldi. Henri loves classical music. A night of feasting began.

We were happy lovers living a dream. Not until our last night on Malta did we speak of what might come next.

We were finishing dinner at a little out-of-the-way restaurant when Henri said, "I'd like to talk about our relationship."

I had been dreading this conversation because of an obvious problem we faced. "I think first we need to talk about your wife," I said.

"I'm not married."

"You may not feel married anymore. But you still have a wife."

"She's not my wife."

"But you call her your..."

"Yes, I say she's my wife, but we aren't married. *We never married.*"

"What do you mean you *never* married?"

It was a moment of comic relief. A woman usually doesn't express stunned disbelief when she learns her lover isn't married.

Henri took my hand. "*Chérie*, I'm yours."

But that started an intense discussion about the meaning of the word *yours.*

Henri was open to us having a romance. He suggested that I move somewhere close to Giverny so we could see each other often.

"But do you see us as a couple?" I asked him.

"You mean a married couple?"

"No. An unmarried couple."

The thought of that gave him pause. And then he did something I'll never forget. He crossed his wrists, as if they were lashed together, and said, "I never want to feel like this."

"Like a prisoner?"

"*Oui*, like a prisoner."

I shook my head. "No."

"Why do you say no?"

"No, I'm not interested in moving to France so that we can have a fling."

"But I want a relationship with you."

"Then you need to stop thinking that I'll be the rope around your wrists."

I didn't sleep well that night. I hadn't slept well all week because of Henri's snoring. But that night, snoring wasn't the issue. It was the image of tied wrists that kept me awake.

If Henri wanted a relationship with me, he needed to step up. It's a huge undertaking and a big expense to move to another country. I needed to know he was committed to making this work.

I gently nudged him to roll over. Instead, he pulled me close to him and within a few seconds was snoring in my ear.

Henri and I were good travel companions. We meandered down cobbled side streets and stopped along the way for refreshments. We didn't like to rush. We didn't have a checklist of must-sees. We liked soaking up our surroundings. More than anything, we wanted to savor our precious time in Malta together.

On our last day, we had the entire afternoon to get to the airport. But cryptic signage and our baffled GPS failed us along the way. GPS on Malta is very spotty. One day, we ended up on top of a hill with a half dozen other travelers in rental cars. Google Maps had led us all astray to a dead end.

Our unplanned detour on the way to the airport led us in a huge circle back to where we started, in an area that wasn't exactly scenic. I could feel the bliss of our holiday fading away.

We were both on the same flight to Rome, where we would then go our separate ways. After we checked in at the Malta airport, we had time for a drink. We hadn't spoken of our conversation the night before, which meant we hadn't resolved the "couple" issue. Or maybe in his mind, we had. Henri's idea of a relationship was no strings attached. Mine was something more. I wanted to know I'd have a partner in this.

I knew Henri had never been to Florence and I asked if he'd like to visit me sometime.

"*Bien sûr!*" Of course.

The forcefulness of his answer surprised me. He seemed to see a path forward, but it wasn't clear to me where we were headed.

We were sitting opposite each other at a little table in an airport cafe. He was looking at me intently. His lifted his eyebrows and the muscles in his forehead contracted. I wondered if he might be having a stroke. And then his ears started wiggling. As he pumped his eyebrows, his ears wiggled more.

I burst out laughing. "How long have you had this skill?" I asked.

"Since school days," he said, his ears still wiggling. "I loved doing this during business meetings with clients."

"And with women you're wooing?"

"Not so much." He laughed.

I kissed his cheek. "You saved the best for last."

As our flight lifted off the runway, I gazed at the twinkling lights along the shoreline below. I remembered the same scene from my arrival only a week earlier. That day, my heart had been in my throat as the plane touched the tarmac. On this night, it ached a little.

Henri leaned into me to see the view out the window. His cheek was just inches from mine.

"Kiss me," I whispered.

We made out like a couple of teenagers on that flight to Rome.

At the Rome airport, we had a glass of prosecco at a chic bar. When his flight to Paris began boarding, I stood next to him in line. We kissed one last time before he approached the gate. I stood to the side watching him enter the jetway. But the man who doesn't like good-byes didn't look back. And then he was gone.

~⁓

Over the next few months, Henri visited me several times in Florence. He fell in love with the city, which I enjoyed sharing with him. I took him to my favorite places and introduced him to my friends.

I could easily see having a wonderful life with Henri. We were so comfortable together. We never ran out of things to talk about and were so good at making each other laugh.

I avoided the subject of our future. During one visit, he asked me what I thought about a real estate listing he had sent me for an apartment in Vernon, which was several miles from Giverny. He thought it might be a nice place for me.

"I'm not looking for an apartment in Vernon," I told him.

He clearly was still struggling with the idea of having a woman in his life again. I often wondered if he was still in mourning for the woman he had lost.

Then one night as we were getting ready to go out to dinner, something changed.

Henri walked into the bedroom, where I was still wrapped in a bath towel from my shower.

"I wish I had known you had been in the shower," he said.

"Why's that?"

"Couples usually wash each other's backs."

"Do they?" I murmured as he kissed me.

He loosened the towel. "Yes, they do."

Chapter 4

My future with Henri hung in the balance one March day in 2018, as I walked across Piazza Farnese in Rome to the French Embassy. Whether he and I would share a life together in his beloved Giverny would be decided by a total stranger in the embassy's visa office that day.

My documents were in order – precise order. The instructions stipulated that I must present the 10 required items in a designated sequence. God forbid that document #6 was in the stack ahead of document #5. Among them was a statement from Henri inviting me to reside at his address. For good measure, he had included a sworn statement called a *déclaration sur l'honneur* – affirming his birthdate, address and signature – signed by the mayor of Giverny. I love that Henri had asked the mayor to vouch for him.

On the train from Florence, I had rehearsed my answers to a dozen questions that I thought I might be asked during my interview. I had written out the responses in French, with the help of a translation app. But I wasn't sure how to explain my reason for wanting to live in France. Yes, I loved its beauty, art, culture and croissants. But should I also say I had fallen in love with a Frenchman named Henri, who unwrapped me from my bath towel one night and said *oui* to being a couple, no wrist ropes attached. I scratched out most of that answer – perhaps a bit too risqué even for the French. So I went with: *I've fallen in love with a wonderful Frenchman who has asked me to make a life with him in beautiful Giverny.*

I had even practiced how to introduce myself and state the reason for my visit, which was a good thing because I had to announce myself into an intercom speaker at the building's entrance. I got an approving nod from the female police officer on duty at the door. "*Très bien*," she said with a smile.

After I went through security, I was escorted to a room with a big table and comfortable chairs. There were books and magazines, toys for children to play with, and vending machines for coffee and snacks. So civilized compared to the immigration hellhole in Florence known as the *questura* – an enormous hall at the police headquarters. During my time in Italy, I had seen hundreds of people crowded into that space – babies crying, children running wild – sitting on broken benches splattered with pigeon shit from the flock that resides there. On sweltering summer days, with no ventilation, the stench from body odor and dirty diapers is overwhelming.

There was no filth and despair in this room. I nervously checked my packet of papers one more time.

I was summoned into an adjoining room where I sat in a cubicle in front of a glass barrier and slid my dossier through the space beneath it. The woman who interviewed me was very nice and spoke perfect English, which was a relief. When she asked about my reasons for wanting to live in France, I decided not to speak of Henri. I spoke about my love for Giverny and the books it had inspired me to write. She was impressed. She liked the certificate from Giverny's mayor, embossed with his official seal, and gave it back to me as a keepsake.

At the end of the interview, I asked how long it would take for the embassy to make a decision.

She shrugged and said, "Unless we find out you're a criminal, your application will be approved."

I was stunned. In my experience in Italy, visa decisions often took weeks.

She said I would receive final confirmation by e-mail the following week, and then she took a photo of me that would appear, along with my visa details, in my passport.

And just like that, my life changed in the span of an hour.

When I texted Henri with my good news, he wrote: *All my congratulations on your success at the embassy. You must be relieved of a great weight! Now you have a new base of life. It's up to us both to do everything to prolong this happiness. We are not entitled to an error. I love you, Rebecca.*

⁓

Three weeks later, I arrived in Giverny for my debut as Henri's new girlfriend. I was the guest of honor at a dinner party of his closest friends, some of whom I already knew. I think everyone was pleasantly surprised by this dramatic turn for Henri. They raised their glasses to us, in a toast to our happiness.

Henri's family was warm and welcoming. When I met his 45-year-old son, Alex, at the family's Easter gathering, I reached out to shake his hand, but he said, "That's a bit formal. You're my father's girlfriend."

"Do you think that's weird?"

He shrugged and then kissed me on both cheeks.

I attended a birthday lunch for Alex's darling four-year-old son, Luc, the next day. At Luc's request, the main dish was homemade French fries.

When I asked Henri if there might be some ketchup in the fridge, Alex informed me that Luc didn't know about ketchup and he wanted to keep it that way.

"What? Fries with no ketchup?" I asked.

"That's very American," Alex said. He wasn't being unkind, but he had strong feelings about protecting French customs and culture from foreign influences. No ketchup.

In the middle of the party, a frail elderly woman arrived. She was pencil thin and looked unwell. Her face was badly disfigured from surgery that had removed part of her lower jaw. I was shocked when Henri introduced her as Pauline, his former wife – the woman who had washed our teacups and tended the laundry as we lay in bed on the day of my arrival.

She turned to me and said something in English, but with her speech impediment, it took me a moment to understand her. And then I realized she was saying, "I brought you eggs."

"*Merci*, Pauline," I said. "They were delicious."

Henri's sister Bernadette had made Luc a beautiful cake adorned with flowers from the garden. As he blew out the candles, Pauline stood at Luc's side, with her arm around his shoulder.

After everyone had been served cake except for Pauline, I whispered to Henri, "Pauline doesn't have a plate."

"She can't eat," he said, as if I should have known that by looking at her.

I wondered why Henri hadn't told me anything about her. It was a lot to take in at a four-year-old's birthday party.

~⁓

Henri had been leading a curious bachelor's life. His daily needs – meals, house cleaning and laundry – were handled by Bernadette, Pauline, and Sofie, the housekeeper. Pauline sometimes prepared meals that he could freeze and use as needed. But it seemed he had dinner most evenings with Bernadette, who cooked for him.

Henri and Bernadette were very close. During our trip to Malta, Henri called her daily, just to check in. As a souvenir, he bought her a Maltese lace doily, just like one I had selected for myself. "Bernadette will like this," he said as he made the purchase. The doilies weren't expensive – about $10 each. I thought it was odd that he didn't also pay for mine, as a gift.

I sensed something horrible had happened to Henri when his partner of many years, Camille, fell into the grips of dementia. I later learned that because they weren't married, he had no legal authority to take charge of her care. Her family put her in a local nursing home and Henri moved from their house in the village into the apartment.

He never spoke of that period in his life. But he did tell me that after she stopped recognizing him, he couldn't bear to see her anymore.

I didn't know if Henri had dated other women after that. He was a big flirt and had a wandering eye. He once said to me, "Just because I'm on a diet doesn't mean I can't look at the menu." My reply to that was, "I'm not a diet. I'm a feast. And if you look at the menu too long, the feast will disappear."

I was dealing with a Frenchman with an ingrained chauvinistic streak. *Chauvinisme* is a French word, after all, and a cornerstone of the culture.

But it was more than that. I could tell from his childhood stories that Henri had been coddled and adored. His was the eldest of six and ruled the roost. In a photo with his siblings, taken when he was about 10, they all look cherubic except for Henri, who's sticking out his tongue at the photographer. Henri was an incorrigible rascal and smart as a whip. He often had to stay after school and help the teacher clean the chalkboards as punishment for his mischief. One day, she made him sit at his desk and write "I will do better tomorrow" 100 times. He tied two pencils together and wrote it 50 times.

These were important things to know about Henri that would come into play as our problems began.

We hit our first snag as we tried to figure out how or if my things would fit into his apartment. There clearly wasn't room. The closets and dressers were packed with his stuff. His expectation was that I'd move to Giverny with a couple of suitcases and a few boxes of books.

"I have a space above the museum where we can put anything you need to store," he told me. "But flying mice live there."

"You mean bats?"

Henri burst out laughing at my horrified expression. Forever after that, he loved teasing me about his flying mice, which he said were a rare species.

Henri had offered to give me his bedroom, where the bed with the memory-foam mattress had been installed. That room was bigger than his guest bedroom at the back of the apartment. The windows of the smaller bedroom looked out on the grimy corrugated plastic roof that kept the rain off the engines in the museum hall below. The front bedroom had a wide set of windows that faced the apartment's front lawn and the wooded hillside beyond. It would be a perfect place to set up my desk. I'm a writer who loves an inspiring view.

Henri was doing his best – or at least, what he believed to be his best – to accommodate me. But for the previous six years he had been a single man who hadn't needed to accommodate anyone.

He had a fixed daily regimen that began with a 7 a.m. breakfast, followed by a shower. He went back to bed for an hour and then started his day by walking his dog and having coffee with Olivier and Maxine at the moulin. He spent the rest of the morning running errands or doing paperwork in his office. Lunch was often a full meal, always followed by a nap. He spent the afternoons in his workshop with his team of mechanics, restoring old engines, either for clients or for the museum collection. During the summer season, Henri would often give tours to visitors. At about 6:45 p.m. each day, work stopped for a ritual Henri called the "washing of hands." It took a good 10 minutes to scrub through the layers of grit and grease, but with Henri, I often noticed that fingernails didn't get much attention. The museum closed at 7 p.m. during the tourist season, which was the appointed hour for "*apero*" – a time for an aperitif and snacks with friends and family.

Everyone congregated in the big kitchen next to the museum or in the adjoining garden. After dinner, around 9, Henri retired to his office to answer emails. By 10, he was in bed, reading a book or watching his favorite YouTube videos on his tablet. He especially enjoyed opera performances and film clips of working steam locomotives. Henri is a man of eclectic tastes and interests.

I began to wonder where I would fit into Henri's schedule. Forget the scarcity of closet space and dresser drawers. Was there room for me in his *life*?

One comment he made came as a gut-punch when he spoke of the family's long-standing Christmas tradition. Every year, on Christmas

Day, a group of them fly to Ibiza, where Henri and Camille used to own a house. Henri sold the place after Camille became ill, but the tradition of going to Ibiza continued. In recent years, the group had dwindled to Henri, Bernadette and a friend of hers named Valérie. The house they stayed at had no heat and a limited water supply that meant they had to ration showers. Henri spent a lot of time chopping wood and slept on the sofa in the living room so that he could stoke the fire during the night.

"You wouldn't like it there," he said to me. "Maybe you should spend Christmas in California." Then he added, "Bernadette needs me."

"Needs you for what?"

"To take care of things there. She won't want to be in Ibiza without me."

This conversation happened as we were on a day trip to a lovely village called Gerberoy, which Henri wanted me to see. The landscape was beautiful – a patchwork of farm fields that were showing signs of spring. The image of that is etched in my mind along with Henri's words: *Maybe you should spend Christmas in California.*

I suddenly felt that I wasn't really Henri's girlfriend. I felt more like a mistress. Bernadette, in fact, was the "wife."

A bad French movie, indeed.

～⁊

Gerberoy is called one of the most beautiful villages in France and is known for its lush sprays of roses that climb the arbors and walls of its storybook cottages. Every June, a rose festival in Gerberoy is a well-attended event.

But on the day of our April visit, Gerberoy was deserted. We wandered the cobbled streets as I took some photos, but we didn't linger. Storm clouds were gathering, which I should have taken as an omen.

We had traveled to Gerberoy in a rental car that Henri had arranged for my visit. He wanted me to have the freedom to go off on my own and knew I was uncomfortable driving a car with manual transmission. He had found an automatic at a Hertz location about 20 miles from Giverny and had paid a premium. I asked him several times to cancel the reservation. I had come to spend the week with him, not wander off on my own. I had spent plenty of time wandering during my research trips to Giverny in rental cars I had picked up at the airport, at a much cheaper rate. But he insisted.

He also insisted on the day of our Gerberoy visit that I drive, which didn't thrill me. I would have preferred gazing at the scenery rather than navigating busy traffic circles and maneuvering narrow country lanes.

When we arrived in Gerberoy, I was able to park in the center of the village, which saved us from walking in from a visitor car park down the road. But I didn't realize, as I pulled next to the curb, that a metal drainpipe imbedded in the concrete had sliced the sidewall of the rear tire.

Henri had no apparent interest in driving that day at all, so I was back at the wheel as we headed home in the rain. Within minutes, I realized something was wrong with the car and pulled over just before we reached the main road.

For the better part of an hour, in a torrential downpour, Henri struggled to change the tire with a jack that didn't fit the car. With me standing over him trying to hold onto an umbrella, he finally got the spare in place. It didn't look roadworthy to me, but Henri said it would get us home. The manual said it was rated for 80 kilometers per hour (48 mph). I handed Henri the keys. I was done driving.

The rain had let up, but the roads were soaked. Henri drives too fast in good conditions, but that day, he showed no caution. When I saw the speedometer hit 109 kilometers per hour (65 mph), I asked him to slow down. He eased off the accelerator, but within a few minutes he was speeding again.

I was furious. "Henri, slow down! I don't care how you drive when you're by yourself, but when you're with the woman you supposedly love, I would think you'd care about safety."

I hadn't seen this defiant side of him. He clearly didn't like a woman telling him how to drive. But I wasn't going to let him endanger us both.

As we rode in silence, I thought about the e-mail he had sent me just a few weeks earlier, celebrating my success at the embassy: *We are not entitled to an error*, he had written.

I couldn't bear the thought that this was all a huge mistake.

~

On our way back to Giverny, we stopped at a gardening center, where I bought Bernadette a beautiful hydrangea plant, as a thank you for her hospitality during my stay. I wanted to have a good relationship with her, though I knew it would be difficult to forge a friendship when we didn't have a common language. She knew only a few words in English and my high-school French wasn't enough to close the void between us. But I felt it was up to me to make an effort to befriend her. I was intruding in her space and in her relationship with Henri. I couldn't afford an error with her.

Bernadette was in the downstairs kitchen when we returned and loved the hydrangea. I had asked Henri to make the selection – he chose blue, a color she adored.

She pointed to three jars of homemade jam on the kitchen table and told me Pauline had brought them as a gift for me. I appreciated the gesture, but I wondered if Pauline was worried that she might lose her paycheck from Henri now that I was on the scene. Was she trying to win favor with me much like I was trying to do with Bernadette?

I suggested to Henri that we keep the jam at his apartment until my return in June. I said I was worried that the jars might break in my suitcase, but Bernadette insisted they'd be fine and told me how to pack them. I listened politely while imaging a shoe filled with gooey cherry jam.

That night, Henri and I had dinner at the Baudy. It was my last night, but I wasn't in the mood for a romantic farewell. I needed to draw a firm line with him.

He looked a bit sheepish when I said to him, "What happened today was unacceptable. I asked you twice to slow down, but you ignored me. Don't think for a minute that this wasn't a warning sign for me."

He seemed contrite, like a child who had just gotten a good scolding. I could easily imagine him sitting at his school desk, with pencils tied together, writing, *I will do better tomorrow.*

On my first day back in Florence, I had an appointment with my Australian chiropractor who noted an unusual amount of tension in my neck.

I regaled him with the highlights of my trip. As he gently massaged the knots in my neck and shoulders, he dispensed some sage advice: "Don't eat the jam," he said. "Leave it out for the bats and see if they die."

Chapter 5

In early May, Henri came to Florence one last time, to help me pack up. He was a man on a mission and arrived with a tape dispenser in his suitcase. He took charge of the packing list and meticulously numbered the boxes. He kindly didn't say anything about the ever-growing *number* of boxes.

Back in Giverny, he had ordered a large IKEA wardrobe for my use and was planning to build a special storage room for my things that he promised would be sealed off from flying mice.

He was making a big effort, which I appreciated.

During my last days in Florence, I said good-bye to my friends and took a farewell stroll along my favorite streets. Florence had been a haven and an inspiration for me. I hoped Giverny would feed my heart and soul like Florence had.

I had coffee with a friend a few days before I left. As I told her the story of Henri, she sensed some trepidation beneath my cheerful optimism.

She squeezed my arm and said, "I hope everything turns out fine. But take a magic carpet with you in case you need to fly away."

On my last day in Florence, a dear friend named Lorenzo took me to lunch at our favorite neighborhood trattoria. We had a long history together that had started one winter evening several years earlier when he followed me out of a Florence bookstore, eager to speak with me. At first, I tried to ignore him as he walked along beside me. I finally stopped and turned to him. Lorenzo does a funny imitation of the dirty look I gave him as he tried to convince me to meet him for coffee the next day.

We spoke for about 10 minutes on that chilly January night. He told me he was a photographer and had lived in Florence all his life. He had learned English in school and loved American movies. When he heard I was from California, his face lit up. He told me how much he had enjoyed his visit to Yosemite. He had climbed Half Dome and said it was the most harrowing experience of his life. He had expressive eyes when he spoke and a sweet smile. I agreed to meet him for coffee.

We exchanged business cards that night and by the time I got home an hour later, he had sent me this message:

Ciao, Rebecca. Sono (I am) *Lorenzo. We met this evening near Piazza della Repubblica. We spoke about cinema, fotografia and creative writing, and I told myself how marvelous it would be to become a friend to this interesting woman. I really hope to see you again and to condivide our life activities, our passions, our ideas. Ciao et...buona serata.*

At the time, I didn't know the meaning of "*condivide*," but I soon learned it's a form of the Italian verb "to share."

Lorenzo and I shared many happy moments together. We had a brief dalliance as lovers, but after a break, we came back to each other as friends.

He lived a few blocks from me and would spontaneously call to see if I wanted to go to IKEA. I loved my trips to IKEA with Lorenzo. For a few hours on those expeditions, I experienced what my life might be like with an Italian husband. We once spent a half hour in the curtain department as he tried to find a fabric that would keep out Florence's horrible tiger mosquitoes (that purchase was a total fail). On another trip, he was in search of the perfect vegetable steamer, but became overwhelmed by the choices and didn't buy one. We'd visit the closet department and he'd ask me if I had suggestions about how to organize his socks. On almost every visit, he'd linger in the bookcase-and-armoire section and get a dreamy look in his eyes. He labored over decisions and in the end wouldn't buy anything or he'd make a purchase and end up with severe buyer's remorse by the time we got home. My favorite IKEA trip was when we went to buy a mattress for his bed-ridden mother. We tested every one, discussing the pros and cons of each while lying next to each other on the beds.

One hot summer's night, he called about 11 p.m. and asked, "You want to go out for gelato?" Five minutes later, I heard his car coming up the street, with his James Brown CD blaring. Lorenzo, who has an amazing voice, loved singing while driving. And so we were off in our own Italian version of Carpool Karaoke, looking for a gelato shop still open at that hour. It was after midnight when we finally found one. It was the best gelato I'd ever tasted and enjoying it in the summer moonlight with Lorenzo added to the pleasure.

Lorenzo, who was 47 when I met him, had never married and had lived in his childhood home all his life. He was the classic *mammone* – the Italian word for "mama's boy." He was so pleased to introduce me to his *mamma*, who, at 79, was showing signs of dementia. She took a good look at me and said to Lorenzo, "She's prettier than her photo."

Lorenzo tenderly cupped his hands around her face. "Oh, *Mamma*," he said with such love in his voice.

He split his sides laughing when he later explained that she had confused me with a Swedish porn star whose photo he kept by his bed.

I was going to miss Lorenzo.

After our trattoria lunch on my last day in Florence, we stopped by his place so he could show me the redecorated living room and his new bedroom furniture. I recognized the IKEA display cases, bookshelves and closet units he had been dreaming about for years. It had all come together beautifully.

Lorenzo put on some music and with a gentle hand on my back, danced me around the living room. He was a skilled dancer and much in demand as a partner at local dance clubs. Sometimes when we'd be walking together through a piazza with music in the air, he'd become Gene Kelly and trip the light *fantastica* with me across the Roman cobblestones. As he spun me around his living room that afternoon for our last dance, it was the perfect, cinematic ending to my life in Florence.

A couple of hours later, I was in a taxi headed to the airport. And by sunset that evening, I was with Henri on the terrace of the Hôtel Baudy, raising our champagne glasses to our new life together.

~᠑

I arrived in Giverny in the middle of June, in time for a garden party that promised to be the event of the summer.

The hostess was an Australian woman named Megan who had moved to Giverny a couple of years earlier. She had been a journalist for years and had lived in London and then Paris, before moving to Giverny. She had extensive connections in government and business circles and organized off-the-record gatherings of thought leaders and influencers at private venues in Paris. I liked Megan at first. We were close in age, and with our journalism backgrounds, I imagined we might become good friends.

Megan had been planning her garden party for months and had enlisted her local cadre of friends – which included Henri – in the preparations. But a rail strike made a mess of the arrangements. Many of the guests who were coming from Paris canceled because of the strike. Those who were coming by car needed overnight accommodations. Megan couldn't put up everyone at her house, so she asked Bernadette if she could provide a room for an American friend flying in from London.

Henri's museum and apartment were part of a sprawling complex that adjoined a large house, built in the 1950s, known in Giverny as the Old Lodge. Henri's family rarely used the Lodge except for large holiday gatherings. But with seven bedrooms, it was an ideal place to host occasional out-of-town visitors.

Bernadette's plan was to put Megan's American friend in the Lodge. But apparently there was a problem, which she discussed with Henri while the three of us were enjoying evening *apero* in the garden. I was having trouble following the conversation, which, of course, was in French. But I kept hearing my name mentioned.

When they seem to have resolved the issue, I turned to Henri and asked, "What's this about? I seem to be involved."

"We're going to say the American woman is your friend. *Pourquois pas?* You're part of the family now."

"I don't understand. Who are you going to tell?"

Bernadette went back inside, leaving Henri to explain their plan.

Their sister, Lucile, ran a B&B in the village and didn't like Henri and Bernadette putting up guests at the Lodge. Lucile said it took away potential business from her and she didn't like that Henri and Bernadette might be making money on the side from their visitors.

"So you're going to lie to Lucile and basically throw me under the bus?"

"What bus?"

"I'm not okay with this, Henri. I don't even know this American woman. Why is Bernadette pinning this on me?"

"It's easy to say the American is your friend. It's not a problem."

"Yes, it is a problem. I want to make a good start with your family. You're not being fair to me."

"Okay. I will talk to Bernadette, but I must do it now. She's leaving soon to talk to Lucile."

Henri disappeared for a few minutes and then returned. "*Bon.* Everything is fine. Shall we go get some dinner?"

It was only my second day in Giverny and already Bernadette had shown herself to be untruthful and no friend of mine. And Henri wasn't exactly innocent in all this.

~~

Turns out, the American woman – Angie from Texas – was delightful. Her natural drawl was tempered by an acquired British accent. In her mid-50s, she was an attorney specializing in international law who split her time between London and Midland, Texas, where her family was in the oil business. Angie and I hit it off instantly and we hung out together at the garden party. It was a relief to be able to speak English to someone other than Henri. I ignored a comment from a local woman at the party who walked by and scolded me for not speaking French.

Despite the lower-than-expected turnout, the party was a success. The food was delicious and the musicians were fantastic. Megan had certainly impressed everyone there with her hostess skills. She was the queen of the afternoon and cut an attractive figure in her tangerine-colored mini-sheath that showed off her slim tanned legs. I marveled at the intricate twists of her blonde hair that had been pulled back tightly in a classic French chignon at the nape of her neck.

The next day, while Henri and I were having coffee at the Baudy, Angie and Megan happened to walk by and joined us. I thanked Megan again for the wonderful party. But she seemed on edge and told me she was trying to stop smoking. Henri, sitting next to her, put his hand on her knee and told her not to be too hard on herself. He, too, had been trying to quit. Their conversation quickly switched from English to French, and I sensed they were talking about more than cigarettes. I couldn't help but notice that his hand lingered on her knee for most of their conversation.

Megan started scrolling on her phone to see what trains were running that day. Angie was hoping to spend the afternoon in Paris.

It was supposed to be a non-strike day, but apparently many trains had been cancelled. "I didn't think that was allowed," I said to Megan.

"They can do anything they want. This has been all over the news. Don't you girls know what's happening in the world?" Megan clearly needed a cigarette.

I later learned from Henri that during their chat *en français*, Megan had been dissing Angie to him. He didn't give me the details. But it was unbelievable to me that she had the nerve to do that in front of us, knowing Angie didn't speak French and assuming my French wasn't good enough to follow their conversation.

Before I moved to Giverny, Henri had told me wonderful things about Megan. But I suddenly realized I might need to watch my back with her, too.

~⸲

The next big event on our summer social calendar was an annual cabaret show put on by the voice students of a local *chanteuse* who was a good friend of Henri's. Every year the show is staged in the museum hall – which is a huge undertaking for Henri and the museum volunteers who must move mega-ton engines with forklifts to make room for the stage and audience seating.

It's a big family-night event. The hall was packed. I greeted the few people I knew and then took a seat in the back. After turning down the lights, Henri came and sat next to me. He slipped his arm around me and smiled. "Who needs opera in Paris when you have this?"

I really enjoyed the performance. The singers – who ranged from teenage to middle age – were at varying stages of their vocal development. But I loved that they all sang their hearts out. It was a wonderful evening.

Afterward, Henri and I were invited to the cast party, which was at the home of one of the singers, just down the street from the museum. There was loads of food. We heaped our plates and sat down with a group of Henri's friends at one of the big round tables in the garden.

Megan was at the table, but sitting on the far side opposite me. She was speaking in French to the people on either side of her. I wasn't paying attention, which I think she realized. Raising her voice a notch, she said to me, "Rebecca, what do you think?"

"About what?" I replied.

"I think children shouldn't be allowed to attend these events. It's very disrupting for the singers, with kids running around during the performance. Do you agree?"

I didn't agree with Megan. It was a popular show and families were welcome. But I knew if I disagreed with her – and I sensed she was baiting me – I would be drawn into an argument I wasn't interested in having.

So I deflected her question and said, "I'm reminded of Jeremy Irons."

I told everyone the story of an unflappable Jeremy Irons during a sold-out event one evening at the Odeon Theater in Florence. As he read from Machiavelli's *The Prince*, a cell phone rang in the back of the theater and an argument broke out when the person with the phone took the call. Despite all the shouting and shushing, Jeremy kept going, not missing a beat. Then up in the balcony, a baby started crying. Only then did Jeremy stop. He looked up at the parents and asked, "Newly born?" He made a quip about introducing children to great literature at an early age and continued reading.

I looked across the table at Megan. "In Shakespearean tradition, even when the audience is pelting actors with rotten tomatoes or kids are running in the aisles, the show goes on."

In my telling of that story, the attention at the table had turned to me. People wanted to know about my life in Florence and my first impressions of Giverny. I was the new New Girl in the village – a distinction Megan had enjoyed until my arrival.

That night, I didn't dwell on the consequences of that. Henri reached over and held my hand. He looked at me with such love in his eyes.

I leaned toward him and whispered, "Let's go home."

We made love that night into the wee hours. In those days, we couldn't get enough of each other.

Chapter 6

What I especially loved about Henri was his spontaneity.

One morning, I was cutting shelf paper for his pantry cupboard when he came bursting into the apartment from his morning walk with his dog, a black Labrador named Facel (after Henri's favorite French sports car, the Facel Vega).

"Come with me," he said, taking my hand. "You have to see this. Bring your camera."

Henri drove me down a dirt road behind the moulin where bright red poppies had blossomed overnight in a field of wheat. It looked like a scene Monet had painted. I could easily imagine Monet at this very spot, at his easel shaded by an umbrella. His thin, arching brushstrokes would have rendered the wheat stems bending in the breeze, with random flecks of red capturing the dancing motion of the poppy petals.

Henri and I waded into the waist-high stalks, walking along a tractor's tire tracks. I have a photo of him looking back at me and smiling, as if to say, *How lucky are we?*

~~~

Sometimes Henri would close the museum early and take me for a drink at the *boulangerie,* the village bakery-cafe, where locals gathered on the patio for the evening *apero* hour. It was a lovely time of day, when quiet descended on the village after the hordes of tourists had gone.

I was a curiosity in those days – Henri's new woman. He had told me I was a hot topic of gossip when word got out that he had gone to Malta to meet me. I was already known in Giverny because of my many visits there for my book research. But our appearance together as a couple turned heads wherever we went.

I struggled to put names with faces because introductions aren't the norm in Giverny. Even though I'd introduce myself, I'd rarely get more than a *bonjour* in reply.

Henri would often say to me, "You know who I'm talking about. You met him at the *boulangerie*."

"I've met lots of people at the *boulangerie*. But they don't tell me their names." I often wondered why Henri didn't properly introduce me.

An American friend of mine, who often brought painting groups to Giverny, had noticed the same custom. "I don't think it's rudeness. I think sometimes they don't know or remember each other's names," she told me, which made me laugh.

Although it took me awhile to be on a first-name basis with many of the locals I'd see every day, I felt welcomed as a newcomer. I was the new girlfriend of one of the most well-known and highly respected men in the village. That, in itself, made my entrée easier.

One summer's night, we were at a dinner party hosted by a long-time friend of Henri's, a Japanese woman named Yuka, who also had been a close friend of Camille's. Yuka raised her glass to me, saying that she looked forward to getting to know me and how delighted she was that Henri had found happiness again.

That meant the world to me.

⁓

Soon after my arrival, I had to present myself and my documents at the French immigration office in Rouen, about an hour from Giverny. A medical exam and a chest X-ray were required, which surprised me. Henri also had to submit paperwork, not as my financial sponsor, but essentially as my partner and landlord. He had to verify that I was staying at his address and prove he was the owner by showing his utility bills and tax records. I'd never had to do that in Italy. I rented my apartments there through a real estate agent who kindly helped me fill out my paperwork. But otherwise, I went through the immigration process on my own.

Henri was a willing partner as I settled in. He helped me set up a bank account and internet and cell-phone service. He'd patiently explain forms I had to fill out. He went with me to the social security office so that I could sign up for medical coverage.

I had no doubt of Henri's love for me. He used to come up from his workshop during the afternoon to check on me. I'd often be sitting on the sofa with my laptop in a corner of the living room where I could piggyback on the neighbor's wi-fi (it took three months to get my own service set up at Henri's apartment). Henri would stand in the doorway smiling at me, as if he couldn't believe his good luck. *"Ça va, chérie?"* How's it going, darling?

When I look back at the photos of Henri and me during our early weeks together, we both look so happy. In one photo, taken on the patio of the *boulangerie*, we're holding hands, looking like a couple of newlyweds. I've cupped one of his hands in both of mine, as if I've found a treasure. I look younger than my age in that photo, with a dusting of summer freckles on my rosy cheeks and a tousled mop of auburn curls. I have that dreamy look that comes from having sex daily. I wondered if that was obvious to everyone. Henri, wearing one of his Pink Floyd T-shirts, looks like a pumped-up poster boy for Viagra.

~∼

I wasn't worried initially when Henri and I started having problems. We had been single for a long time. Rough patches were bound to happen as we found our comfort zone together, I told myself.

But comfort, in fact, was the first big issue. After a few nights on that memory-foam bed, my back started bothering me. I hated to say anything to Henri because I knew it had been an expensive purchase. He'd already had the bed for a few months, so I knew he couldn't return it. I wondered if it would fit in the small back bedroom, where Henri was sleeping on a double bed. The memory-foam bed was queen size. I took some measurements to be sure it would fit before I asked him if we could switch the beds.

"The new bed won't fit in that room," he said.

"Actually, it will. I measured," I said. "Henri, I know this was a big purchase, but I wish you had taken me with you. I need a bed that's comfortable for me." It suddenly occurred to me that the bed had been Bernadette's choice – like the charcoal bedding.

I could tell he was annoyed.

"My back is bothering me. I need a spring mattress."

He suggested we swap rooms temporarily until we could move the beds. He assured me that the bed in the back room was comfortable.

It wasn't. Henri had said the mattress was fairly new, but later admitted it was more than 10 years old.

I slept on the bed in the back room for a week and Henri never made mention of making a change. So one day, on my own, I went to the local furniture store to look at new beds.

That evening, Henri asked what I'd like to do the next day.

"I'd like to go buy a bed for me."

"You don't like the bed in the back?"

"The mattress is sagging. And that room is depressing. It smells like a gas station back there." The windows in that room overlooked the museum hall, which reeked of diesel fuel and cast iron – a scent that, to Henri, is perfume.

Henri and I were butting heads over this, but I wasn't going to back off.

We went to the furniture store together. The manager, a friendly young man named David, recognized Henri from his visit with Bernadette a few months earlier.

I tried every spring mattress in the store, as Henri and David looked on.

I said to them both, "I feel like the Princess and the Pea."

David laughed. "*Oui*, I know that story. You are Rebecca and the pea."

Within an hour, Henri was buying a bed for me and arranging for its delivery.

Our new relationship was getting expensive for Henri. But my expenses were quickly mounting as well.

The next week, my boxes arrived from Florence. (The FedEx shipping bill was more than $1,000.) Henri off-loaded the truck himself and randomly stacked the cartons in the living room. I hadn't planned to unpack them all at once. In fact, my plan was to store some of them and unpack only what I needed.

My back got worse as the unpacking began. I asked Henri if some of his museum volunteers could help me organize the boxes, but that didn't happen. Within a week, I was limping. A trip to IKEA nearly did me in. I didn't have room in my rental car for some of the items I needed – a desk, an office chair and a bookcase. It would have taken a few weeks to have them delivered, so I asked Henri if he'd come with me in his truck.

I didn't think my back would tolerate the truck ride, so I suggested I drive separately in my car. The IKEA store was a half hour from Giverny.

For some strange reason, he insisted that I ride with him. He became angry and said, "Bernadette rides 500 kilometers in that truck without a problem."

"I'm not Bernadette," I said calmly, "She doesn't have a back problem."

The next morning, Henri pulled up at the front door in the truck and opened the passenger-side door. He clearly expected to win this argument. The muscle spasm in my low back was so bad that I couldn't lift my left leg high enough to get into the cab.

I was near tears. "I can't do this." I turned away and went to my car. We drove separately to IKEA.

As I lay on a heating pad in bed that night, Henri sat next to me and said, "*Chérie*, I could see the pain on your face this morning. We'll find you a doctor."

~~~~o

I had been under chiropractic care for back and neck problems for many years and kept myself in alignment with maintenance appointments once or twice a month. I knew I had done too much heavy lifting during the move and Henri's uncomfortable beds hadn't helped.

Henri had been seeing a physiotherapist for a disc problem and thought we should start there. The therapist was a young Spanish guy named Jose who had a pain clinic a short distance from Giverny. He was multi-lingual and spoke excellent English. I liked his jovial manner, but I soon discovered that inflicting pain was his specialty. He had state-of-the-art equipment and used electric stimulation in his treatments. He also had thumbs of steel. During one deep-tissue massage, I cried out in pain. He proceeded with the treatment. But it was too much. I begged him to stop and started sobbing.

The sobs were releasing something deep inside me, I knew that. Jose asked me to come into his office after I got dressed. As I sat at his desk, I couldn't stop crying. He said sometimes in the process of relieving pain, the memory of pain from long ago is released. He said he would not put me through anything I couldn't tolerate and asked me to tell him when I was at my limit.

When I got back in the car, I didn't think I'd ever see Jose again.

I cried all the way home. Henri was stunned at the distraught state I was in when I arrived back at the apartment.

"*Chérie*, what happened?"

I couldn't speak. He held me in his arms for a long time as I cried like a baby.

Ironically, it was Megan who told Henri about a chiropractor she thought might be good for me. Several months earlier, she had fallen off a ladder and broken her forearm. It was a bad break that had required surgery and a long rehabilitation program. She was pleased with the therapy treatments she was getting and suggested Henri book an appointment for me.

On the day of my first visit, Megan happened to be there, finishing up a therapy session. She introduced me to Jean-Raymond, the chiropractor, who spoke a little English. Henri had come with me to translate, but asked Megan to speak to him instead.

I felt awkward having Megan translate my chiropractic history for me. I hardly knew her. But given the circumstances and the pain I was in, I was glad to have found a chiropractor who could help me. I had Megan to thank for that.

~～⁹

I was still trying to find my footing with Bernadette.

Early on, I had asked Henri if she would appreciate my help in the kitchen. He said, "She would appreciate if you *offered* to help, but that's it."

One evening for *apero*, Henri had asked me to make Aperol Spritzes, which I had introduced him to in Florence. Aperol is a bright orange Italian aperitif made from rhubarb, oranges and various herbs and roots. When mixed with prosecco and sparking water, it becomes a Spritz. Twists of orange slices are the finishing touch.

Aperol Spritzes are served on ice, which Bernadette brought from the kitchen fridge to the garden where several friends had gathered for a party after France had won the World Cup soccer championship. I had set up a little bar at the table and was mixing the drinks when Bernadette did something that amazed me. She leaned her body into mine, trying to push me aside so that she could chop up the orange slices I had already cut. I said, "No, like this," as I made a thin cut through the center of an orange slice, which I then slipped onto the rim of a glass.

I paid a price for that moment of audacity.

During dinner, she warned me about croissants. I thought she was telling me not to feed croissants to Henri's dog, who loved croissants. Henri said something to Bernadette in French. I thought he said, "He didn't have a croissant today."

But what Henri actually said was, "*She* didn't have a croissant today." Henri was in the habit of bringing home croissants from the *boulangerie* every morning for our breakfast together. By the time he had arrived at the *boulangerie* that morning, they had already run out.

Bernadette pretended to grab a roll of fat at her slim waist and shook her finger at me. She was telling me croissants would make me fat.

A few minutes later, she told me I needed to find another place to park my car because it was in the way of delivery trucks that needed access to a storage space next to Henri's apartment. The storage space and Henri's apartment were on the opposite side of the property, far from her turf. It really was none of her business where we parked our cars and to my knowledge, there hadn't been any problems with deliveries to the storage space.

The "wife" clearly was pissed off that Henri had asked me to play hostess and bartender at the *apero* party.

~

My summer project was to plant a flowerbed in the lawn area in front of Henri's apartment. I had ordered some English roses from the nursery of famed rose hybridizer David Austin, in Shropshire, England.

A month after I had arrived in Giverny, the roses were still in their containers waiting to be planted, along with perennials I had purchased locally as companion plants.

I had also bought an edging tool to cut the shape of the bed, which I had staked out with pegs and string. I needed someone with a rototiller to break up the thick layer of sod and turn over the topsoil.

Henri kept dragging his feet, telling me there wasn't anyone who could do the work. How can that be, I'd argue. We were living in a village famous for its gardens.

Finally, he asked an older man named Gabriel who lived down the road to come help me. Gabriel was an avid gardener and owned a rototiller. He prepped the bed, but then went off on holiday for a few weeks.

My roses and perennials sat in their pots, wilting in the July heat.

I felt myself wilting from exasperation.

~

Henri had been in the habit of leaving his apartment unlocked. Before I moved in, there wasn't much of value in the apartment. Henri said there wasn't a problem with house break-ins in Giverny, so we didn't need to lock the doors.

But I had brought things of value. My computer and camera equipment alone were reason enough to lock the doors. I had seen tourists wander onto Henri's property to look at the ram and the goat in the corral beside his driveway. Tourists can be very intrusive in Giverny and regard the entire village as though it were Disneyland.

I also wanted some privacy. There were two doors to the apartment. The back door was the main entry for friends and family, who never knocked before entering. I was on the toilet one day when one of Henri's buddies came in the back looking for him. I was surprised he didn't open the bathroom door to see if Henri was on the pot.

The only lock on the back door was a deadbolt that had to be secured from inside the apartment. So I got in the habit of securing the bolt and locking the front door when I was out. That meant Henri had to carry a key to the front door to get into the apartment.

He made a big fuss about that. He said he wasn't used to carrying a key. We had a shouting match about this one night after he couldn't get into the apartment because he had misplaced the key.

"You're not in California," he yelled at me. "There's no need to keep this apartment locked. We don't have a problem in Giverny."

"You keep your office locked downstairs because you have things of a value there. Why can't I do the same? You don't care about my security and privacy."

"You don't get to make the rules!"

"Why are you so upset with me?"

"I don't like the way you speak to me," he said. "No one *ever* speaks to me this way."

"What about the way you speak to me? You walked in here mad as a bull."

"A what?"

"A bull."

He shook his head. "You can express yourself in your own language. But I can't tell you how I feel in mine."

I went into my room and shut the door. I sat on the end of the bed and looked out at the lovely view. The blue shadows of twilight blanketed the hillside, as the treetops caught the last light of day. In the distance, cuckoo birds sang as they settled in for the night.

My life in Giverny had started as a dream come true. But for the first time, I let myself face the reality I had made a horrible mistake.

A short while later, there was a faint knock at the bedroom door. "Come in," I said.

Henri walked over to the bed and sat down next to me. "We're fighting a lot these days," he said, putting his arm around me. "Are you unhappy being here with me?"

I didn't know what to say. I felt the air go out of him.

That night from my bed I could see the light of the moon. It was the day after the longest lunar eclipse of the 21st century. It had caused a phenomenon called the Blood Moon. The "blood" was actually a reddish-brown hue on the moon's surface, created by the refraction of rays of sunlight as they passed around the edge of the Earth during the eclipse.

I couldn't sleep, so at one in the morning, I slipped outside in my nightgown and slippers. There was a light breeze, which felt good.

I stood next to my still-unplanted flowerbed, looking up at the sky. We hadn't been able to see the eclipse the night before because of cloud cover. But oddly, there still seemed to be a tinge of red – the color of dried blood – in a ring of clouds around the moon.

I jumped when I heard a noise in the grass near my feet. It was the neighbor's cat, Mimi. Her fur rubbed my leg, and she looked up at me as if to say, *You're not alone.*

As the moon disappeared behind the clouds, I sent up a little prayer to my angel friends on high: *Help!*

Chapter 7

One evening at a dinner party, I met an American woman named Rosalind – she went by the nickname "Roz" – who was renting a place in Giverny for the summer. She was attractive and vivacious, in her late 70s, and was from the Central Coast wine-producing region of California, where for many years she had owned a well-known restaurant. She had published a cookbook and was interested in opening a cooking school in Giverny.

"Tourists need something to do here if they're staying for a few days," she told me. "After they've seen Monet's gardens and visited the Impressionist museum, what then?"

I thought that was a great idea. Many of my American friends love to take cooking classes when they travel. In Italy, entire holiday packages are built around cooking classes at a Tuscan villa with daily shopping excursions for ingredients at local markets. I could easily see something like that here.

Roz was looking for a venue and was in negotiations with a Giverny businessman who was buying a property that she hoped to rent from him. She was bubbling with ideas for her new venture and when she heard I was a writer and photographer, she wondered if I'd be interested in working with her. She was planning a website and had ideas for another cookbook.

We met one day for tea at the house she was renting, a beautifully renovated historic property known as La Villa des Pinsons that had been owned by Monet and where members of his family had lived.

As I sunk into a comfy chair in her living room, she asked how

I was enjoying life in Giverny. It was the first time I had said this to anyone, but I decided to be honest. "I love our surroundings here, but I've not had an easy time."

Roz had met Henri at the party and apparently knew a bit about him and his family. "Has the family been welcoming?" she asked. I could tell by her tone that she knew something about them.

"For the most part." I didn't want to mention Bernadette. "The language barrier has been a problem. No one in the family speaks much English, so I'm lost when they speak fast French and feel left out if Henri doesn't translate for me."

"He doesn't do that?"

"Sometimes, but not often enough."

"Are you taking French lessons?"

"I've had a few sessions with a tutor who comes to the house."

"I need a tutor as well. Maybe we could take lessons together."

I liked Roz's enthusiasm and positive outlook. She was going back to California for a couple of months to organize things she wanted to ship to France. I admired her spirit of adventure, especially at her age, as she envisioned a new life for herself in a foreign country.

"Don't try to shoulder too much," she advised. "Find people who can help you." Roz had found a local driver to take her on errands and to Vernon on market days. She had a housekeeper who came three days a week. "I love to cook, but I don't do dishes," she said with a laugh. "I was born with a golden spoon in my mouth."

Not a silver spoon, as the saying goes, but a golden spoon. What an odd thing to say. Bragging about wealth can work against you as an American living abroad. But maybe she truly didn't need to care about money.

She served a delicious lemon tart that she had bought that morning at the Saturday market in Vernon.

"I've found this wonderful young woman from Senegal who's a marvelous pastry chef. She just graduated from a culinary school in Paris and wants to open a shop in Vernon. I want to help her." Roz took a bite of the tart. "Isn't this divine?"

It was divine. As I listened to Roz's big plans for her cooking school in Giverny, I took some inspiration from her. She wasn't going to let anything stop her. "I give my desires to the universe," she told me. "And I know what's meant to be will happen."

Roz sent me home with half of the lemon tart, which I brought to Sunday lunch with Henri's family the next day. Bernadette had made a delicious plum tart, but the lemon tart was a big hit. I told them the story of the pastry chef and how she was looking to set up shop in Vernon. Bernadette took one bite and then laid down her fork. She asked me if I knew the name of the culinary school in Paris the young woman had attended, as if questioning her credentials. Bernadette appeared to be unimpressed – and perhaps a bit miffed at being upstaged.

~

The weather turned beastly hot in August and Megan invited a group of us for a pool party at her place one Friday evening. The most remarkable aspect of the pool, enclosed in a glass conservatory, was a 10-foot poster, propped against one wall, of Megan in a glamour pose with her long blonde hair flung over one shoulder.

Megan had become known for her Friday night gatherings, which she held every few weeks for a dozen or so of her closest friends in Giverny. She called these evenings "Shabbat Night." Megan's Friday-night soirées had nothing do with the sacred Jewish observance of Shabbat that begins on Friday evenings with a meal in honor of the Sabbath. Jewish friends of mine had once included me in their Shabbat dinner and it was one of the most beautiful meals, filled with prayer and song, that I've ever experienced. Megan wasn't Jewish. When I asked Henri if anyone in the group was offended by this, he just shrugged.

Megan's "Shabbat" menu typically was finger food and lots of wine. Everyone brings a dish and a few bottles to share.

"Megan likes Margaux," he told me. Margaux is a highly rated red Bordeaux that, at the low end, costs around $20 a bottle. Henri took two bottles to the party that evening.

I made a pasta salad. It wasn't finger food, but I brought serving utensils and plastic forks.

After Henri and I had greeted everyone on our arrival, we joined Megan at the far end of the long table she had set up on her patio. Henri sat between us. A handsome, middle-aged man named Stephan sat down beside me. He spoke fluent English, so I was glad to have someone to chat with.

Megan was speaking French to Henri and looked over at me. In English, she said, "How much of this do you understand?"

"Is there going to be a quiz later?" I asked sarcastically.

Henri shot me a glance.

"No, I just want to be sure you feel included in the conversation."

I wasn't buying it. I had an ominous feeling it was going to be a long evening.

The problem with "Shabbat Night" is there's too little food and too much wine. So after a few hours, inhibitions and filters fall away as the alcohol kicks in.

Megan was chain-smoking and at one point, offered Henri a cigarette. "Smoke with me," she said. She lit his cigarette from her own. There was something comfortable and casual about the way this happened between them.

That wasn't what surprised me. It was the first time I had seen Henri smoke since before our trip to Malta. He had told me while we there that he had given up smoking. "I know you're not a smoker," he had said. "I want to do this for you." I knew it wouldn't be easy. He'd been a smoker since he was a teenager. In the past few months, he had been using nicotine patches, but found they made him shaky. Most of the time, he relied on willpower, but I knew it was difficult for him when he was around people who were smoking. I was furious with Megan. She knew he had been trying to quit. I wanted to grab the cigarette from Henri and snuff it out on her plate.

Henri had a different persona when he was smoking, I discovered that night. At one point, he stood to tell a funny story to the group. With a cigarette in hand, his presence was more commanding, his long inhales and smoky exhales added dramatic punctuation. He exuded confidence, even a sexiness I hadn't seen before. He didn't look at me once during the telling of his funny story. It was hard for me to watch his performance. I felt he was breaking a promise to me, intentionally. I looked over at Megan and could tell she was loving every minute of it.

Darkness had fallen when the worst part of that "Shabbat Night" unfolded. Out of the blue, Megan turned to Henri and said, "Rebecca needs to rewrite your sign at the museum – the one above the donation jar."

"What's wrong with the sign?" he asked her.

"What does it say – something like, *Thank you for your support...*"

Henri finished her sentence, saying, "*We are pleased to share our passion with you.*"

Blowing a plume of smoke in the air, Megan said in a louder voice, "I don't think you should be asking for donations." She turned to the rest of the group. "What do you all think? I think Henri should charge admission."

This was Megan's modus operandi. Throw a grenade and watch everyone react.

Henri's Japanese friend Yuka, who was sitting at the far end of the table with Bernadette, enthusiastically said, "I agree!"

Then Megan turned to me. "What do you think, Rebecca?"

"That's for the family to decide," I said.

Megan loves debate and discussion – that's what she does for a living at her high-priced Paris luncheons with heads of government and industry. That night, after more than a few glasses of Margaux, she was looking for debate and discussion with me.

"Surely, you have an opinion," she said to me.

"Megan, next time you're at the museum, read the guest book," I said. "Last week, an American woman wrote that she was fairly certain her teenage son had decided to become an engineer that day because of the tour Henri had given them."

Megan flicked the ash off her cigarette. "Then she should be willing to pay for that experience."

"How do you know she didn't leave a 20-euro note in the jar?"

"How do you know she did?"

"It doesn't matter, Megan. Many people give generously and make up for those who don't. Regardless, Henri and his volunteers love sharing the collection with anyone who comes through the door. I've seen so many kids in that museum mesmerized by those engines. You can't put a price on that experience."

"I disagree."

I looked at Henri. "It would be sad if families wouldn't come to the museum because they couldn't afford admission. Remember the little boy who was telling you how he was going to invent a car that could drive on water?"

He nodded. I could tell Henri appreciated I was taking his side.

What worried me was that Megan was translating what I was saying for Bernadette, who was the only one in the group who didn't understand English. And Megan knew I didn't understand French well enough to correct her translation.

There was discussion around the table. At one point, I heard Bernadette say, "*Rebecca dit...*" Rebecca says...what? I couldn't hear what Bernadette thought I had said.

I turned to Henri. "How is my position being presented here? Does Bernadette understand that I'm not agreeing with Megan?"

Henri was inexplicably quiet. He hated confrontation.

Stephan, the man sitting beside me, leaned toward me and said, "If you think you're going to make changes in the family you're now a part of, good luck."

"But I'm not the one wanting them to change this. It's Megan."

It was a baffling end to a horrible evening. When Henri and I got in the car a short while later, I said to him, "I don't know what just happened there. But I'm done with Megan. Please explain to Bernadette that I didn't agree with her."

After that, my new nickname for Megan was Mean Girl – or "MG" for short.

MG's "Shabbat Night" pool party was a game changer for me. I remembered what my mom used to say if I'd come home from school complaining that someone hadn't been nice to me. Her wise advice: "Find someone else to play with."

I saw Roz a few days after the "Shabbat Night" pool party and told her what had happened.

"*Shabbat* Night?" she asked incredulously.

"I know. Unbelievable."

Turns out, Roz had met MG when she had been looking for an apartment that summer. MG had a guest unit that she offered on Airbnb.

"I didn't have a good feeling about her," Roz said. "She seems to be a very unhappy person."

"And she likes inflicting her misery on others."

"Stay away from her. And keep up your French studies so you can be part of the conversation." Roz went over to a bookcase and took an enormous French dictionary off the shelf. The book's spine was the width of my hand. "I give this to you as a gift," she said. "There are way too many words in this book for me to learn at my age."

A few days later, Roz was getting ready for her return trip to the U.S. and I offered to bring her a few shipping boxes from my move to Giverny.

Her front door was open when I arrived. She was on the phone and motioned for me to come inside. She disappeared into another room, but I could hear her side of the conversation. There seemed to be a problem with the Giverny property where she had planned to set up her cooking school.

When she finally got off the call and joined me in the living room, I asked if everything was okay.

"I'm not sure," she said. "There are some complications."

She didn't give details and I felt it wasn't my place to ask. I helped her pack up the boxes that she would be storing in Giverny until her return.

"I'm so looking forward to seeing you when I get back," she said. "I think we're at the start of a wonderful friendship."

She looked so serene that day, standing barefoot in a patch of sunlight. Her tousled graying blonde hair beautifully framed her face. I could easily envision her as a much younger woman.

Over cups of tea, we spoke of our hopes for our new lives in Giverny. My hopes had been badly shaken, but I wanted to be optimistic.

When I got up to leave, she took my hands and cradled them between hers. "May I say an affirmation?" she asked.

I smiled at her. "I'd like that."

Roz closed her eyes and said, "In this time of acclimation, please make it possible for Rebecca to share the beauty of her spirit in this place, her new home. Amen."

Chapter 8

Henri and I reached a breaking point a couple of weeks after MG's pool party. He was smoking again, though not in my presence. He seemed to think he was camouflaging his habit with breath mints and chewing gum, but he reeked of tobacco smoke. He kept saying he had given up cigarettes. But one day, I saw a pack of pencil cigars in his car, tucked behind the visor.

One night, he slipped into bed next to me and wanted to make love. I pulled away as he tried to kiss me. I hated the taste of him.

"What's wrong?" he asked.

"You promised me you'd try to stop smoking. I know it hasn't been easy. But you don't seem to care anymore. You smell like an ashtray. "

"Why are you so hard on me?"

"I want to help you, Henri. I see that you're struggling. But you knew from the beginning that this would be a problem for me. I was so relieved and grateful that this wasn't going to be a wedge between us. But now, it is."

There had been a worrying change in Henri's behavior. As our disagreements had escalated over the summer, he had begun acting out.

It had started with passive-aggressive goading. I had purchased some pretty French linen tea towels that I had hung in the kitchen by the sink. They were meant to be used for drying hands. But Henri started using them as if they were paper towels.

One day, he wiped tea residue from a cup, leaving a dark stain on the linen.

"I won't be able to get that out," I said.

"That's because you don't know how to use the washing machine," he retorted.

"I didn't know you were a laundry expert," I said. "Please show me how to use the washer." Henri had never done a load of laundry in his life. His mother, sisters, partners and housekeepers always had done it for him.

The very next day, while I watched, Henri wiped tomato juice from a glass with another linen tea towel – and when he saw my look of dismay, he laughed.

This had moved beyond tea towels.

"Are you sorry you've invited me to come live with you?" I asked.

He asked what "sorry" meant and then wanted me to spell it. He knew full well the meaning of the word.

"Do you want me to leave?" I asked. We were standing opposite each other at the butcher-block counter in the kitchen. I ran my finger along a knife cut in the wood. "I've spent the last five months packing and unpacking. I can pack up everything again. No problem."

We stared at each other for a minute.

Finally, he said, "No, I don't want you to leave."

I took the tea towel, with its bright red stain, and threw it in the trash. "We'll use paper towel from now on. You clearly don't appreciate nice things."

~~⁓~~

I began to see that if I was going to make a happy life for myself in Giverny, I needed to find my independence. I needed to have my own activities, my own circle of friends.

One day, Marie Noëlle – the charming Madame Red Shoes – stopped by the apartment with the man who owned the Pierre Bonnard house near Giverny. He was planning a weekend open house for Patrimony Days, a national event each September that celebrates French heritage. He wanted me to sign copies of the book I had written about Bonnard and be part of the festivities he was planning.

A door opened to me with that invitation. I couldn't imagine a better book-signing event, in the room where Bonnard had painted his famous views of the Seine.

Henri had come up from his workshop to say hello and Marie Noëlle invited us for dinner the following Saturday. She had lived in Vernon for nearly 50 years and loved bringing her friends together for soirées in her garden. I knew it would be a wonderful evening.

In fact, it was. But it didn't go exactly as planned. Fifteen minutes before Henri and I were due to leave for the party, he came up from the downstairs kitchen and said his plans had changed. His son Alex had arrived with food and drinks for an impromptu barbecue.

"But we're supposed to be at Marie Noëlle's in half an hour," I said.

"What am I supposed to do? Alex brought all this food."

"Tell Alex you already have plans this evening."

"I can't do that."

"But Marie Noëlle is expecting us. We said yes to this a week ago."

"You go alone. I have no choice."

"Yes, you do have a choice in this."

He put up his hands as if to say *"I don't want an argument"* and went back downstairs to join the family.

When I arrived at Marie Noëlle's, one of her sons greeted me at the front gate. "Where's Henri?" he asked.

"Something came up at the last minute. I'm so sorry."

Marie Noëlle looked surprised when I apologized for Henri's absence. It was then that I realized Henri and I were intended to be the guests of honor.

She knew I was embarrassed and gently tucked her arm in mine. "Come, let me introduce you to the others." I could tell that she also knew there was more to this than I was letting on.

It truly was a lovely evening. Everyone at the table spoke some English and I was able to follow their conversation in French, if they spoke slowly. *Lentement, s'il vous plaît.* Slowly, please. I had become aware that I needed to speak English more slowly, too. Bridging a language gap is a lot like a slow dance.

One woman in the group commented on my excellent diction. "It is very easy to understand your English because you speak clearly and slowly," she said. "And your American accent makes it's easy, too. I can't understand a word when I'm talking to someone who's British."

"I usually watch British films with the subtitles on," I said, which made everyone laugh.

Slowly, slowly. I will find my way, I told myself on the drive home that night. The evening had been a success. I had held my own, without Henri.

When I got back to the apartment, it was about 11. Henri was already asleep in his room. For the first time in many nights, I slept like a baby.

In the early weeks of the summer, I had been driving an automatic I had rented, for $750 per month – twice the cost of cars with manual transmissions. Henri thought I should learn to drive a stick, so he took me for a test drive in his SUV. In a moment of spontaneity, he had pulled over on a country road next to a field of beetroots and said to me, "You can take us the rest of the way home."

We were only a mile from his place, with an unlikely chance of encountering another vehicle. But I could feel my palms getting clammy as I gripped the steering wheel. I lurched from first to second and then got us into third.

We left the beetroots behind and entered a forest. I knew the road well. I called it the Tree Tunnel. The overarching branches formed a lush green canopy that fractured the sunlight. I always had the feeling I was a character in a Grimms' fairy tale on that road. Wild boars and deer roamed in the woods. Local hunters had a cabin there where they slaughtered their Sunday spoils. (Hunting in Giverny is allowed only on Sundays.) I tended to speed up as I'd pass one particular giant tree that reached out from the edge of the forest. At the top of its enormous trunk, a tangle of vines twisted the leafy top branches into a grotesque, beastly face – as if to warn children they shouldn't wander here alone.

I wasn't thinking about fairy tales as I maneuvered the bends in the road. At the edge of the forest, a sign marking the boundary of Giverny appears. And just a few hundred feet beyond that is the entrance to Henri's driveway.

There's a slight incline at the driveway entrance, which proved to be my undoing. I stalled four times, to Henri's amazement. He clearly had no idea how impaired I was at stick-shifting.

I persevered and triumphantly pulled up at the front door.

"Not bad," I said, turning to Henri for his assessment. "On a scale of one to 10, how did I do?"

"I'd give you a two."

Henri cast a wide net online, looking for an automatic for me to buy. It was early August at that point, only two months after my move to Giverny. I was feeling uneasy about making this financial commitment to my new life that seemed to be going sideways. I still had boxes I purposely hadn't unpacked. Emotionally, I took great comfort in knowing I had a magic carpet tucked away if I needed to fly away.

I definitely needed a car. Giverny is a tourist village with no food stores, banks, gas stations, pharmacies, or shops that sell more than souvenirs. Wheels are essential. The nearest grocery store is five miles away.

Previously owned automatics were extremely scarce and new ones were costly and usually had to be ordered. Henri's local mechanic had a used automatic that was so compact I could barely slide my legs under the steering wheel. Finally, a Citroën dealer in Vernon called Henri to say he'd just gotten an automatic on a trade-in.

It was one of the ugliest cars I've ever seen. A white SUV, it had black rubber side panels that looked like giant Legos. The previous owner had commuted to Paris in it and the body was badly scraped. It looked like it had been in a combat zone.

I couldn't sustain the cost of a rental, so I decided I would put a third down on the Lego-mobile and finance the rest through Henri's bank, where I had set up an account. But when we met with Henri's personal banker, he said the loan committee wouldn't review an application from me because I was a foreigner. I got the impression that being a foreign *female* was part of the problem. In the blink of an eye, the banker drew up loan papers in Henri's name and arranged for the monthly payments to be transferred from my account to his. I didn't like that our finances were now entangled – Henri and I had agreed from the beginning that we wouldn't co-mingle our funds. But Henri didn't mind the loan arrangement and I had little choice at that point if I didn't want to pay full price for the car.

We went to the dealership to pick up the car in late August. Henri knew the salesman, a pudgy middle-aged guy who exuded a lube-oil slickness. The two of them chatted in French as I signed the papers. What escaped my attention, largely because Henri's translations were vague, was that, at Monsieur Lube Oil's suggestion, Henri's name went on the title along with mine because of the financing arrangement.

I handed the salesman a cashier's check, drawn from Henri's account where the loan funds were on deposit, for 11,000 euros (about $12,000 at the time). The salesman gave us a bottle of champagne as a thank-you gift from the dealership. It was close to lunchtime and French businesses typically close for two hours during the middle of the day. The salesman handed me the keys and gave us hurried instructions about the car's features. The Lego-mobile had a dashboard computer system that would allow me to take calls. My phone had lost its charge, so I plugged it in while the salesman programmed

Henri's number into the system. He then shook hands with Henri and went back inside.

"What about *my* phone?" I asked Henri.

"You can come back another day and he'll take care of it."

I noticed my plugged-in phone was functioning again. "I want him to do it now."

"*Chérie*, they're closed for lunch."

I could see Monsieur Lube-Oil inside the showroom with a group of colleagues, congratulating themselves on a good morning.

"I just handed him a check for 11,000 euros," I said firmly to Henri. "He can do this now."

A guy from the dealership's repair shop came out holding a ring of keys, intending to close and lock the front gate. He looked at me and then at Henri.

"He wants us to go so he can shut the gate," Henri said to me.

"I'm not moving this car until your buddy comes out here and programs this phone."

Henri mumbled something and went inside to get the salesman, who looked unhappy that my request was interrupting his lunch break.

I didn't give a shit. In fact, in that moment, I couldn't have been happier. I had three Frenchmen looking rather unhappy with me as I got the customer service I deserved.

In my trial-by-fire during my early months in Giverny, I had learned a lot about French chauvinism and arrogance.

When Gabriel, the gardener, finally returned from his holiday to finish the work on my flowerbed, he didn't hesitate to question my methods for planting roses. Henri, who knows nothing about roses, agreed with him.

I held my ground that day and literally dug my heels in with them. I knew a vast amount about growing roses. I had become a certified rosarian at the Los Angeles County Arboretum, after completing a comprehensive course there in rose horticulture. I'd had a beautiful rose garden of my own. I became a big fan of David Austin roses when they burst on the scene in the U.S. and read volumes about their growth habits and care.

When Gabriel and Henri suggested that I didn't know what I was doing as we were planting my David Austins, I stared at them defiantly and said ENOUGH.

Chapter 9

To curb my growing exasperation with the challenges I was facing in my new life, I turned my attention to the beauty around me.

I loved photographing Monet's garden and often wished I could depict on canvas what I saw through the camera lens. Sometimes I felt like a painter as I composed a shot, trying to capture the essence of Monet's vision. I'd squint at the landscape, seeing the interplay of color and light that inspired not only his work but a painting movement that marked the beginning of modern art.

The unique light of the Seine Valley was what captivated Impressionists. The air has a vapory quality, tinged with morning mist and evening fog. The Impressionists were *plein-air* painters – they painted in the "open air," adapting to changing light and weather conditions. Giverny experiences ever-changing weather, as fronts move across Normandy, eastwardly from the Atlantic and from the English Channel, to the north. One day, in the span of an afternoon, I photographed Monet's lily pond under brilliant sunshine, stormy skies, a gentle rain and then dewy twilight.

A year earlier, I had tagged along with a painting group organized by American artist Caroline Homes Nuckolls and her photographer husband, Rich, the founders of Art Colony Giverny, whose week-long sessions in spring and fall gave artists an opportunity to paint in the gardens and on location elsewhere in the area. I hadn't painted since I was in first grade and loved learning how to mix colors and properly hold a brush. Caroline sent me home with several tubes of paint, but they ended up in a drawer.

I found them in a box I had shipped from Florence and asked Giverny artist Christian Avril if he would give me a painting lesson in the gardens. Chris, much beloved in Giverny, was often seen around the village at his easel, in his *artiste* attire. In his mid-60s, he presented a youthful persona in brightly colored floral shirts or sometimes, a more dapper ensemble: flax-colored trousers with a matching vest, under a linen jacket. A loose-fitting tie and straw hat – his essential accessories – completed the look.

In those days, it was possible to buy a *Billet Artiste* – an artist's ticket – that gave painters and photographers access to the gardens after hours, from 6-8 p.m. The cost was €9.50 (about $11), the same price as admission during the day. After 6, the gardens would go quiet as the security guards ushered out the last of the day's visitors. The painters and photographers were then free to set up their easels and tripods and immerse themselves in the golden hours of evening.

At the appointed hour of my painting lesson, I met Chris at the front steps of Monet's house. As I followed him to the lily pond, I asked where he had gotten his vintage wicker painter's trolley.

"On the internet," he said. I loved the irony of that.

My painting kit was cobbled together from odds and ends I had found in the storage space next to Henri's apartment. I felt inspired carrying an easel that had belonged to the late Gale Bennett, who for many years was Giverny's well-known American-artist-in-residence and whose studio had been on the other side of what is now Henri's living room wall. For a decade, Gale had rented the Lodge to accommodate participants in his plein-air painting program. Henri had been his landlord.

Chris made quick work of setting up our gear on the little bridge at the far end of the pond. He laughed at Gale's easel. "There's a part missing here," he said, jerry-rigging the top clamp.

Painters usually carry fresh water to clean their brushes. Chris' method was more organic. He swung a twine rope, tied around the neck of an open-ended plastic container, high above his head. On the downswing, he leaned over the bridge railing and scooped up water from the pond. I imagined little tadpoles swimming around the bristles of our brushes.

The subject of my first painting was to be Monet's iconic Japanese bridge, cloaked in dark green wisteria vines, at the opposite end of the pond. At 6 p.m. in mid-September, the sun is low and the light fades fast. Chris asked me to outline in blue paint – a blueprint, essentially – the scene I intended to paint. He handed me a pad of paper to use as a palette and gave me a paint-mixing lesson.

"This is how you make the green of the bridge," he said, swirling some cadmium yellow with phthalo blue.

"Okay, begin," he said, grinning. "Good luck."

I pretty much had no idea what I was doing. Occasionally, Chris, who was working on an immense canvas that had somehow materialized out of nowhere, would check on my progress. Looking at my tentative brush strokes, he said, "Gale Bennett would say, *Don't be bashful with your brush. Be bold.*"

So, I became more emboldened. And slowly but surely, the magical alchemy of the color wheel began. I was boldly brushing cadmium yellow and Monet green on whorls of violet and magenta, creating the sun's glow on the wisteria canopy. A daub of titanium white on a dash of pink and – *voila!* – a water lily was born.

It was a warm evening, with no chill in the air to warn me that the sun was setting. When Chris said, "Okay, the last thing you must do is paint the bridge," I realized it had disappeared in the fall of night.

I conjured up my memory of it and carefully painted its outline against the foliage. The bridge is barely discernible in the finished work – true to my *plein-air* experience.

We quickly packed up, cleaning our brushes in the little tub of pond water. I laughed when Chris slipped his huge canvas into a nearby clump of bushes. "I'll finish it tomorrow," he said. I wondered if Monet had stored his works-in-progress in the bushes, too.

I loved my first lesson and went back a few days later. I was the only artist in the gardens that evening – a surreal experience – and decided to paint the rose arbors spanning the *Grande Allée*. I set up near the front steps of Monet's house. The *allée* stretches down to the main gate from the walkway in front of the house. During the summer, nasturtiums, planted along both sides of the *allée*, creep toward the middle and meet in the center by fall. They were nearly at their meeting point and had formed a thick carpet, dotted with orange and yellow blossoms.

As I drew my "blueprint" on my gessoed board, there was the sound of a vacuum cleaner and laughter in the house as staff closed up for the night. By the time I was filling in the details of the dahlias and the sunflowers an hour later, the sun was setting fast. When I put down my brush, I felt I had more to do (and so much more to learn), but I liked that the picture captured a fleeting moment as the sunlight vanished down the *Grande Allée*.

I laughed to myself remembering my first painting lesson in the garden with Caroline the year before. I had set up my easel in the same place, facing the *Grande Allée*, when all of a sudden, a wind kicked up. As my easel tipped toward me, I grabbed the canvas, but dropped my palette that was covered with blobs of paint. It landed face down on the pebbled walkway.

My impressionist imprint was about the size of a placemat. The paint was acrylic, so I poured water from a large bottle in my supply bag and made a very colorful puddle. I started dabbing it with paper towel when I noticed the head gardener, renowned English horti-culturalist James Priest, was coming my way, on his evening rounds.

I had been hoping to meet him all week. But not exactly under those circumstances.

I quickly pressed more paper towel on the spot and then covered it up with a sheet from my sketchpad. I set my little tub of water on top of everything, concealing the evidence.

My picture had sustained only minor damage. I quickly put it back on the easel and got back to work. Thankfully, Mr. Priest turned down another *allée*. He walked with metal crutches then because of a knee problem, so it was easy to keep track of his movements as the crutches clacked on the pavement.

I was sweating paint pellets by the time Caroline returned. When she started critiquing my painting, I whispered to her, "We have something more important to discuss."

Her eyes grew wide when she saw my sidewalk art.

Caroline, a proper Southern Lady to her core, always impressed upon her students the rules of decorum when painting in the gardens. Caroline's groups had special permission to paint in the gardens not only in the evening, but during the early morning, which is a magical time as dew blankets the flower beds and mist rises above the lily pond.

Much of the work in the gardens takes place in the early morning, so it was important for us to stay out of the way. Just before the gardeners arrived at 7 a.m., Caroline would gather her students across the street from the large green service-entrance doors used by the gardening crew. We'd stand behind a white line painted on the pavement for delivery trucks, waiting for the gardeners to arrive. They had pseudo-rock-star status in Giverny. I have a great photo of them walking down the street. It was more of a strut, with attitude. I tried not to laugh as Caroline asked someone in the group to step *behind* the white line – their foot had ventured over the line onto hallowed ground. It was as if we were witnessing the passing of royalty. I looked to Caroline to see if we were supposed to bow our heads in respect. I thought I saw a nod from her as they passed. I couldn't see her face, which was hidden under a big straw hat that complemented her painting attire – a billowing long denim skirt with a blousy white shirt.

Caroline, under pressure, had the coolness of a mint julep. She quickly began flushing my sidewalk painting with water and dabbing it with paper towel.

We worked as a team for ten frantic minutes. She pulled out an expensive boar-bristle paintbrush from her bag and used it like a scrub brush. *Mon dieu!*

And then she said to me, "We need more abrasion. Get some dirt."

"Seriously? You want me to scoop dirt out of a Monet flower bed?"

Caroline handed me a painter's trowel from her bag.

I casually sauntered over to the nearest flowerbed and pretended to be inspecting a dahlia as I scooped up a clump of richly composted soil.

The dirt helped. "We need more," Caroline said.

As I went back for another scoop, I saw Mr. Priest clomping toward us on his crutches.

It was a Lucy-and-Ethel moment in Monet's Garden. We were busted. But how would we charm our way out of this?

Caroline jumped to her feet and intercepted Mr. Priest – she knew him as James. I couldn't hear what she was saying, but I caught the lilt of her sugary Southern drawl. She stalled him long enough, so that by the time they reached the scene of the crime, the spot was spotless.

I apologized to him, fearing the group might lose painting privileges in the garden. I knew he would be attending a party that night at the moulin where the program participants would be showing their work.

"I hope to redeem myself this evening," I said to him.

"And how do you plan to do that?" he asked me. "Do you sing?"

I liked James instantly. He was so *English*, with his boyishly tousled graying hair and sunburnt nose. I could tell by the sparkle in his eyes he was enjoying my profuse apology.

"I do sing," I said earnestly. "But I've also put together a slideshow of the gardens that I think you'll enjoy." I had spent my free time that week culling more than 3,000 photos I had taken of Giverny and the gardens, for a photo book I was planning to publish.

It all ended well. It was a thrill for me to share my photos with James Priest that evening. He asked me questions about how I was able to achieve certain effects, especially with the reflections on the lily pond. That made me smile. I had nothing to do with it.

"Monet used the pond as a mirror. I used his toolbox of special effects – the clouds, the ethereal light, the breeze rippling across the pond," I told him.

"I've never seen anyone photograph the gardens like this," he said approvingly.

It was a great evening. I met Chris at that party. He told me he'd had a similar mishap in the gardens. We agreed that Grand Master himself surely had tipped over an easel or two in his time.

~~~

When my photo book of Monet's gardens was published a year later, I had the honor of presenting it to James in person. We met at the front steps to Monet's house, on a sunny October day.

I looked at the spot, a few feet away, where my paint palette had left a nearly indelible impression on the front walkway.

"I've come back to the scene of the crime," I said.

James laughed. "Have you been losing sleep over this?"

I told him I had written a cathartic blog post about the incident, which made him laugh harder.

It was the final days of the season. In just over a week, the gates would close until the following April, for the annual winter respite. The gardeners would immediately rip the planting beds bare. The meandering nasturtiums would be loaded into wheelbarrows. The autumn profusion of dahlias would quickly become just images on tens of thousands of photo memory cards.

The soil would be tilled and enriched with compost. Spring bulbs would be planted and tucked into their beds for a long winter's nap. Hopefully, weather permitting, they would spring awake by April 1. At least hope springs eternal.

I'd had the great fortune of seeing Monet's garden in spring, summer and fall. James asked me which I liked best.

On my first visit in Spring, I had witnessed the bloom of the wisteria, which draped the Japanese bridge with a cascade of lavender blossoms. I stood on the bridge that day with tears in my eyes. For years, I had seen Monet's paintings of this scene, but for the first time I was experiencing its soul-stirring beauty – and the heavenly scent of it – for myself.

"Spring here takes my breath away," I told James. "But there's something about the final frenzy of fall."

I looked around at the wild tangle of blooms that nearly choked the pathways and leapt up the arbors.

"It's like the frantic climax of an opera. The diva dahlias are nearly spent – but they hold on to their glorious high notes until the last breath of autumn."

"I love that you see the garden as an opera," James said.

Amazingly, with winter closing in, we were still surrounded by tender dahlia buds that were about to burst open.

"Look at them. They're so lovely and delicate," I said sadly. "They don't know the curtain will come crashing down on them soon.

James smiled. "Their beauty is in their innocence."

It's no wonder this place is paradise on earth, I thought, with a master gardener whose vision allows for both spectacle and the grace notes of innocence.

I was pleased James liked my book. As he leafed through the pages, he said, "I'm going to use this as my planting guide next season."

I finally felt redeemed.

Chapter 10

After my difficult summer with Henri, I hoped we could recover in time for the big event of his year – an antique engine show he hosts in September on the fairgrounds below the Hôtel Baudy. Exhibitors come from around Europe and Britain, bringing their engines by truck and, for the Brits, by ferry across the English Channel. The show typically draws a thousand visitors during the course of the weekend.

The preparation for the show begins weeks in advance. Henri, who's extremely organized, has a schedule set in stone. Promotional materials and souvenir plaques for exhibitors are ordered at least two months in advance. By early August, posters go up and flyers are in local shops and at the tourist office. The week of the show, Henri and his team erect small tents for each exhibitor and a big food tent where they set up kitchen equipment, along with picnic tables. Henri's younger son, Paul, who lives in Switzerland, handles the food service and is a master at feeding a crowd.

Bernadette is in charge of the show's floral decorations. Wildflower arrangements are her specialty. For the show, she uses large old metal milk cans for stunning bouquets of cosmos, daisies and whatever is in bloom in the prairies around Giverny. She enlists the wives of the exhibitors to help her hang floral garlands in the food tent. The show is called *Le Moteur est dans le Pré* – The Engine is in the Meadow. Bernadette creates the meadow.

Exhibitors start arriving a few days before the show opens. Many come with trucks that are also outfitted as campers, which are parked in a grassy area next to the fairground. Other exhibitors book B&B rooms in the village and leave their trucks and vans, once they've been unloaded, on the large lawn in front of Henri's place. One day, I sat at my desk by my bedroom window and watched the arrival of the vehicles. I briefly feared for my flowerbed as flatbed trailers were unhitched and maneuvered into place. I quickly realized this wasn't the first rodeo for these steam-engine cowboys.

I went down to the fairground with my camera on that Friday, the setup day. Photography is more than a hobby for me and I had the idea that I could do a photo book of the show for Henri. He had many digital photos and videos of past events, but not an actual book he could enjoy.

I knew I would be a "woman of interest" to this crowd. Most of the attendees are old friends, who meet up at engine shows around Europe. The biggest show of the year happens in the Netherlands, in the town of Nuenen where Vincent Van Gogh's parents once lived. Henri has told me stories of those Nuenen shows. He and his team of mechanics sleep in the back of his truck, a notch above sleeping in the rough, in my opinion. Bernadette goes on these trips, too, but according to Henri, she sleeps in a car they take to the event. The exhibitors bring favorite native dishes to share in what sounds like a wonderful three-day party. Henri springs for hotel accommodations and a restaurant meal for his crew on the last night before the six-hour drive back to Giverny. That year's Nuenen show had taken place a month before my move from Italy. The news of me and my upcoming arrival was a story heard round a few campfires, I'm told.

I had just begun my walk around the fairground, where engines were being unpacked and unveiled, when I noticed that an early-bird group, sitting at a long table, was already enjoying cocktails and snacks. They instantly figured out who I was and waved for me to come join them. I had just met the Dutch Camp.

The wives in the Dutch Camp took me under wing. The Dutch generally are multi-lingual, so speaking English was no problem for them. I really appreciated their warm hospitality. One woman in particular, Anne-Marie, was especially gracious. At one point during the weekend, she confided that her husband would be receiving results from medical tests when they returned home. I could see the worry in her eyes. The doctors feared he may have cancer.

Every year, Henri's show has had the blessing of beautiful autumn weather. Only once in 15 years had it rained on his parade and it was only a brief overnight drizzle. Henri is an *imprésario extraordinaire*. He loves speaking to a crowd, whether he's giving tours at his museum or doing a demonstration at a county fair. I once watched him enthrall an audience with his description of a machine that made wooden clogs, like those worn in parts of Normandy and Brittany. The kids, hanging on the ropes in front of his exhibition tent, were amazed as they listened to Henri and watched his machine carve a wooden shoe out of a birch log.

Henri was in his element as his comrades gathered on the fairground. He looks forward to this weekend all year. In the antique-engine world, he is revered. He has been featured on the cover of magazines and is a leading expert on steam-engine restoration. Henri's museum is one of only five of its type in the world that has a workshop in operation.

I have such happy memories of that weekend. Henri's close friends Martin and Jacques had arrived earlier in the week. The three of them are known as the Musketeers. Several months earlier, they had spent a few weeks driving around Pennsylvania, Ohio and New York State, visiting steam-engine museums and collectors. Henri, who had spent many years of his career as a mechanical engineer working on projects in the U.S., was their fearless leader. He introduced his pals to Mexican food, which they loved, and guided them through the streets of Manhattan. One night, they ventured into a gay bar and still laugh about that. "It was the only place open near our hotel and we were hungry!" declares Henri.

The two musketeers obviously knew about me. On the day Martin arrived, I was sitting in the downstairs kitchen as he strode across the room with outstretched arms. I felt very well received.

During the show weekend, Henri treats his exhibitors and their spouses to dinner at the Baudy – a big expense covered by visitor admissions to the show. It's a huge dinner for 100 people in the upstairs dining room. Henri and Bernadette, along with Henri's brother Charles who's a vital part of the museum's mechanics team, carefully deliberate over menu options provided by the Baudy's owners. They want to present their guests with the best of Normandy cuisine and the Baudy delivers an impressive spread.

Before the big dinner, the crowd gathers on the large patio outside the museum where a steam engine that once belonged to Henri's father, himself a mechanic, has pride of place. A long table filled with foods brought by the exhibitors becomes a scrumptious buffet. Wine flows. Toasts are made. Friendships are celebrated. That evening, I took a photo of Henri with a glass in hand and a smile that spoke volumes. This man, who had once seemed to me to be so very sad, couldn't have been any happier.

From the museum, it's a short walk to the Baudy. As the guests made their way to dinner, I hung back to walk with Henri. He held my hand, clearly glad to have me at his side. As always, Henri's dog, Facel, trotted along beside his master.

As Henri and I climbed the Baudy's back steps to the party room, his phone rang. He waved me on and told me to sit with the British Camp, which I thought was odd. I had looked forward to meeting the Brits, but that hadn't happened yet.

The dining room was packed, with very few empty seats at that point. There were none available at the British table. I walked toward the middle of the room, feeling conspicuously out of place.

Henri's son Paul and his wife, a lovely Lebanese woman named Leisha, had entered the dining room just ahead of me. Paul's cousins, who had helped out at the food tent that day, had saved them seats, but there wasn't room at that table for me. Leisha turned toward me, sympathetically. She, too, had come to this family and their way of life as an outlander. That afternoon, she and I had had a long talk at a picnic table in the food tent. She loved Henri dearly, having lost her own father some years ago. But not all of the family had embraced her. She told me some of Henri's family had refused to attend her and Paul's wedding. I could see Leisha's pain when she told me the reason: "They said it was because I am an *Arab*."

I appreciated Leisha in her moment of hesitation. She didn't want to leave me alone, with nowhere to sit.

Just then, Anne-Marie, who was sitting with Dutch friends at the far end of the room, saw me and waved. There were three empty seats at their table. I waved back, motioning that I would join them.

I went looking for Henri, who was just coming in the door with Facel. I took his arm and told him Anne-Marie had saved us a place. What I found especially odd was that none of his own family had reserved a spot for him.

I could tell that wasn't lost on Henri either, as he scanned the room. When we sat down at the Dutch table, Anne-Marie motioned for Bernadette, who had been greeting friends at our end of the room, to take the empty seat next to me. Bernadette shook her head and pointed to a vacant chair at a nearby table.

Apparently, Henri wasn't accustomed to being shunted into a corner. Whatever had been past tradition hadn't happened, for reasons I couldn't fathom. Between courses, he would leave the table to make his rounds, ever the Master of Ceremonies. That would have left me with an empty chair on both sides. Anne-Marie moved to the seat she had offered Bernadette earlier so that I would have a dinner companion. I appreciated her kindness.

On the final night of the show, after all the visitors have gone, it's a long-standing tradition for the exhibitors and their families to gather in the food tent for one last feast. They serve up all the foods they've brought from home, most of them indigenous to their regions. The Brits unwrap the Stilton, the Germans slice up chunks of sausage and dish out heaps of potato salad. The Dutch are known for their buttery cookies and sweet treats. The French pull out the stops with regional cheeses and charcuterie. What's left of Paul's roasted pig and Bernadette's pear tarts are devoured by the end of the evening.

What I loved about that final evening was the camaraderie of the group. After dinner, one of the French exhibitors played his accordion. I sat with the Brits, who were great fun. One man and his wife travel from their home in England in an enormous bus that has been kitted out as his display booth. He calls himself the Yorkshireman.

I was sorry to see everyone leave the next day. The front lawn at Henri's place looked sad and bare when the last flatbed was hauled out the driveway.

Henri had started doing these shows when he was in his late 50s. A lot of his pals are about his age – all now in their mid-70s – and still going strong. But from behind the scenes, I saw all the work involved. Henri's team wasn't fazed by all the heavy lifting. They were like kids at a carnival riding forklifts around the fairground as they loaded engines, refrigerators, and tables and chairs into trucks for the short trip back to the museum.

When it was all over, I asked Henri if he ever imagined not doing it anymore.

"Not yet," he said. "Not yet."

~

Henri's 75th birthday was coming up, a couple of weeks after the show. I put in some late nights, after he went to bed, working on my book of photos from the show that I would give him as a birthday gift.

I was pleased the photos captured the spirit of the event. I had asked many of the exhibitors to pose with their engines. I had wonderful pictures of Henri. I took a beautiful photo of Bernadette standing by one of her milk-can flower arrangements. I devoted an entire spread in the book to her and her flowers.

I had spent the better part of the weekend roaming the fairground with my camera. I became fascinated with the components of steam engines and how they worked. I made a fun photo collage of engine control dials that looked like faces. I loved the shapes and styles of the engines' glass oil bulbs and included shots of a number of them in the book.

I learned the importance of patience when photographing steam engines. To capture a plume of steam escaping from a smokestack, I had to anticipate when the belly of the beast was getting ready to belch. And if I wanted to show the steam plume bending in the breeze, I had to listen for the wind in the trees AND anticipate the belch. It took me ten tries to capture that moment with one engine, but it turned out to be one of my favorite photos in the book.

During the show, the fairground is filled with the sound of engine clatter – sputtering valves, clanking armatures and purring gears. All goes quiet at lunchtime when the exhibitors take a break. But before too long, the show resumes – often with the toot of a steam whistle – and the clatter starts again.

I assumed a big party was being planned for Henri's 75th. When I asked how he'd like to celebrate, he said, "I know Bernadette will do something."

I wondered if I should ask her if I could help with preparations. Was she planning a surprise or a big family dinner? I thought about having a gathering of friends at Henri's apartment, but didn't want to step on her toes. Henri seemed certain she was in party-planning mode.

On the eve of Henri's birthday, I gave him the photo book, which I'd had printed by a high-end online publishing service. I had ordered premium paper, which made the images pop off the page. Henri was over the moon. He looked through the book, then went back and studied each photo, page by page, telling me stories about some of the exhibitors and the rarity of certain engines.

The next day, a Sunday, the family – about eight in all – gathered in usual fashion for lunch in the downstairs kitchen. Henri had bought the champagne for his own birthday celebration on his run to the grocery store earlier that morning. I thought someone at the table should have made that effort. They all lifted a glass in his honor and drank his champagne.

Henri had brought the photo book to show everyone at lunch. I watched Bernadette as others at the table expressed amazement at the book itself. They gathered round, poring over the photos. Bernadette stayed in her seat at the head of the table. She has a way of literally looking down her nose, through her bifocals, while lowering her chin in what comes across as an expression of disdain. Fortunately, I had placed the photos of her with her flowers in the first pages of the book. She seemed pleased to see that. As she thumbed through the pages, I could tell she was impressed.

There was no birthday cake for Henri at lunch. I assumed Bernadette was saving that for the big finish at the evening meal or whatever celebration the family was planning. Bernadette was known for her spectacular cakes – covered with fresh flowers and candles – like the one she made for little Luc's birthday during my Easter visit.

While Henri was in the workshop that afternoon, I decorated his bedroom with Pink Floyd posters I had purchased online. I wrapped a Pink Floyd coffee mug I had gotten from the same website and put it on his pillow. Henri is a huge Pink Floyd fan. On the first night of our "honeymoon" trip to Malta, he came to bed in a T-shirt Paul had given him that read: Never Underestimate an Old Man Who Listens to Pink Floyd. That really made me laugh.

There were five of us at the family dinner that evening. Any minute, I expected a throng of people to come bursting through the door, singing "Happy Birthday" and bearing gifts.

But nothing happened. We had leftover dessert from lunch – a delicious apple tart Bernadette had made. Charles' wife, Amélie, cleared the dessert plates and joined Bernadette, who was partially hidden behind a high counter that separates the kitchen's food prep area from the dining space. I couldn't see what they were doing, but I suspected they were lighting candles on Henri's cake.

But a few moments later, they both walked out from behind the counter empty-handed. Amélie put on her coat and Bernadette did the same.

In the moment I realized they were leaving, I glanced at Henri, who was sitting next to me, and could see his disappointment. When Amélie, Charles and Bernadette said their good-nights and shut the kitchen door behind them, he didn't make a move to get up. I reached over and rubbed his back.

"Let's go upstairs," I said. "Your birthday isn't over yet."

It was a chilly night. I was wearing one of Henri's oversized, old jackets and pulled it tight around me as we walked through the museum hall. It always seemed like a spooky place, with huge flywheels casting enormous shadows on the cinderblock walls. My favorite engine, an enormous diesel-powered machine that had come from a 19th-century chocolate factory in Paris, towered over us. Rudolph Diesel peered down at us from a photo that hung on one of the valves.

"Ooo, this is scary," I said to Henri, slipping my arm through his. "Ghosts live here."

Facel, who flanked my other side, pressed himself against me and gently took the hem of the jacket between his teeth – as if to say, "I'm Super Dog. I'll protect you."

Henri was amazed by Facel's sensitivity to me. Still holding the hem of the jacket in his teeth, Facel led me up the back stairs of the museum hall, with Henri lighting the way with his phone. Even when we got to the boiler room outside the apartment's back entrance, Facel kept hold of the jacket hem. Not until we were inside the apartment and in the warm security of the kitchen did he let go. I rubbed his head and gave him a little treat.

"What a wonderful dog," I said to Henri.

I didn't have a cake for Henri, but I had bought a couple of lovely pastries at the *boulangerie* earlier that day. I had some birthday candles on hand. I took a lemon tart from the pastry box and put a candle in it as I sang "Happy Birthday." I filled the kettle and we ended the day with tea and tart.

As Henri headed down the hallway on his way to bed, I waited in the hallway for him to open the door to his room. When he flicked on the light, the kaleidoscopic colors of the Pink Floyd posters greeted him.

Henri was delighted. "*Chérie*, when did you do this?"

"After that long nap you took this afternoon."

He saw the little package on his pillow. "And what is this?"

"Something for your bedtime tea and morning coffee." I sat down on the bed next to him as he unwrapped the box.

It seemed like inadequate compensation for the blow he had been dealt downstairs by his own family. But I think it helped ease the sting of that.

We made love that night. It had been a while. A few weeks earlier, Henri had noted our "retreat from intimacy," as he had described it.

That night, I felt we took a turn together, into uncharted waters to be sure. Everything he knew to be true had shifted. The Sister-Wife, as I would come to call Bernadette, was behaving like a jilted spouse. I was the Girlfriend Troublemaker who had arrived on the scene and upset her apple cart.

I knew I'd likely have hell to pay for stealing Henri from her. But for that moment, that night, I felt protected from all harm, with Henri and Super Dog at my side.

~~~

A few days later, Olivier and Maxine had a belated birthday dinner for Henri at the moulin. They also were belatedly celebrating their 15th wedding anniversary from a few weeks earlier. Maxine showed me a framed faded photo, partially hidden by a coat rack, on the wall of the dining room. She, in her bridal dress, rode next to Olivier on a tractor he drove after the ceremony. I was struck by how attractive Maxine was in her twenties. She had lost the beauty of her youth – the ravages of her smoking habit that had left her looking older than Olivier, who was 15 years her senior and still handsome in his late fifties.

I enjoyed getting to know two friends of theirs who joined us

that evening – a friendly woman named Céline, a physical therapist whom I'd met a few times at the *boulangerie*, and her husband
Georges, a forensic pathologist in the prefecture's coroner's office.
His stories were both fascinating and revolting. He'd been on the
scene when they fished a body out of the Seine, not far from the
moulin. Thankfully, he spared us a graphic description of the corpse.
Georges seemed so mild-mannered for a guy who dealt daily with
horrors of the flesh. I wondered what his dreams were like.

Maxine brought out a cake she had made for Henri. When he
blew out the candles, I asked him what he had wished for.

"I would like 75 more years," he said. "There's so much more I
want to do in this life."

"Like what?" I asked.

Henri thought for a moment. "I want to ride a spaceship around
Mars."

That got a chuckle at the table. But I could tell he was serious.

"Mostly, I want to ride a locomotive to the moon," he said.

"How will you do that?" I asked him.

"I will first lay tracks for the locomotive to ride on."

My inquisitive mind was now fully engaged. "And what will
support the tracks?"

Henri's eyes twinkled. "That's the secret." He leaned close to me
and said in a loud whisper, "I will suspend them with balloons."

That got a cheer. A toast was made to "Henri and his train ride
to the moon!"

A week later, Henri showed me a piece of mail he had received
from Georges, in an official envelope from the coroner's office. Inside
was Henri's death certificate, which Georges had filled in with great
detail. On his date of death, Henri was 150 years old. The cause
of death was a heart attack he had suffered when a buxom Russian
beauty sat on his lap at his 150th birthday party.

I knew then I'd need to keep an eye out for Russian babes in
Giverny.

Chapter 11

In mid-October, Roz returned to Giverny. I had kept in touch with her during her time back in the States. In one email, she told me the deal for the cooking-school property had fallen through. She was looking for a place to rent – a small house would do, she said, but she needed a kitchen with a gas stove.

That didn't seem such a tall order until Henri and I started making inquiries. The first problem was that there weren't many long-term rentals because most owners were cashing in on the Airbnb market. And surprisingly, many kitchens had electric cookers.

Shortly before her arrival in Paris, Roz sent me a message asking if I'd meet her flight and take her to a place she had rented for a couple of weeks in Vézelay – a two-and-a-half hour drive from the airport. She invited me to stay with her there. Henri and I already had plans that week, so I sent her my regrets that I couldn't meet her flight.

I met her train in Vernon a couple of weeks later, after her stay in Vézelay. A young man helped her onto the platform and then carried her luggage off the train. She had two huge suitcases, with assorted parcels dangling off the handles. I wondered how she had managed all that on her own.

She waited for me to come to her on the platform and warmly embraced me. The young man wished her a pleasant stay and walked away.

"Who was that? He's very cute," I said.

She laughed. "Just one of my travel angels. I meet them every-where. They just appear and help me with my luggage or get me a cab. Where are you parked?"

I pointed down the platform. "I can't wait to see your new car," she said. She started walking down the platform, leaving her luggage behind. I then realized I was her new travel angel.

Roz was thrilled to be returning to Giverny. As we crossed the bridge over the Seine, she looked down at the river cruise boats docked along the shore. "I have so many marvelous ideas!" she exclaimed. "I want to get a boat. I'll do cooking demonstrations for tourists on the river cruises. Isn't that a marvelous idea?"

It was a marvelous idea. Cruise lines are always looking for unique excursion packages.

I was surprised to learn Roz had arranged to rent an apartment below a small community theater venue in Giverny. The building and the theater were owned by Henri's nephew Denis, who always looked a bit disheveled, as if he spent most nights sleeping in his clothes and not necessarily in a bed.

I asked Roz what had happened to the other property she had hoped to lease in Giverny. But she said it was a story for another day.

Denis' rental apartment was a bit grim. It needed a good scrubbing. The bathroom was a mess and the kitchen stove had electric burners. "I'm going to pay for a gas stove," she told me, gazing out the kitchen window. "Look at this garden!"

It was a cottagey garden with possibilities. Roz clearly imagined what vegetables and flowers she would plant. "Can't you just see it, Rebecca?" she asked breathlessly.

Her enthusiasm felt like a gust of fresh air.

She wanted to hear how things were going with Henri and the family. She pulled a couple of tea bags out of her purse – more like a Mary Poppins carpet bag – and filled a kettle that was on the stovetop. "I have some cookies I bought at the most divine bakery," she said, rummaging through her bag.

We made a little tea party in the sitting room. Roz looked around the room. "I see the potential here...I'll need to get a desk. Do you know where I could find one?" she asked.

"Not offhand. But I'll ask Henri."

"Do you think he has one?"

I laughed, thinking about the vast storage spaces that surround the museum hall. "I haven't ventured into Henri's storerooms. He tells me flying mice live there."

"Flying mice?" Roz burst out laughing as she got the joke. "Oh, Rebecca, how are you holding up?"

She sincerely wanted to know, so I shared some of the highlights of my difficult summer. Roz was sympathetic and assured me things would be different now that she was back in Giverny.

"We're going to have such fun," she said, affectionately squeezing my arm. "You're going to love my ideas. The first thing we need to do is find a boat. Do you know of anyone with a boat?"

"How big of a boat? I know of a man who has a little sailboat he uses to take artists on painting trips along the Seine."

"I need room for my cooking supplies and a big table for demonstrations. And a little kitchen, too."

"His boat wouldn't work for that. It's very small. He can take a half dozen people, tops."

"I need a big boat, a flat-bottom boat that can hold 30 people. We need to find a boat, Rebecca."

I suddenly felt an undertow, like the pull of a rip tide at the beach.

"Will you do that for me?" she asked.

"Find you a boat?" I stifled a laugh.

"Yes! Good, good. Please look into that. I can't wait to tell you all about my plans."

~

I stopped by to see Roz the next morning, a Wednesday, but Denis told me she had gone into Vernon to the semi-weekly market. I wondered how she had gotten herself there, but I figured a travel angel had appeared.

She called me that afternoon and suggested we go to the *boulangerie* for coffee. I swung by to pick her up.

"The gate's unlocked," she called out when I rang the bell.

She was in the kitchen, eager to show me all the fresh fruit and veg she had bought that morning. "I've gotten some wonderful recipes I want to try for the most delicious tarts." She looked at me as if she'd just been struck by lightning. "I need to talk to you about *recipes*. I could use your help with those."

A boat, now recipes. Given my severe challenges in the kitchen, finding a boat seemed like an easier project.

Roz walked into the *boulangerie* like she owned the place. It was her favorite luncheon spot and she had made herself a fixture there during her earlier stay in Giverny. The staff and the young owner, Antoine, were happy to see her, greeting her with hugs and kisses.

Roz was in fine form. She admired the new artwork on display and inspected the pastry case to see the latest additions.

"What is this divine concoction?" she asked, pointing to a swirl of meringue and caramel, topped with a sliver of fig. She ordered two.

She and I sat on the outdoor terrace under a lime-green umbrella. There was a smoky scent of autumn in the air. It was one of the moments you want to memorize – a quintessentially perfect end-of-the-season day in Giverny.

I waited for Roz's verdict on the pastry chef's creation. As she let the caramel and meringue melt on her tongue, she closed her eyes, discerning the ingredients. "There's something unexpected here," she said softly. "I'm not quite sure. We must find out the secret."

Roz's use of "we" was beginning to alarm me. I tucked my fork into the meringue, hoping she wouldn't ask my opinion. I made great s'mores as a Girl Scout, but my cooking merit badge didn't cover French pastries.

She sipped her cappuccino and looked at me with great expectation. "So here's what I want to talk to you about," she began, cradling her cup. "I want to do a book about the chef at the museum restaurant – have you eaten there?"

I nodded. Giverny's Impressionist museum had a bistro that

opened to a stunning garden. The menu was a bit pricey, but the food was good. The restaurant was popular with museum visitors who had time to linger in Giverny – a cut above the tourists who were on half-day tours and didn't have a chance to enjoy more than a boxed lunch on the bus.

"Ivan is a charming young man from Bulgaria," Roz said. "He studied in Paris and is going to have a big career. I see a Michelin star in his future."

I imagined a scene in a movie with Roz looking into a crystal ball.

"I want you to write his story, Rebecca. Wouldn't that be marvelous? We'll include his recipes, which I'll work on with him. You can do the photos – I love the photos you take. You'll say yes, won't you?"

So there it was...a book about a Bulgarian chef named Ivan. How badly could this go wrong, I asked myself.

The next day, Roz and I had lunch at the museum and Ivan came to our table with a petite, cast-iron, lidded pot. It was empty, which I thought was odd. Silly me. Ivan presented it to Roz as a gift. She was thrilled.

She chatted away, effusively telling him her BIG IDEA – a book all about him and his fabulous recipes. He looked to be in his late 30s and I knew would be photogenic with his dark, good looks. His English was marginal, which would make my work a bit harder. But this book would be mostly about his recipes. Roz said she was going to handle that part, though with her very limited French, I wondered if she'd understand his instructions.

I didn't sign up for anything that day. I spoke to Henri that evening, mostly about his impression of Roz. He had met her only once, at the summer garden party when she told us about the property she was hoping to rent for her cooking school. Henri hadn't heard any murmurings in the village about what had happened with that.

There was another matter I wanted to discuss with Henri. I

wondered if he thought Roz might be a good tenant for the Lodge. He seemed interested in what I had to say.

It pained me to have this conversation because I once had hoped he and I could live at the Lodge. A few months before I moved to Giverny – when I knew we'd be facing a tight squeeze at his apartment – I had gently broached the subject. He said the Lodge was too big for us and would be too expensive to heat. I suggested that we seal off the upstairs bedrooms and use only the downstairs. There was a spacious bedroom suite with an adjoining sitting room that I could use as an office, a large eat-in kitchen and a big living room that opened onto a terrace with a lovely view of the village. He could rent out his apartment and we'd rent the Lodge. He and three of his siblings owned the Lodge, so as investors, they would profit from the additional income.

For years, the Lodge had been rented year-round by Gale Bennett, the American artist from Florida. When he passed away, a gallery rented the downstairs space for a couple of seasons. But for the past few years, the Lodge had sat empty and had become a financial drain.

Henri said he'd discuss my idea with the family. He was the primary stakeholder, but he didn't hold a majority share. He alone couldn't make the decision.

I began visualizing our life there. I imagined friends gathered at the big table in the kitchen. How wonderful it would be to have friends come stay with us. The expense of opening some of the upstairs bedrooms during the summer season wouldn't be too costly, I thought. I let this fantasy carry me away, which set me up for a big disappointment.

When I arrived for my Easter visit, Henri was pleased to show me not only the bed he had purchased for the room that would become mine, but also a large print he'd had custom made of a Theodore Robinson painting of Marie called *Val d'Arconville*. It's a beautiful scene of her reading a book on a hillside of wildflowers, with a sweeping view of Giverny rooftops and the Seine Valley beyond. The print had been mounted on sturdy cardboard and split into two sections to cover a large double window, next to the bed, that overlooked a dingy corridor that led to the apartment's back door. I appreciated that Henri had gone to some effort and expense to ensure my privacy, in what clearly was a grand gesture to accommodate me. But in that moment, my heart sank as I realized this was his passive way of telling me that we wouldn't be moving to the Lodge.

A couple of days later, I asked Henri what the family's response had been to my idea. He waffled a bit, saying there were other issues and it wouldn't be possible, at least for now. Even then – new as I was to Henri's waffling – I took that as a pretty firm no.

I soon had other ideas for the Lodge. I saw it as multi-use venue for activities that would appeal to tourists. I could give talks about the American artists who had followed Monet to Giverny. We could have a gardener at the Monet Foundation talk about how to create a Monet-like flowerbed. And if men in the groups weren't interested in art history and flowers, they could go downstairs and tour the museum.

Henri liked my American thinking when it came to marketing. Soon after my move to Giverny, he asked me if I'd be willing to write a proposal that he could present to the family – to Bernadette, Lucile, and his brother Charles, whom I hadn't met at that point. Charles split his time between Giverny and southern France and would be returning to Giverny in early August.

When Charles returned, I waited for Henri to give me the nod, but I was careful to keep my ideas to myself when I was at family gatherings.

And then one night later in August, while Henri and I were having drinks before a rare dinner alone, he informed me that Lodge was for sale.

I was stunned. "When did this happen?"

"A few days ago."

"Why?"

"The family wants to sell."

"Do you?"

"No," he said, swishing ice cubes around in his Spritz. He poured himself another shot of prosecco.

"But you're the main shareholder."

"I have only 46 percent."

I didn't know how the pie was split – but assuming they each had a healthy slice, the other three had voted against him.

"But you love the Lodge."

Henri shrugged. "I don't want to go against my brother and sisters."

Henri was a benevolent family patriarch. He once told me he had purchased the Lodge hoping Lucile would use it as a B&B. But when she found out how expensive it would be to heat the place and keep the lights on, she lost interest.

Henri said they weren't going to list the property. They wanted the word to get out in the village. He seemed optimistic they'd get an offer. They were asking 750,000 euros (about $825,000 at that time), which, given all the work it needed, I thought was much too high.

"What's your bottom price?" I asked him.

"We know it needs rewiring, a new heating system and new windows. We'd come down 80,000 euros," he said.

The price would still be too high, based on what I'd seen advertised in the area.

"The Lodge has a big problem," I said. "It's not a freestanding property. It's attached to the two apartments in the back and the downstairs kitchen area below. Other than the terrace – which is wonderful – it has no outdoor space. And there's no parking."

"We've talked to an engineer who says we can cut a driveway through the front hedge. There would be room for parking there."

It surprised me that they had talked to an engineer. This wasn't a plan that had been hatched a few days earlier.

"Do you envision giving up some of the space here – like the lawn area?" I said, looking at the kitchen window.

"No, no. This all will stay as it is."

I could see his deflation. His family had overruled him. I wondered why he hadn't gone into this arrangement with a majority share.

An offer came in two weeks later at 500,000 euros. They'd be crazy not to take it, I thought. There's an old adage in real estate that your first offer is usually your best offer. But sellers with an inflated sense of a property's worth often turn it down.

"You're going to accept it, aren't you?" I asked Henri when he shared the news.

"Absolutely not."

"Is it a clean offer? No contingencies?"

"They'll do an inspection. But they know what they're getting. It's an old property."

"With a lot of problems." I knew it wasn't my place to insert myself in this.

"We're not in a hurry to sell. We'll wait. Sometimes properties sit on the market here for three or four years. But in the end, you get your price."

That sounded totally insane to me. But it was none of my business.

The family rejected the 500,000-euro offer in early September and there hadn't been another offer since.

But now Roz was back. If she couldn't find her boat, I wondered if she might like to rent the downstairs of the Lodge for her cooking classes, with the proviso that the Lodge would stay on the market while she was a temporary resident there. She had mentioned she intended to go back and forth between Giverny and California where her family lived. Even on a short-term basis, the Lodge would at least be bringing in some income while the family waited for an offer.

"Do you trust Roz?" Henri asked me.

"Do you think I shouldn't?"

"Well, you don't know her well. She seems to be putting a lot on you with all her ideas."

"I can handle that part. But she's heard the Lodge is for sale. She asked me about it the other day."

"Will she want to buy it?"

"I don't know. She may be interested in renting the downstairs for her cooking school. She could live there as well." It hurt to say that. *I wanted to live there.* "Maybe it would be a good interim solution if she doesn't mind that the property is on the market and you'll be showing it. A buyer may like that there's a tenant in place."

"*Pourquoi pas.* Bring her to see it. There's no harm in that."

Two days later, Roz sent me an early-morning text saying that she'd like to meet for lunch that day at the *boulangerie.* She said she'd see me there at noon.

It was a chilly day, so we took a table inside. There were only a few other customers. No one I recognized. I was becoming more conscious about being discreet in my conversations with Roz when we were out in public. Gossip in a small village spreads like a brush fire. I knew she was a bit of a curiosity in Giverny, especially after her real-estate fiasco. She still hadn't told me what had happened.

Roz was crackling with excitement. I had barely sat down when she asked, "Are you free tomorrow afternoon? Ivan would like us to come to the museum. He's going to make his fabulous duck recipe. It's his signature dish, you know."

"I had no idea."

"His sauce is divine – honey with Szechuan pepper. I can't wait for you to taste it. We should be there by 2. Could you pick me up around 1:30?"

I agreed to do that. I wasn't on board yet with Roz's book project, but I wanted to see her in action. She was so American, with her brashness and big ideas. She could be off-putting, but I was intrigued with her because she was such a *character.*

Moments after we ordered lunch, our conversation turned to the Lodge.

"I'd like to see it," she said. "Have they had any offers?"

"One."

"Are they in negotiations?"

I shook my head. "The family turned it down."

"What was the offer?"

"I shouldn't say. I'm privy, but not at liberty. Are you an interested buyer?"

She lowered her voice. "I have a friend in California who's looking for a possible cooking-school venue."

"She's stealing your idea?"

Roz smiled. "No – she'd buy the property and I'd run the school."

"It needs upgrades. Lots of them."

"Money isn't an issue. She's very well off."

I wondered about Roz's financial situation. I remembered her saying she had been born with a "golden spoon" in her mouth.

"When could I come by?" she asked.

"I'll need to speak with Henri."

~♪

The cooking session with Ivan the next day turned out to be a lot of fun. He adored Roz. He gave her an apron and put a chef's toque on her head. I got a wonderful photo of them together at the stove, with his arm around her as she stirred "Ivan's Sauce Divine," as she called it.

In the middle of the session, Antoine, from the *boulangerie*, walked in the back door with a bread delivery. He seemed surprised to see Roz and me in the kitchen. I didn't think much of it, but Roz whispered to me after he had left, "Did you see the look on his face? I think we have a problem."

Ivan served up the duck for Roz and me and we took our plates to a table in the dining room with a view of the garden. I was already visualizing the photos I would take of this place for Roz's book.

Ivan's sauce was truly divine. "Can you taste the secret ingredient?"

Roz asked, scribbling in her notebook. "It's *flamed cognac*. I need to double-check the measurement." She peered at me over her reading glasses. "Rebecca, are you on board with this project?"

I was relieved, in a way, that she was acknowledging I hadn't yet said yes.

"Tell me exactly what you're envisioning and what my role will be."

"Initially, I thought this book should be all about Ivan," she said. "But today, when we saw Antoine, I wondered if he would be offended if we did a book about this restaurant and not his."

I thought about that for a moment. We were two American women who had to tread carefully with a project like this. There were a number of restaurants in Giverny – one with a Michelin star – that were worthy of inclusion. We didn't want to offend anyone by focusing on some and not others. But it was October 20. The season ended November 1. Restaurants would soon close and be boarded up for the winter. Even the *boulangerie* would close for the winter after its *Beaujolais nouveau* party in mid-November. How could we possibly gather everything we needed for a recipe book in 10 days?

Roz and I discussed the options. We'd approach the major restaurants in the village – six in all – and tell them about the book. We'd ask them to contribute a couple of recipes tailored to home cooks. I saw this as a book we'd market mostly to tourists. Roz liked that idea. She had found very few cookbooks featuring Normandy cuisine with recipes in English. We'd need to write it in a way so that phone apps could easily translate the text from English to other languages – no American cookbookese with ungrammatical sentences. (*Whisk in oil to make dressing.*) My job would be to write an introduction for each restaurant and handle the photography. Roz assured me she'd handle writing the recipes with the help of the chefs.

I explained to her I had other writing projects coming up, including a new novel that would be published before year's end. I would need to focus on that soon, I told her. I was willing to work with her on the recipe book, but we'd need to move quickly so that I could complete the photography before the restaurant kitchens closed for the season.

When I told Henri of this new twist at dinner that night, he again raised a bushy eyebrow. "Are you sure about this?" he asked.

"Not exactly." In fact, I was anything but sure.

But I felt it was worth a shot. The recipe book would showcase local restaurants, which could sell the books to their customers. If we tapped into Giverny's huge tourist market, the book could be a big success. Thousands of visitors roam the streets of Giverny on a typical summer's day, and I'd say most of them are crazy about French cooking.

The next day, Roz and I began calling on restaurants. We were on a mission, presenting our best American selves to the chefs of Giverny.

Chapter 12

Henri and I were enjoying a time of peace in our relationship that I truly hoped we could sustain, especially after our rough start. We were settling into more of a routine as a couple. With the summer season ending, there were fewer family gatherings for *apero* and dinners. I liked having more time for just us.

But Bernadette was still ever-present. Although she lived in Vernon, she came every day to the museum property, tending the flowers and feeding the animals. She had a pet goat in the corral named Praline. A few years earlier, a baby ram had come to live in the corral. Henri's grandson Luc had named him Dou-Dou (pronounced "Doo-Doo" in English). I laughed at first, thinking the name in French, like in English, meant *poop*. But Henri explained *dou-dou* means a cute, cuddly thing.

Bernadette rarely came to "our" side of the complex. She could enter the corral from the museum side of the property. Occasionally, she'd pick fruit off the trees on the lawn in front of our apartment. But I rarely saw her except during family meals in the downstairs kitchen.

One day, Bernadette came to collect a wheelbarrow that our neighbor Léo, who lived in the apartment next to ours, had borrowed. Léo was in his early 50s and worked as a security guard at the Impressionist museum. He was wiry, with wild curly gray hair, and always had a treasure trove of items he had scavenged from flea markets in the back of his van. As part of his rental agreement with Henri and the family, Léo mowed the lawn. He used a push mower because he liked the workout, he said. He was very meticulous. I had noticed during my Easter visit, when dozens of naturalized tulips were popping up in the grass, how he carefully mowed around each one of them.

Léo had been doing other gardening work on our side of the property and Henri had suggested he use Bernadette's wheelbarrow to haul away debris. She was away and wasn't using it. No harm in that, I thought, especially since Henri had given Léo permission. For a few days, it stayed near the garden wall by my flowerbed. I had been doing some fall planting and had put some of the discarded plant containers in the wheelbarrow, intending to take them to the recycling bin.

I was working in the flowerbed one afternoon when Bernadette came from around the front of the property. Her face looked pinched. I could tell she wasn't happy. She walked over to the wheelbarrow and tossed my containers onto the driveway and then grabbed the handles backwards, pulling the wheelbarrow behind her. My rotator cuffs ached at the thought of the strain on her shoulders. The raised veins on her forearms looked like a 3D roadmap.

She paused to inspect my flowerbed. She walked along the edge of the bed, naming the plants. Many of them she knew. But a few were unknown to her. I wished I'd had enough French to engage her in a conversation about gardening. It was our common interest. But I could tell she wasn't interested in lingering. I watched her walk away, pulling the wheelbarrow behind her, in Alpha female mode.

~‿∂

A recurring problem Henri and I were having was his habit of forgetting to tell me when he had made plans that involved me. He'd often have lunch downstairs with his team of mechanics and Bernadette, who fed them well, and they'd discuss plans for dinner. At 7:10 or so, after everyone was sitting down for *apero*, he'd come running upstairs to tell me dinner would be served in 20 minutes.

One night, early in the summer, he came bursting in, saying, "We're waiting for you."

"Waiting for what?" I asked. I was still in work clothes from a day of unpacking. I wasn't ready to go anywhere.

I could see by the look on his face that he suddenly realized he had forgotten to call me or come up to let me know what had been decided hours earlier.

At first, when I was new on the scene, I thought sometimes he honestly forgot he had a girlfriend living upstairs. He had been alone for six years and had a set routine that didn't involve telling a woman his whereabouts or plans he had made.

I didn't make a big deal about it at the beginning. But when this forgetfulness became routine, I asked him to give me more advance notice. I told him I'd like some time to take a shower, especially if I'd been working up a sweat – the summer days in Giverny can be hot and we had no air conditioning at the apartment. At the very least, I needed a chance to change clothes and freshen up.

But that all seemed to fall on stone ears. Henri was hard of hearing to begin with, but he could also be selectively deaf. He once told me, tugging on his left ear lobe, "I'm blind in this ear."

He could easily charm and cajole his way out of these face-offs, but soon the head-butting began.

Early one evening, Henri's Japanese friend Yuka and her partner Marc had stopped by our apartment on their way home from a walk. It was nice having people come by to see us for a change. Usually, visitors congregated in the downstairs kitchen. A popular hiking trail went past the museum side of the complex. The kitchen door was usually open and friends would gather at the long table there for drinks and snacks.

It was not the custom to invite friends who've come for *apero* to stay for dinner, which I found awkward. Because Yuka and Marc's visit had been spontaneous, I had nothing to offer them for a proper meal. But Henri suggested they come downstairs. He said Bernadette had made a big lasagna for lunch and there would be plenty of leftovers.

They said they'd return home to get wine and would come back in a bit. The timing was a bit vague. After Yuka and Marc left, I asked Henri if I should come down to help. He said no, Bernadette was downstairs and would get everything ready. He told me to be there in a half hour.

When I arrived, Yuka and Marc were already at the table. Dinner wasn't quite ready. Bernadette was sautéing chanterelle mushrooms Henri had found on his walk that morning.

It was a fun evening. Yuka and Marc spoke English, so I felt I was part of the conversation, which was a nice change.

The next day, Yuka called me and asked if I'd like to come over to her place for tea that afternoon. Marc was out working in the garden when I arrived. Yuka and I sat at the table in her cheery kitchen and she served a sponge cake she had made. As the sunlight streamed through the window above the table, I could see age lines etched in her face. She was just a few years older than I, but I could tell she had known the wear-and-tear of an expat's peripatetic life.

I really appreciated her invitation. I didn't have a girlfriend yet in Giverny. Yuka was warm and very empathetic with my situation as a foreigner who didn't speak the language. She asked how my French lessons were going with the tutor. I confessed I had been really busy with my new novel, which was in the last phases of production. The final proofreading had been time-consuming. I didn't mention the book project with Roz that was moving into high gear.

"How are things going with the family?" she asked casually.

I hesitated, which gave her an entrée to what she asked next. "Are you having trouble with Bernadette?"

Had Yuka noticed something at dinner the night before, I wondered. "Why do you ask?"

Yuka replied, "She said something last night."

"At dinner? I didn't hear that."

"No, before. When Marc and I came back with the wine. I asked where you were. Bernadette said, 'Rebecca is always late.' "

"Actually, I was on time. Henri told me to come down in a half hour."

"You don't come down to help before dinner?"

"Henri says Bernadette prefers to be alone in the kitchen. I set the table, clear the dishes, slice the bread. That's about it."

Yuka poured tea into small ceramic cups.

"Bernadette is not an easy person to know. She can be hard. But she is a good woman." Yuka gently placed her hand on my arm. "I wonder if it would be a good idea for the three of us to go away together for the day – maybe to the seaside. We could have a nice lunch and talk together. I would translate. You need to understand each other."

Yuka's offer was extremely generous.

"I don't want you to have a problem with her," Yuka continued. "Bernadette was hard on me – so was Amélie – when I first came to Giverny. They made fun of my clothes and my way of speaking. But one day, Bernadette and Amélie came to Paris, where I had an apartment at the time. They saw me in my surroundings. My clothes were suddenly chic to them when they saw me in Paris. They saw me in a new way."

I knew a little bit about Yuka's background. She had worked in Beverly Hills at Fendi, the Italian fashion house. At her summer dinner party, she told me, "I also *lived* in Beverly Hills," making the point that she had immersed herself in that lifestyle, which most people in Giverny couldn't begin to imagine. Yuka had had a big career in fashion and now worked as an emissary at the Impressionist museum where she was a valuable asset when Japanese dignitaries, in government and the art world, visited Giverny.

"So why are you always late for dinner?" Yuka asked.

"Because Henri forgets he has a girlfriend and doesn't tell me until the last minute."

That made Yuka laugh. "We must train him to do better. He's a very good person, but he must change his ways. He has been a single man for a long time now."

Yuka then began telling me the fascinating story of Henri's former partner, Camille.

Henri had told me about how he and Camille had grown up together in Giverny. They were playmates as children and went to school together. He used to have lunch at her big family house where her English grandmother had a strange way of cooking, at least to his palate. He especially hated her pumpkin soup.

I knew Henri and Camille had gone their separate ways after they married other people. In fact, their weddings had happened two weeks apart, at the Giverny town hall. Camille and Henri's ex-wife Pauline had been schoolmates and good friends, according to Henri.

But Yuka said that wasn't so, not after Henri and Camille became a couple.

"Pauline was terrible to Camille," Yuka said. I suddenly was glad I hadn't eaten Pauline's jam. "Camille didn't have an easy time in Henri's family. Camille's family was wealthy. Henri's family – they are peasants."

It surprised me to hear Yuka say this. I hadn't viewed his family that way. They were provincial in many ways, but they were well traveled. They weren't highly educated by American standards. Henri had gone to technical school to become an engineer. I wasn't aware that any of his siblings had continued their education beyond high school. But they had been successful in their livelihoods and were living comfortably in their retirement years. They certainly didn't fit my preconceived notion of "peasants."

I remember Henri once telling me that Camille's mother didn't like him. "Not at all," he had said. "She thought I wasn't good enough for her daughter."

I found that puzzling. By the time he and Camille had become a couple, he was well into a very successful career.

But what Yuka was saying made sense in a way. His family was from "peasant" roots. For generations, they had farmed the land and raised livestock. To me, some of Henri's childhood stories were from a distant century. As a young boy, he would accompany a 17-year-old female cousin into the hills above Giverny where their grandfather, in his later years, tended a large flock of sheep. They brought him food and provisions. He camped out with his flock and moved them from place to place.

Henri's father, a mechanic, repaired farm equipment and ran an old mill, where Henri and his siblings grew up. He remembers how the kids slept in one room, always with the lights on. Generating electricity kept the paddle wheel from turning too fast. He told me that story one night, after I had turned off his bedside lamp. "I'm afraid of the dark," he said, pulling me close. He was only half-joking.

His parents were intelligent and progressive. They had one of the first telephones in Giverny. They subscribed to newspapers and even "Mickey Magazine," as Henri called it, published in French by a Disney-affiliated company in Paris in the 1950s, that he and his siblings enjoyed. They lived well with a worldly view, but they weren't part of well-heeled society. I sensed even in the French microcosm I was living in, there was a divide between town folk and country folk.

Henri enjoyed sharing with me boxes of old photos Camille had organized of their trips together. They spent a couple of months every winter at their home in Ibiza. Their property there adjoined the grounds of a villa owned by her parents. Henri and Camille's house was simple and rustic, with a terrace shaded by olive trees. Henri had put a lot of sweat equity into that place. He loved showing me photos of the stone walls he had built and the beautiful garden they tended there.

We had spent hours looking at those photos. I often wondered why he wanted to share them with me. Many seemed so personal. Sometimes I felt like I shouldn't be seeing Camille sunbathing topless on the beach.

I had no doubt that Camille had been the love of Henri's life. He told me they had met up again, after all their years apart, on the French Riviera. She and her-then husband ran a professional yacht-delivery service for clients who needed their boats delivered to different ports around the Mediterranean. Henri had a lot of business in Nice at the time. He and Camille began an affair. She was unhappy in her marriage and Henri was divorced from Pauline. Two childhood playmates fell in love later in life.

I could easily imagine the stir that caused back in Giverny. I hadn't yet pieced together the story of Pauline. I knew it was a sordid tale. She had become an alcoholic and during divorce proceedings, lost custody of Paul and Alex. The boys had moved around a lot during their childhood and their care was the reason Henri curtailed his international travels so that he could raise them. He eventually decided to move back to Giverny. His father had passed away and Henri assumed his role as patriarch of the family.

When Camille's dementia symptoms began, she knew her fate. Her father had suffered early-onset dementia as well. She and Henri owned a little cafe in the heart of Giverny, where she sold ice cream, pastries and light lunches. Camille was not in denial about what was coming for her. She insisted on selling the cafe and its furnishings so it wouldn't become a burden for Henri.

I actually had met Camille on one of my early visits to Giverny, though I didn't know her by name. I had visited the cafe a few times and noticed a rack of vintage postcards on the counter. One of them – a photo of an old moulin – caught my eye. I asked her if it was Olivier's moulin, the B&B where I was staying, and she said yes. Of course, I didn't realize the family connection and she didn't elaborate. I bought the postcard and 12 years later, it appeared in my book *The Secret of Marie*.

Henri's stories of his wonderful life with Camille were heart-wrenching in a way, especially when you knew how their love affair would end. When her family took her to a dementia-care facility, I don't know if Henri had tried to stop that or whether, by that point, he was too exhausted to object. He told me that on his last visit to Ibiza with Camille, she wandered away from him at the Barcelona airport and he frantically had raced through the concourse before he found her.

Yuka and Camille had been close friends. What Yuka said next shocked me. "Camille did not have an easy time with Henri. She used to tell me that his priorities were his dogs and his engines. She came third."

I didn't know what to say. This went against everything Henri had told me about his relationship with Camille. He had such loving memories of her. From the start of my relationship with Henri, I never expected I could replace her. And now I'm hearing that despite his lovelorn stories, Camille didn't feel more important to him than his dogs and his engines.

"I know Henri loves me. I'm sure of that," I said.

Yuka suddenly realized she had rattled me. "Rebecca, there is no doubt of that. You can see that in the way he looks at you. He's a different man now. He's so happy. He stands taller." She pulled her shoulders back and sat taller in her chair. "The old Henri is back. We're all so happy about that."

But in that moment, I felt gutted by Yuka's revelation. I could never tell Henri I knew this about Camille. I was sure it would crush him. He couldn't make amends now, not with her in a dementia-care ward, sitting in a wheelchair and barely able to lift her head. Her much-younger sister had recently come to visit and had moved her to another facility. She had given Henri a full report about Camille's declining condition.

I wouldn't be able to shake off this story as I looked at my own relationship with Henri. Did I already know this to be true about him? Was I deluding myself thinking I was his number-one priority? In fact, I could well be farther down his list than Camille was – dog, engines, Sister-Wife, family – and then me?

Had Yuka really been a friend to me to tell me all this?

In my French lessons, my tutor had cautioned me about "false friends" – words in different languages that look or sound similar, but have very different meanings.

The meaning of friendship loomed large for me that day. Was Yuka truly a friend – a person whose stories I could trust, whose interest in me was sincere, and who would hold what we talked about in confidence? Should I worry she might be a *faux ami*.

That night, Henri asked if I'd had a nice visit with Yuka. I told him she was concerned that there was friction between Bernadette and me.

"How would Yuka know that?" he asked.

"Last night, before I arrived for dinner, Bernadette told her I'm always late for meals." I let that hang in the air for a minute and then told him about Yuka's proposed day trip to the seaside. "She wants Bernadette and me to get to know each other better – in a pleasant, relaxed setting. Yuka would translate for us."

Henri didn't say anything.

"Do you think it's a good idea?" I asked. "Would Bernadette be willing?"

He shrugged in his quiet way of saying no.

A few days later, Henri and I joined Yuka and Marc at the Baudy for *apero*. I hadn't seen Yuka since our visit in her kitchen, so she didn't know that Henri wasn't receptive to her lunch-at-the-seaside suggestion. I was surprised when she suddenly turned to Henri and scolded him for not giving me more notice of family dinner plans.

"A woman needs time to get ready and comb her hair." she said.

"I don't accept that," Henri replied.

Yuka glanced at me, realizing Bernadette wasn't my only problem.

Chapter 13

Roz and I had decided to call our book *A Garden of Recipes from the Restaurants of Giverny*. We envisioned a collection of recipes from local chefs – inspired by the culinary traditions and bounty of Normandy – and presented with lovely photos I had taken of Giverny and its gardens.

We quickly got several restaurants on board and began discussions with the chefs about which of their dishes to feature in the book. We wanted to mix traditional Normandy cuisine with new variations of old recipes and needed a full range of starters, mains, salads and desserts that ideally could be made in home kitchens without too much angst.

The chef at the Baudy prepared an elaborate luncheon spread for Roz and me so that we could sample the menu favorites. Roz knew the owners of an old hotel in the village called La Musardière, known for its *crêperie*. They kindly shared their family recipe for Crêpe Normande and the chef served it to us with great flourish, igniting a ladle of calvados as he poured it over the caramelized apple topping.

Antoine at the *boulangerie* was enthusiastic. Roz wanted to do a special section in the book about the art of making a French baguette. Antoine gave us a demonstration of the bakery's ovens, which produced as many as 1,000 baguettes daily during high season. The chef and sous-chef welcomed us into the kitchen to watch the preparation of several dishes that we were considering for the book.

Roz and I had lunch one day at Le Jardin des Plumes, a luxury hotel with an elegant restaurant that had been awarded a Michelin star a few years earlier. Roz was interested in meeting the new head chef, who was adding his creative flair to the menu. She chose his recipes for guinea fowl and homemade gnocchi served with butternut squash velouté. When he gave us the recipes, written in French, I could see how complicated they were. We'd not only need an English translation but a detailed explanation of the preparation steps.

From the start, I had made clear to Roz that I wasn't a cook. She assured me she would take charge of the recipes. A few of the chefs spoke some English, but I worried she'd be in over her head since she knew very little French. She had decided to give ingredient measurements in both metric and U.S. equivalents, and I wondered if she could handle that.

I worked out a production timeline. Our goal was to have proof copies ready to show the chefs and Giverny gift-shop vendors by the following March, before the start of the tourist season in April. I told Roz she would need to finish the recipes by early December, which was just a month away, so that I could start laying out the pages. She didn't see that as a problem.

Roz wanted to include at least one recipe from Monet's household cooking journals and was considering a fish creole dish made with an Atlantic cod called *cabillaud* in French, which she would prepare.

"It should be beautifully plated," I said to her.

Her eyes lit up. "They sell Monet's china pattern at the garden gift shop. Shall we go take a look?"

"Those dishes are beautiful, but so expensive."

"I can afford it," she said.

Monet's gardens and gift shop would close for the season in a few days, so we went to take "a look."

The dishes, made of Limoges porcelain, replicate the dinner service Monet designed for his home in Giverny. The pattern is simple, but striking. The white center of the plate is rimmed by a wide yellow band, with a thin cornflower-blue border at the edge – a perfect complement to his bright yellow dining room and blue-tiled kitchen.

An attentive saleswoman opened the glass display cabinet as Roz asked my opinion about what to buy. A dinner plate, which cost about $120, and a salad plate would be enough for our purposes, I said.

"What about a soup bowl?" she asked.

"Do we need a bowl?"

"It would complete the set. Actually, I should get two sets. What good is only one?"

I quickly did the math. "Are you sure? That's a big purchase."

Roz nodded to the saleswoman and then linked arms with me, leading me to the register. "Just look away."

After the saleswoman tallied the items – the total was 550 euros (about $660) – she looked to me for approval. I wondered if she thought I was Roz's daughter.

Roz pulled a credit card out of her wallet and asked that the items be bubble-wrapped and put in a sturdy box. A man emerged from the stockroom and Roz asked him to carry the box to the car. Roz was adept at enlisting her flock of angels.

I carried the box into Roz's living room, and at her request, put it in the corner next to the sofa.

"Mission accomplished," Roz seemed pleased as she took off her coat. "Let's have some tea." As if stricken by an afterthought, she asked, "Should we have gotten cups and saucers?"

~

Roz was actively looking at Giverny properties for her cooking school and asked me to set up an appointment with Henri. He wanted me to handle the showing, which was fine. I didn't want to get the family involved unless Roz's friend was serious about making an offer.

On the day we went to see the Lodge, I could tell Roz wasn't feeling well. She was pale and had a crackling cough that she dismissed as a "little cold."

Henri had left the front door of the Lodge unlocked. As Roz

and I entered the foyer, there was a chill in the air and a noticeable old-house smell. Not a good first impression.

Although the house was built in the 1950s, it appeared to be much older. The expansive living room, with its dark wooden ceiling beams and big stone fireplace, was charmingly old-fashioned – decorated with an assortment of antique pieces and a large, well-worn oriental rug.

As if on cue, sun streamed through large windows that flanked a set of French doors, which opened to the front walkway.

"What a lovely room," Roz remarked. She ran her hand over the top of an old library table. "I have a Tiffany-style lamp that would look beautiful here."

Roz spent most of our visit in the kitchen, envisioning what could be. "It needs a lot of work," she said, inspecting the outdated appliances. "But it's a nice open space with lots of possibilities." She especially liked the outlook onto the terrace. "Can't you just imagine summer-night parties there?"

I nodded, trying not to think about my own disappointment in all this.

We did a quick tour of the six bedrooms upstairs. The furniture was covered with sheets and half of the light bulbs were burned out.

"I can't believe they haven't changed these bulbs," I said.

The big shock came when we walked through the bedroom suite downstairs. On a table in the cold, dingy sitting room, Bernadette had placed boxes of apples she was storing for the winter.

"This is unbelievable," Roz murmured. "How do they ever expect to sell this place?"

We sat down in the living room, which Roz agreed would be perfect for large gatherings.

I was up front with her about the problems with the property. Henri had gotten an estimate of 30,000 euros (about $36,000) to repair the rotting window frames.

"I could cover that," she said.

I sensed a shift in Roz's plans. "Why would you pay for that if your friend wants to buy the place?"

"If that falls through, I could lend the family the money they need to upgrade the property while I live here, which would enable them to get a higher price. They could pay me back when it sells," she said. "I don't think this place is going to sell quickly. It's priced way too high, considering all the work it needs."

I knew in that moment that I didn't want to present a proposal from Roz to the family. I sensed a slippery slope. Roz's ideas didn't always seem rooted in reality. Although she didn't appear to have money worries, I knew nothing about her resources. I thought it best not to tell Henri about her offer to pay for the window repairs.

I could see that her energy was flagging. "Let's get you home," I said. "You need to get some rest."

~

That evening when I called to check on her, Roz sounded much worse. Henri and I had just arrived at the *boulangerie* for dinner, and I told her I'd ask Antoine to make her a plate and I'd bring it to her. She said she'd be waiting for me.

When I arrived at her place, she was wrapped in a blanket, sitting next to a space heater by the front door. She held my arm tight as I led her into the kitchen.

"Roz, I'm really concerned. We need to find you a doctor."

As she sat down at the table, she looked at me with panic in her eyes. "I need to talk to you about something, Rebecca." She reached for some papers on the table.

What transpired in the next several minutes was astonishing. She told me she was on her third pacemaker and didn't want to be put on life support if she ended up in the hospital.

"This cough is affecting my heart," she said. "I can feel it."

She showed me the documents, which would authorize me to withhold life support.

I was stunned. "I can't sign these. This is for your children to decide."

"I don't want them making the decision," she said firmly. "They keep their dogs alive too long."

I assured her I would take her to the emergency room if she needed to go. I warmed up her dinner in the microwave. It was a new dish on Antoine's menu. Even in her dark hour that night, Roz recognized it was a culinary tour de force – a baked phyllo pastry filled with andouille de Vire, calvados-flavored apples and slices of camembert cheese, served with a cider-cream sauce. After one bite, she said, "We *must* get this recipe."

I was a mess when I got back to the *boulangerie*. "Henri, you won't believe what happened," I said as I sat down. "She asked me to pull the plug – or keep them from plugging her in."

"What plug?"

"To her life-support machine!"

"*Chérie*, calm down." He pushed a glass of wine he had ordered for me across the table.

Just then Henri's nephew Denis, Roz's landlord, walked in.

"Denis, I need to talk to you!"

Denis looked askance at me because I had skipped the pleasantries of *Bonsoir, ça va*? (kiss-kiss).

"*Doucement, doucement*," he said. Don't get excited, say hello first.

I explained that Roz was sick with a bad cough and had a serious underlying heart problem. "She might need to go to the hospital tonight."

Denis spoke a little English and assured me he'd take her to the emergency room, if necessary. He then went over to the bar and ordered a drink.

Maxine and Olivier were sitting at the next table. When Denis was out of earshot, Maxine turned toward me, curling her fingers in a fist that she twisted around her nose.

"What does that mean?" I asked her.

She shook her head. "He'll be too drunk to drive anywhere tonight."

It was an ominous beginning to what turned out to be a fraught partnership with Roz. If I had known how bad things would get, I would have slammed on the brakes then.

Fortunately, she didn't need to go to the hospital that night. A friend got her in to see a doctor the next day. Within a week, she was feeling better and ready to resume work on the recipes. She couldn't stop talking about the fabulous dinner Antoine had made for her. "Croustillant with Camembert, Apples & Andouille de Vire" was a delicious addition to the book.

Chapter 14

Every November 11, on Armistice Day, Giverny residents gather at the local cemetery to remember their fallen heroes. It was the 100th anniversary of the Armistice that year, so despite the miserable rainy weather, there was a good turnout. As we huddled together under umbrellas for the ceremony, I thought of my mother's father who had fought in France during World War I. He had grown up in the Smoky Mountains of Tennessee and probably couldn't have imagined a granddaughter making a life for herself in France. But I felt his hand at my back that day.

It's the village tradition after the Armistice ceremony for villagers to go to the *salle des fêtes* – the community center were exhibitions and parties are held – to officially welcome newcomers who have taken up residence in Giverny that year. There were seven of us who were asked to step forward as the mayor read out our names. I could tell it was a proud moment for Henri. And it was a wonderful moment for me.

A woman on the village council came over to talk to us and said how happy she was that I had decided to make my home in Giverny. In French, she asked Henri if we'd be adding to the elementary-school enrollment. When Henri translated for me, I burst out laughing. I typed into Google translate: *Madame, that ship sailed long ago.*

A week later there was an embroidery fair at the *salle des fêtes*. I enjoyed perusing the display tables, which were overflowing with beautiful handmade items. France has a rich embroidery tradition that spans many centuries. It was wonderful to see so many local women keeping this art form alive.

I met two lovely French women named Brigitte and Madeleine who were members of a cross-stitch embroidery club that met every Tuesday in the nearby village of Vernonnet. They called themselves *Deux Mille et Une Croix* – 2001 Crosses – because the group had formed in 2001. Brigitte and Madeleine proudly showed me some of the projects the group had produced for a recent exhibition. Among them was an exquisite cross-stitch rendering of Monet's house on finely woven linen. I was delighted when Brigitte and Madeleine invited me to come to their next meeting.

The cross-stitch ladies were very welcoming. A few of them spoke English and could translate for me when I'd ask questions about their projects. Madeleine had been an English teacher before her retirement and took me under wing. Her son lived in southern California, where she had visited often, so she and I had a lot to talk about.

Meeting this group was a turning point for me. But meeting one particular woman in this group changed everything.

Sometimes you just know when a new best friend appears in your life. I felt that way about Sarah, the minute I met her. I'll never forget that Tuesday afternoon. As soon as I walked in the door, she got up from her seat and came to greet me. She had just come back from a holiday and had heard from Madeleine about the group's new American member. Sarah was clearly happy to meet me.

She invited me to sit next to her and wanted to know all about what had brought me to France. She was English, originally from Cornwall, and had spent most of her adult life in France. We were the same age. Divorced, mothers of sons. We both loved gardening, traveling and sewing. I could tell Sarah had a chic sense of style. She wore a tailored embellished jacket that day and gold-sequined sneakers – "trainers," as she called them. Her wavy brown hair was stylishly cut. She had a strip of white along the part line. I couldn't tell if she was going natural or going for a Look.

Sarah was an accomplished seamstress, but new to cross-stitch. She showed me her not-so-secret Santa project that would be part of the group's Christmas gift exchange. She was embroidering squares with colorful cross-stitched figures of women from around the world in native costumes. She said, "I'm not sure what I'm going to do with them. Maybe a cushion cover?"

She saw the corner of a wooden frame sticking out of my tote bag. "What are you working on?"

"I've inherited this project," I said, smiling at Madeleine who was sitting across the table from us.

I pulled the frame from the bag and showed Sarah the unfinished needlepoint canvas attached to it. The design was a basket of flowers. The basket and a few of the flowers had been stitched in, but the rest of the pre-printed canvas was unfinished.

"I've not done cross-stitch before," I said to Sarah. "I'm not sure my eyes are strong enough. Madeleine thought I might give this a try."

I looked around the room at all the women peering at their work through magnifiers attached to their embroidery hoops. Some actually wore magnifiers that clipped on to their eye glasses. I spent so much time staring at my computer screen that I didn't relish taking up a hobby that would cause more eye strain. Needlepoint would be much easier for me. The holes in the canvas were large. A tapestry needle had an oversized eye that would be easy to thread.

Madeleine flipped up the magnifiers attached to her glasses. "How are you coming along with that?"

"I'm still figuring out a color scheme."

"Where did this come from?" Sarah asked.

"It was for sale at the embroidery fair, but no one bought it," I said.

"There's no kit or color chart? No yarn at all?"

I shook my head, fingering some sample strands of yarn in various colors that dangled from the edge of the canvas. "This is all I have."

Madeleine said, "I'll check in the boxes that came back from the fair. Maybe we'll find something."

"I belonged to a quilting group when I lived in California, and we called our unfinished projects UFOs…"

Before I could explain, Sarah said, "Unfinished objects."

I laughed. "Apparently, it's a global phenomenon among women who stitch?"

Sarah rolled her eyes. "You have no idea. You should see my sewing room."

At the fair, there had been a box full of felt patches in the shape of flower petals, in a rainbow of colors, each of them edged with a decorative buttonhole stitch. The vendor thought they may have been made as epaulets for military costumes. A woman standing next to me guessed they were meant to be decoration for an abbey prayer rug. *We really should leave notes with our UFOs,* I thought.

An afternoon ritual at the embroidery meetings was afternoon tea, served at 4. The room accommodated two long tables – one for working on projects and the other for teatime. Home-baked goodies often materialized on the tea table, along with tins of tea in exotic flavors. An assortment of pretty mugs appeared from a storage cupboard. On a busy afternoon, 20 women would gather round that table. I loved listening to their chatter in French, even though they spoke much too fast for me to understand most of it.

On that particular day, I asked the group if they knew the original owner of my inherited UFO.

"She's dead," one woman said.

"Does anyone know her name?" I asked.

After some discussion, someone remembered: Madame Souliman.

That evening, back at Henri's apartment, I hung Madame Souliman's UFO tapestry on my bedroom wall. It looked lovely just as it was, even in its unfinished state. The wooden stretcher framed it beautifully. The yarn strands were telltales of the palette she had envisioned. I ran my fingers over her neat stitches. Maybe it wasn't for me to complete her project. There was something appealing about *imagining* what was meant to be.

Tuesdays quickly became my favorite day of the week. I had found a niche to call my own in this new place I called home. And I had found a new best friend named Sarah.

Chapter 15

As the recipe-book project got underway, it soon became apparent that Roz was not equal to the tasks she had told me she could handle. She had no computer skills. Absolutely none. She delivered the first recipe to me in longhand. It took me an hour to decipher her wobbly handwriting, which meandered across the page in faint pencil.

She said she wasn't comfortable typing on her laptop and asked me to find her an electric typewriter. "Could you find me an Olivetti? I like that brand."

"That's not going to help, Roz. We need to share *digital* files so that we can make revisions."

"Then I'll need to find someone to type for me."

Roz found a young woman who lived close by and knew enough English to type up the recipes, which she'd then email to me. She made a lot of grammatical and spelling errors, but that was the least of my worries.

I began to see discrepancies in Roz's measurement conversions from metric to U.S. equivalents. One day, I was sitting at her desk and asked to see the conversion table she was using.

"I use my phone," she said matter-of-factly. She googled "almond cream" and without opening the link, pointed to a measurement that appeared at the end of the text block on her screen, which she hadn't bothered to read.

"Roz, that's the conversion for tahini," I said, pointing to the word TAHINI. "Don't you have a book of equivalents? A cooking encyclopedia like Larousse? Surely, Julia Child covered this."

When she shook her head, looking very sheepish, I instantly realized the enormity of what had gone wrong.

We were already a few weeks into the project and had finished about a dozen recipes. All that time, she had been randomly and carelessly pulling numbers off her phone. As it turned out, her math was pretty spotty, too.

We had to begin again with the conversions on all of the recipes we had completed to that point.

I found a website with an extensive conversion chart that covered 6,000 ingredients. I had no idea that salt and sugar, for example, don't have the same equivalents as flour, which in the book of conversions, is its own sub-genre. And then there were the oddities of French measuring implements such as soup spoons and coffee spoons, which can be imprecise. We needed measurements in grams for dry ingredients and milliliters for liquids before we could determine the U.S. equivalents.

I enlisted Henri to help me figure out the conversion for a *bouchon*, which, in French recipe parlance, is the cap of a bottle and is often the measurement for calvados, which flavors many Normandy recipes. Henri took a scientific approach, measuring a capful of calvados into a shot glass that he had already weighed on a kitchen scale, so that he could determine the weight of the brandy. We crossed-checked that measurement with an American cocktail jigger that was marked in ounces and then we poured the contents of the jigger into one of my Betty Crocker measuring spoons. To confirm his calculations, Henri repeated the process, sipping as he went. After several rounds, he declared that a *bouchon* equaled one U.S. tablespoon. But he had imbibed a lot more than that to reach his conclusion.

Compounding the already difficult situation with Roz was her mercurial temper, which came as a surprise to me. She had seemed so serene and at peace with the universe when I first met her. But under that veneer, there was a darker side to her. Even more worrying were signs that her circumstances – as a 79-year-old woman with health problems, living alone in a foreign country where she didn't speak the language – were beginning to overwhelm her.

On the day the Impressionist museum closed for the season, in early November – a few weeks before everything went sideways with the conversion calculations – I had arranged with the restaurant's sous chef, a young Moroccan man named Namir, to take some additional photos of him clipping herbs in the museum garden.

I had arrived about a half hour before Roz was due so that I could complete the photography before she and I met with Ivan to finalize the recipes.

I was seated at a table adjacent to the kitchen, reviewing the photos I had taken, when I looked up to see Roz coming toward me from across the dining room. I could tell she was angry. Her face was red, her hair looked wind-blown. She had her coat and handbag over one arm and was clutching a little aluminum-foil packet, which suddenly split open.

"Shit!" she exclaimed, as several pieces of ham flew to the floor.

She stormed over to the table and threw her coat on a chair.

"Hello," I said quietly, bracing for the fury that was unfolding.

She said nothing as she opened her handbag and tossed a recipe at me from across the table.

She sat down opposite me and morphed into a boss who was about to dismiss an employee. "Rebecca, I'm a former CEO and expect people to do things for me." She was nearly hissing at me. "I appreciate all you've done, but I had no idea you had other commitments."

"I was very clear about that from the beginning. But I've made myself available to you and this project. My other commitments haven't gotten in the way."

"You can have the Monet dishes."

"What – as severance pay? Are you firing me?" I looked over at the ham on the floor. "Roz, what's going on?"

"I need something to eat. Where's Ivan?"

"He's not here. Namir told me he left early."

"I made an appointment with him. He said he'd be here. The restaurant closes today. I need to speak with him." Roz slowly stood up and flagged a young man who was working behind the bar.

When he came to the table, she demanded a menu. "The kitchen is closed," he replied.

"We'll see about that," she retorted.

It was mid-afternoon at that point. Lunch service had ended. In disbelief, I watched her walk toward the kitchen entrance and barge through the doors.

Within seconds, Namir appeared, gently holding Roz's arm. He looked over at me, bewildered. He escorted her to a table in the dining room.

Namir came over to where I was sitting. "I will make her something to eat," he said.

"I'm so sorry, Namir. She's very upset. I'm not sure why."

"It's no problem."

I collected Roz's things and walked over to her table.

I sat down next to her and could clearly see how distraught she was. "I don't know what has upset you…"

"Everything has upset me. My driver didn't show up – I had to walk all the way here. I'm hungry. I've not had lunch."

"Namir is going to make you a delicious lunch. If you'd like to join me, there's a concert starting in a half hour in the museum auditorium. I'd be glad to get you a ticket. Or if you'd rather just relax and enjoy your meal, I'll come by when the concert is over and take you home."

She declined my invitation to go to the concert. And when I came back to the restaurant after it was over, she had gone.

A few days later, Ivan agreed to meet with us at his home to go over the recipes. It was a long session because he had to use a translation app on his phone to explain the preparation steps. Roz kept asking him the same questions. At one point, while I was taking notes, I looked over at her to see if she was following along. She had lost interest in what we were discussing and was cleaning out her handbag.

When I realized a few weeks later that we'd have to re-do the conversions, I sat in my car after I left her house that day, feeling the stress of what was coming. I wanted out, but I felt obligated to keep going. We had enlisted the help of restaurant owners and chefs, who already had spent a lot of time answering our questions and clarifying instructions as we translated the recipes into English. I felt we couldn't let them down. But everything had shifted that day. I knew the weight of this project was squarely on my shoulders.

Chapter 16

Henri was eager to firm up plans for the annual Christmas trip to Ibiza, but there were complications.

Yuka and Marc were interested in joining us, which I thought would be fun, especially if we rented a house where we all could stay. But Bernadette wasn't on board with this, which put Henri in a difficult spot.

I remembered the painful conversation I'd had with him during my Easter visit when he told me I should spend Christmas in California. He knew I wouldn't like the rustic accommodations in Ibiza, in a house with no heat and very little hot water. "The price is right," Henri had told me. "The owner is an old friend who lets us stay for free. But I know you wouldn't be comfortable there."

He had been clear that his priority was Bernadette. *She won't want to be in Ibiza without me. She needs me to take care of things.*

That turned out not to be true. While Henri was still discussing travel arrangements with Yuka, Marc and me, Bernadette and her friend Valérie booked their flights and the house-with-no-heat, apparently unconcerned that Henri wouldn't be there to keep logs on the fire.

Yuka sensed there was a problem. Bernadette pointedly had told Yuka that she and Valérie would be going off on their own, hiking every day.

In the end, Yuka and Marc decided not to come. I was disappointed, but I didn't blame them. "We don't feel welcome," Yuka said to me.

Henri and I spent hours on Airbnb, looking for a place for just the two of us. He wanted to be close enough to the house-with-no-heat, just in case he'd be needed there. His plan was to show me the island by day and then we'd join Bernadette and Valérie in the evenings for dinner.

He was doing his best to find a compromise. But more than that, I could see how eager he was to share Ibiza with me.

We found a lovely two-bedroom house near Henri's favorite village, Santa Gertrudis de Fruitera, which was close to where he and Camille had lived.

"Will you be okay?" I asked him one evening, as he was showing me a guide book of the island. "Aren't you going to be missing Camille?"

He leaned over and kissed me. "No, because I'll be with you."

My new novel, *By Chance*, came out in late November. The postman delivered my author copy just as I was leaving for an appointment with my chiropractor, Jean-Raymond. I tucked it into my bag so that I could show it to him. I knew he'd be pleased. He had worked hard to get the kinks out of my sore writer's neck.

When I walked into his office, I was surprised to see Mean Girl in the waiting room. We exchanged the usual pleasantries – *Ça va? Bien. Ça va?* As I sat down next to her, she noticed the book poking out of my bag.

"What are you reading?" she asked.

"You may know this author. She's local," I said, handing her the book.

"When did this come out?"

"Today."

MG put on her glasses and studied the vintage black-and-white photo on the cover.

"That's my mom and dad on their wedding day," I said.

"What a great picture."

The photographer had captured, in one brilliant click, my mother losing her footing on the steps in front of my grandparents' house as she and my dad were leaving on their honeymoon, under a shower of rice. You see the surprise on her face as she starts to fall. But my strapping, sure-footed father has his outstretched arm around her waist, with a grin on his face that says *I've got you.*

"It was my father's first act of gallantry as a married man."

MG read the synopses on the back cover. "Are you the protagonist of this story – *a divorced, middle-age woman, who regrets that true and lasting love has eluded her?*"

"It's partly my story. But a good bit of it is fiction."

There was a lot of me in my protagonist, actually. When I began writing the book, my biggest regret in life was not falling in love in my youth with a man I'd grow to love even more as we aged together. I often had wondered about the times I'd said no to possibilities and had turned away from a love that might have been. But as the story unfolded, I came to realize I had known love in abundance, even if it wasn't lasting. I had experienced intimacy and tenderness that had given me a gentle heart, and even in the anguish of lost love, I hadn't lost hope that true love would find me.

I dedicated the book to "those longing for love, with the hope that, just *by chance*, the wonder and mystery of it will find you – and delight you – when you least expect it."

I hadn't gone looking for Henri. But the pull of Giverny had brought me to him. In an extraordinary twist of fate, as I wrote two love stories set in Giverny, I found myself in one of my own. What a wonderful surprise that had been.

Love can be fraught with missteps. Although Henri and I were struggling to find our footing as a couple, a great love held us together even as we stumbled.

Henri likes to tell the story of how he flew to Florence to see me during the early weeks of our romance, on the tail of a snowstorm that had swept northern Italy. Undeterred by flight cancellations and delays in Paris, he finally got on a plane bound for Florence. But while he was en route, the Florence airport closed and his flight was diverted to Bologna. He waited an hour in line for a taxi at the Bologna airport and shared a ride to the Bologna train station with a kind Italian gentleman who got him on a train for the 40-minute ride to Florence. Henri had another long wait in the taxi queue in Florence, where several inches of snow had blanketed the city. The taxi driver couldn't make it up the icy slope to my apartment, so she dropped him off on a side street.

I was watching from my living-room balcony window when I saw him come around the corner, pulling his carry-on suitcase through the snow. He was actually *running* through the snow.

I opened the window and called down to him. "You made it!"

He looked up at me and waved, without breaking his stride.

Within minutes, he burst through my front door, looking like a lovestruck teenager. He had been traveling for 12 hours. But none of that mattered to him as he scooped me into his big strong arms.

I will never forget the love I felt for him that day as I watched him running through the snow.

Chapter 17

Winter was closing in on Giverny. I went for a walk one afternoon and didn't see a single soul in the village. Henri had warned me that Giverny was a very lonely place in the winter.

I looked forward to my Tuesday afternoons with the embroidery ladies. I had decided to let Madame Souliman's work-in-progress hang in its unfinished state on my bedroom wall, which meant I needed to find a new project.

At one meeting, Sarah gave me a cross-stitch lesson, but I nearly went cross-eyed. "I really can't do this," I told her.

She laughed. "It's a cross-stitch club. Why did you join?"

"Because I wanted to make new friends. Do you think they'll kick me out?"

"No, you'll be fine. But we need to find you a project."

Sarah and I signed up for a workshop with a woman in the group named Chantal who made beautiful quilts that she embellished with embroidery. The workshops were in her home – a quaint cottage in an ancient quarter of Vernon – which she had decorated with her exquisite handiwork. Although I had been a quilter for years, I was intrigued with how Chantal enhanced her quilts with decorative elements. The choice of embellishments was endless at Chantal's dining table, which was always strewn with silk ribbons, skeins of floss, and packets of sequins, beads, and buttons.

I loved working with silk ribbon and ordered some supplies online. Thanks to Chantal's inspiring ideas, I had lots to work on at the Tuesday meetings. The ladies in the group took an interest in my projects. One older woman, who was skilled at silk-ribbon embroidery, copied pages of instructions from books she had at home so I could learn some of the more complicated stitches.

The cross-stitch ladies had a festive Christmas party at a local hotel. We each received gift certificates to use at a sewing shop in Vernon. We drank champagne and enjoyed an exchange of the secret-Santa projects. Sarah's cross-stitched women of the world ended up, not as cushions, but as pencil-cup covers. As we raised our glasses and wished each other a *Joyeux Noël*, I felt so happy to be part of this group.

~

The big holiday fete on Henri's calendar was his annual dinner for his museum volunteers and their spouses.

The night before the event, Henri's buddies Jacques and Martin arrived and the feasting began early. Martin brought oysters from the coastal village where he lived. A dish that I thought was a gooey coil of chocolate cake turned out to be blood sausage. The *pièce de résistance* was *coq au vin*, which Bernadette served with great flourish. After placing the roasting pan on the table, she plunged a fork into the simmering stew of rooster parts and vegetables. She held up what to me looked like a white mushroom and popped it in her mouth.

Henri leaned into me and said, "That's the cock's testicle."

"Does he have two?" I asked.

Everyone watched in amazement as my fork and I went searching for testicle *numero deux*.

I placed it on Henri's plate and cut it in half. I couldn't tell if Bernadette was impressed or shocked as I followed her lead. Not entirely to my surprise, I felt like I had a mouthful of salty mush.

"Well?" Henri asked.

"I've tasted better."

That got a big laugh.

The party the next evening was held at a lovely restaurant across the river from Giverny, with an outstanding menu of Normandy dishes prepared by skilled chef Benjamin Brisset from his family's recipes. Before dinner, guests gathered for cocktails in a large comfortable lounge by the bar, warmed by crackling logs in an immense fireplace. Bernadette assumed the role of hostess and welcomed everyone, before turning the evening over to Henri, who gave a toast of appreciation to the 20 or so guests.

Most of the museum volunteers – all of them men – stood with their wives. Henri stood with Bernadette. I stood off to the side, taking it all in.

∼♪

One Sunday afternoon in mid-December, I got inspired to decorate Henri's apartment for Christmas. I wanted to surprise him, so I waited for him to go downstairs to his workshop after his nap. He and his mechanic buddies often worked on their projects on Sunday afternoons, so I knew I'd have a few hours to do my magic before he returned for dinner.

I went into the storeroom Henri had built for me – sealed off from flying mice – and found a few boxes of Christmas decorations I had acquired during my travels.

The day before, we had gotten a small tree that Henri had put on a low table to give it some height. It had a gangly top, which is typical of fir Christmas trees in Normandy. But I was equal to the challenge. I had purchased a large patchwork star at Giverny's Christmas craft sale that would nicely nestle into the top branches.

I had an eclectic collection of ornaments that came from England, Italy and the Christmas markets of Berlin. I had purchased my newest ornament at the Monet Gardens gift shop: a miniature felt version of Monet himself, wearing a big floppy hat and holding a water lily. When I showed it to Henri, he burst out laughing. "It's so Mickey." (Mickey – as in Mickey Mouse – was Henri's word for "tacky.")

I carefully unpacked an exquisite German-made, tiered Christmas carousel – topped with windmill blades driven by warm air that rises from lit candles around its base, causing the carousel to spin. Each tier is decorated with hand-carved figures that tell the Nativity story. I was happy to see that the wise men, camels and angels hadn't lost their footing on their journey from Florence.

I had just turned on the Christmas-tree lights when I heard Henri come in the back door. It was 7:30. Perfect timing. I pulled a bottle from the kitchen wine rack.

Henri admired the decorations and sat down at the dining table as I lit the carousel's candles. When the windmill blades began to spin, he smiled. "Thermal engineering."

"My darling engineer, shall I open the wine? I'm not sure what we're having for dinner, but at least the candles are lit."

Henri suddenly looked uncomfortable. "Bernadette is waiting downstairs. She has prepared dinner."

He had made no mention earlier in the afternoon that we'd be having dinner with Bernadette. I had been looking forward to a quiet evening together, just the two of us. I was in comfy clothes and slippers, wanting to curl up on the sofa with a glass of wine and enjoy the Christmas trimmings.

I could feel my anger rising. "Henri, why does this keep happening?"

"I'm sorry," he murmured.

"It's late. Go without me," I said. "I'm not going to rush to get ready. This is so inconsiderate of you."

I could tell he was annoyed, but I was furious. After he left, I heated up some leftovers from the previous night and made myself a salad. I was at the table, still eating, when he returned 45 minutes later. He sat down opposite me and said nothing as I finished my meal. After I cleared my dishes, I came back to the table and was stunned by what happened next. Instead of making amends, Henri shouted, "It's always my fault!"

I slammed my hands on the table as I stood up. "This problem is your fault!"

I went to my room and got ready for bed. I closed the bedroom door, which wasn't my habit. I tried to read, but couldn't concentrate. I could hear Henri in the kitchen making his bedtime cup of tea. I turned off the light and burrowed under the duvet. A short while later, I heard Henri's footsteps in the hallway. He paused at my bedroom door, but didn't knock or enter. I heard his bedroom door close and then all went quiet. It was a silent night of the worst kind.

~୨

The next day, Henri pretended all was fine. That was his way. After an argument, he'd later come back into the room, grinning as though nothing had happened. It wasn't as easy for me to recover and carry on.

In the days before Christmas, I was busy baking and wrapping gifts for a little party I had planned for Henri's family. It would be the first time Henri and I had entertained at his apartment. We had decided to have an afternoon gathering, on a Sunday, two days before Christmas. Henri's son Paul and his family would be arriving from Switzerland earlier that afternoon. We thought it would be a nice way to start his visit.

That morning, as Henri and I made preparations for the party, his phone rang. He took the call in another room and after he hung up, told me it had been Bernadette. He didn't say anything more.

Around noon, I suggested we take a break and asked what he'd like for lunch.

He looked up at the clock on the kitchen wall and said, "Paul will be here in a half hour. We're having lunch downstairs."

"When was this decided?"

"When he called Bernadette this morning to tell her they would be here in time for lunch."

"And that's why Bernadette called you earlier – to tell you that?"

"*Peut-être.*"

"Maybe? You've known this for more than an hour and didn't think to tell me?"

He shrugged.

Henri hadn't forgotten to tell me. He had intentionally decided not to.

He went downstairs to have lunch with the family without me. I still had things to do for the party and needed to shower and get dressed. It was after 2 when he returned. He sat in the living room as I put out trays of food. Just before 3, I lit the candles and dialed up a Christmas playlist on my iPod.

The party was to have started at 3. But by 3:30, no one had arrived.

"Where is everyone?" I asked Henri.

He then informed me that, during lunch, everyone had said they'd come a little later – closer to 4. Once again, I was the last to know.

The party, when it finally started, was a success. Everyone enjoyed the food and their gifts. The only one who didn't thank me at the end was Henri, even though he'd clearly had a wonderful time.

I was at a loss to explain his hurtful behavior and I wondered if he understood it himself.

As I lay alone in my bed that night, listening to a cuckoo that often serenaded me, I closed my eyes and could see Henri on that wintry day in Florence, running through the snow.

What had happened to us?

~♪

I woke up the next morning – the morning of Christmas Eve – to the smell of coffee brewing and heard the shuffle of Henri's slippers in the hallway outside my bedroom.

"Are you awake?" he asked, poking his head through the doorway "Just."

Carrying two steamy coffee mugs, he came over to the bed.

"Good morning." I sat up, propping a pillow behind me.

"*Bonjour.*" Henri handed me a mug. "Did you sleep well?"

"I woke up with a cold nose in the middle of the night."

"It was below freezing this morning." He sat down on the bed next to me. "You'll warm up in Ibiza. I just checked the weather. It's going to be beautiful while we're there."

I wanted to feel the joyful anticipation of a week in Ibiza. But Henri and I were in trouble.

He seemed to read my mind. "I want us to have a good time together on this trip."

Part of me wanted to say yes to that, but the truth won out. "We're not in a good place, you and I."

"*Chérie*, what's wrong?"

"I'm so unhappy, Henri. And you don't seem to care."

"Of course I care about you."

"How can you say that? You exclude me. You disregard me. You yell at me when you know you're in the wrong."

"That's not true."

"You *know* it's true. You've been so unkind and defiant lately. I feel like you're pushing me away."

"I don't mean to hurt you," he said.

"I don't believe you, Henri. Your behavior is hurtful – intentionally hurtful. It seems you're punishing me."

"For what?" he asked.

"For being the rope around your wrists. Remember what you said to me in Malta? The reason you didn't want to be a couple?"

He shook his head. "*Je ne comprends pas.*"

I put my coffee mug on the nightstand and crossed my wrists. "You said you never wanted to feel like this, remember? Is this how you feel? If you want out of this relationship, just say so."

"No, that's not what I want."

"Then this has to stop. I can't do this anymore."

"I don't want to lose you." Henri looked at me sadly. "Can we try to have a nice Christmas? Can we start there?"

In France, the big celebration at Christmas happens on Christmas Eve with an elaborate family dinner. There were 16 of us, including an assortment of relatives, so Henri had decided to open up the Lodge for the festivities. We gathered in the living room where a live potted Christmas tree, which gets dragged in from the garden every year, sparkled with lights, ornaments and tinsel. It seemed Father Christmas had come by earlier to leave gifts under the tree for the children, who were amazingly restrained as they inspected the packages.

The table looked beautiful and was lit by two stunning silver candelabras. Henri's 10-year-old granddaughter had folded the napkins in the shape of water lilies. A leg of lamb roasted on the spit in the fireplace. Henri's son Alex served an appetizer tray of grilled African crocodile, as we drank champagne.

Fresh English-Channel oysters started the meal. It's the French custom to sip the salt water from the half-shell. To cut the briny taste, baguette slices, slathered with sweet butter from Brittany, are served as an accompaniment. (French bread is rarely served with butter, except at breakfast.)

I ventured into the kitchen to see if I could assist with the next course. Naturally, Bernadette was in charge and to my surprise, she welcomed my help as she carefully sliced and plated the *foie gras*. I added the garnish and the teenage girls in the family whisked the plates to the dining table. It was a smooth operation that earned me a high-five from Bernadette. No minor Christmas miracle.

Wine bottles were uncorked with every course. The long dining table turned into a veritable groaning board as side dishes joined the heaped platter of lamb. After the main course, a beautiful cheese plate made its way around the table. And then came the traditional French Christmas dessert, *Bûche de Noël*, a chocolate-cake and ice-cream Yule Log. My contribution was my mom's Peanut Blossom cookies, made with Peter Pan peanut butter and Hershey's Kisses I had ordered from a website that imports American food to homesick expats in France. Knowing how discerning the French can be when it comes to "foreign" food, I was relieved there was a general murmuring of approval. Chocolate combined with peanut butter apparently was a new taste sensation for this crowd.

The kids opened gifts and ran wild, reminding me of being that age and doing the same with my cousins. Henri's dog, Facel, was in heaven, loving the chaos and the scraps that fell not-so-accidentally to the floor. He won a game of tug-of-war that took place under the table, with all the kids pulling on his leash, which he held in his teeth.

At one point during the merriment, Henri, sitting next to me, took my hand. "*Joyeux Noël, chérie,*" he said. "*Je t'aime.*"

~

Our merry Christmas was short-lived. The next morning, Henri woke up with a sore throat and a fever. By afternoon, he was coughing, and by evening we had canceled our flights for the next day to Ibiza. We couldn't get a refund on the house we had rented, but the owner said we could re-book some other time.

Bernadette and Valérie held to the plan. I could see Henri's wistfulness when Bernadette called daily to give him a full report of their activities and the gorgeous weather they were enjoying. But on their last day in Ibiza, while they were hiking on a steep cliffside trail, Valérie fell and broke her leg. It was a severe compound fracture that required surgery they couldn't perform at the hospital on the island. Bernadette made arrangements for Valérie to be medevacked back to Paris. She herself traveled back to France alone.

I knew Henri felt he should have been there to help them. But Bernadette had managed well enough without him.

By New Year's Eve, Henri was feeling better and we celebrated at home with a dear friend of his named Claire Joyes, an art historian and author who lived nearby. We had a lovely evening and drank copious amounts of champagne over a dinner that lasted until 2 a.m.

When I woke up the next morning, I felt fine until I turned my head. Henri was in bed next to me, suffering from the same fate.

"Are you hung up?" he asked.

It hurt to laugh. "I'm probably hung up," I said, gently stroking his cheek. "But I'm definitely hung over."

Chapter 18

While Henri had been busy planning our Ibiza trip that didn't happen, I'd been making arrangements to return to California after the holidays for a monthlong visit. I wanted to see my son and meet his new girlfriend. I needed to purge my storage units, which had gotten exorbitantly expensive. Henri said he'd like to join me for a week. Our plan was for me to leave in mid-January, with him arriving a couple of weeks later. In mid-November, I booked my flights and he said he'd do the same. But after a few weeks, he went quiet about coming to California. When I asked him if that was still his intention, he said, *"Bien sûr!"* Of course.

I had been thinking about shipping some things from my storage units to Giverny and mentioned this to Henri.

"What more do you need?" he asked.

"I have things that are special to me – family heirlooms, photo albums, books, paintings, my beautiful wedding china…"

"I think we have enough dishes."

"My wedding china is Limoges. It belongs on a French table." After slaving over a French recipe book, I was feeling inspired to cook.

"There is nowhere here to put these things."

"Do you ever see us living in a place where we'd have room for your things and *mine*?"

I had begun to fantasize about finding a place of my own in Giverny – maybe a studio where I could spend my days writing. I imagined shelves full of books and a big desk by a window that looked out on a little patio with a café table and pots of David Austin roses. I envisioned Sarah and me sitting there, drinking tea from Limoges cups.

Four days before I was set to leave for California, Henri informed me that he wouldn't be able to come. His excuse was that the electric company needed to dig a trench along the driveway for a new cable to our apartment. We'd been having power outages because of old wiring that needed to be replaced.

I knew if Henri truly had wanted to make the trip, he would have postponed the installation, which he said was scheduled for early February – precisely when he had planned to travel. I seriously doubted the excavation work could even happen then, given the likelihood of bad weather.

"I'll need to cancel a party that friends of mine were planning in your honor," I said. "They've been looking forward to meeting you."

"*Chérie*, I don't want this to hurt our relationship."

I didn't want to argue. Part of me was relieved he wouldn't be there, offering his opinions about the storage purge.

"I'll wear my ball and chain until you return," he said, smiling.

"I'd suggest you go down to your workshop and cut that chain. I'm sorry you feel like a prisoner, Henri."

"I'm making a joke, my dear."

The next day, as I reached for a pan in the kitchen cupboard, I saw Pauline's three little jars of jam tucked away at the back of the shelf. I put them on the butcher-block counter as I considered my options, remembering my Florence chiropractor's suggestion to use them as bat bait. Pauline had gone to some trouble, that was clear. She had handwritten the labels and made fabric lid covers trimmed with ribbons. I wondered about the shelf life of homemade jam – this batch was probably a year old. Overcome by an urge to purge, I put the jars in a bag and paid a visit to the village recycling bin across the road. I felt a twinge of guilt as I dropped them, one by one, into the bin. But mostly, it was a moment of catharsis that I couldn't quite explain.

~~~

Henri drove me to the airport on the morning of my flight. We arrived early and had time for coffee, so he parked the car and came into the terminal with me.

We found a café near the check-in area. I grabbed a little table in the corner while Henri got our coffee and croissants.

I could see his sadness when he sat down next to me. I reached over and squeezed his hand.

"A month is a long time," he said.

"You could still come."

"I don't see how."

"Then look at the bright side. You'll have your old life back for a whole month."

"Is that what you think I want?"

"Sometimes, yes."

It was the first time I'd ever seen tears in his eyes. "I'll miss you," he said.

"I think we need some time apart, to miss each other. That might be a good thing."

When we said goodbye at security, I gave him a hug and kissed his cheek. "*Je t'aime,*" I whispered.

The Frenchman who doesn't like goodbyes said nothing in reply. My heart sank a little when he turned and walked away.

~~~

On the 11-hour flight to Los Angeles, I wrestled with a big decision: *Should I continue living in France?*

I hoped Henri and I could still find our way together despite our many missteps. But as I floated above the clouds that day, I let myself imagine a new life in Giverny, on my own. As a local author, I could do book talks on board the river cruise boats that docked in Vernon and were popular with American tourists. If Roz and I ever finished the recipe book, we could organize cooking classes. I'd need to buckle down and improve my French. I had become much too dependent on Henri as my interpreter. I'd have a lot to manage on my own, but I felt a surge of confidence. At a cruising altitude of 35,000 feet, all things seemed possible.

I wasn't ready to move back to the United States. I loved living in Europe, immersed in its Old World beauty and rich history. Becoming a resident of Giverny had been a dream come true for me. I didn't want to let that slip away.

More than anything, I wanted to make a home for myself. For the better part of a decade, during my vagabond years, I had lived in places furnished and decorated with other people's belongings. If I was going to spend the rest of my life in France, I wanted to have my things with me.

I didn't have much time to ponder this. According to French customs rules, I was allowed to ship personal belongings to France duty-free during the first year of my visa. My first year in France would end in June. Shipments from Los Angeles could take four to six weeks to reach the French port of Le Havre on the Normandy coast. If I missed the June cutoff, customs fees on future shipments would be prohibitive.

By the time I arrived in L.A., I was saying "yes" to France, "maybe" to Henri, and "oh my god" to the monumental task I was facing at the storage facility.

The storage purge took a full month. I had two large units. One contained antique furnishings, paintings, large boxes of quilts and linens, a desk, a few chairs, and an assortment of lamps and odds and ends. The second unit was packed tight with about 100 small boxes, most of which hadn't been opened in 10 years.

I decided to rent an additional smaller unit for a month to use as my sorting and staging area. I set up a long table and put my favorite desk chair into service. I needed to feel organized and comfortable in the face of chaos.

My son, Kyle, who lives in northern California, flew in to help and filled a U-Haul van with his belongings. We sorted the remaining boxes into Yes, No and Maybe stacks. We moved the Maybe boxes into the small unit so that I'd have room to assess what I wanted to keep.

I spent a few hours each day in the Maybe Room. I didn't make a marathon of it. I wanted to pace myself and try to enjoy the process – and amazingly, that's what happened, for the most part.

Forgotten treasures emerged. A blue velvet jewelry box containing my mother's dazzling collection of costume pieces caught my breath. As I opened the lid, I thought I smelled a whiff of her perfume and heard the rustle of an evening dress. When I was a little girl, I loved peeking inside the box, which my mother kept in the top drawer of her dresser. The necklaces, bracelets, earrings and brooches – studded with rhinestones and sapphire crystals – were the epitome of 1950s bling. But to me, at age 5, they were the jewels of a queen.

In a box of family papers, I found photos of my grandfather as a soldier in France during World War I, along with letters he wrote to his future bride, my grandmother. To my surprise, in a yellowed bundle of postcards he had sent to his mother in Tennessee, there was a map of the French town where he had been billeted.

When I found my Tiny Tears doll, dressed in a knitted outfit my grandmother had made for her, I nearly cried tears of my own. Her eyelids opened as I pulled her from the box. I asked her if she'd like to go to France and she said, *Oh yes, please take me with you.*

As I contemplated what I might send to Giverny, I had a nagging thought: WHAT IF the ship sank or the container slid off the deck? I had heard stories about accidents at sea. I started making a pile of what I would take on the plane in my checked luggage – and a tiny pile of what I would put in my carry-on.

My carry-on items came down to this: A rock my son painted for me as a Cub Scout. A little Lalique dish my favorite editor at *People* magazine – where I had worked in New York before marriage and motherhood – had given me as a wedding gift. A clay figure of a Scottish piper that I bought during my student days at the University of Edinburgh. A cobalt-blue vase that belonged to my mother's mother and a journal of her poems that she wrote out for me by hand. My grandfather's letters to her from France. A lovely paperweight that my father's mother kept on her desk. A small pewter oil lamp my father bought for me on a business trip to Antwerp, Belgium. A Christmas photo ornament of my son as a baby.

My most precious things were touchstones of people and places I've loved, and they all fit in a carry-on.

But then there were the big things that I didn't want to part with and didn't want to pay to store. It soon became apparent that I would be shipping more than a few boxes to France. A moving company agent came to give me an estimate: My YES pile would fill 80 percent of a 20-ft container.

When I shared that news via email with Henri, he sent a calculation that my boxes would fill his entire living-dining room to a height of one meter. A war of words started, punctuated with lots of question marks.

He claimed he had no room for the contents of a 20-ft container.

To which I replied: *Look at all you have and all the room you have to store engines, trucks and tractors – and you seem to be able to make room for more and more. When will it be possible for you to make room for me in your life?????? I'm really close to giving up hope.*

He bristled when I suggested that I find a studio space. *Would this mean the end of our life together???* he asked. *How can you imagine that? You absolutely have to tell me your intentions.*

I held firm: *If you want me in your life, you need to make a commitment to finding a home that's comfortable for us both.*

Henri said he wouldn't discuss our future together from a distance. *We arrive very quickly at regrettable remarks, which make me very sad.*

Only your happiness matters to me, even at the cost of a separation that I dread because I love you.

In the swirl of all this, Henri's world seemed to be flying apart: His brother Olivier had been diagnosed with a benign brain tumor that required immediate surgery. Henri's dog, Facel, had killed a neighbor's baby goat that had wandered onto the museum property. And then came the shocking news that Pauline had died. Henri said she had been feeling poorly one morning and was dead by that afternoon. With more than a twinge of guilt, I thought about the jam jars and couldn't unhear the sound of glass shattering as they hit the bottom of the bin.

After Pauline's funeral, Henri wrote to say that he was going to Ibiza for a few days and mentioned he would be staying in the house that we had rented (for which I had paid half). He also mentioned the electrical work had been postponed indefinitely because of bad weather. No surprise there.

~

My son returned to Pasadena for a second visit, this time with his new girlfriend, Julia. He was eager for me to meet her, but told me she was nervous about meeting me.

"She's read your books, Mom."

"That's sweet. But tell her not to be nervous."

"She's kind of shy."

I knew from his Facebook posts that she loved going to Disneyland. She made good use of an annual pass and had an assortment of Minnie Mouse ears to wear on her visits to the Magic Kingdom.

I went online and bought my own Minnie ears. When I picked Kyle and Julia up at Burbank airport, I put them on before I got out of the car.

Julia looked at me warily, as if she were thinking, *He didn't tell me she was crazy.*

I gave her a hug and told her how happy I was to meet her.

"I like your ears," she said.

I decided to play crazy and said, "What ears?"

We had a wonderful weekend together. I had a feeling she was The One.

I remembered one Halloween when Kyle was about six. A girl in the neighborhood, slightly older than Kyle, showed up at our door, in a black leather jacket, with spiked hair and black lipstick.

"Who are you supposed to be?" I asked her.

She seemed insulted that I had to ask. "I'm a biker chick. What does it look like?"

That made perfect sense. Her dad was a biker who added a bit of chrome and color to the neighborhood.

Kyle looked puzzled. "Mom, what's a biker chick?"

"Oh, I'll explain later, sweetie." Or maybe never, I thought.

Just then, the little girl who lived across the street bounded up the porch steps in a Minnie Mouse costume and restored my faith in childhood innocence.

Later that night, as I tucked in my sleeping son one last time, I gently kissed his cheek and whispered in his ear, "Biker chicks, no. Minnie Mouse, yes."

And so it happened that 24 years later, my wish was fulfilled. My dear boy had found his Minnie Mouse.

~༠

In mid-February, I signed a contract with a freight company to ship a 20-foot container to Giverny and was immediately buried in paperwork. I had to translate the inventory forms into French and answer a raft of Customs and insurance questions. I wrote to Henri and told him I needed to extend my stay by two weeks.

He had returned from Ibiza, where apparently he'd had a pleasant visit by the looks of several photos he had sent me. I hoped his time away had helped him decompress. He had kindly answered some of my translation questions and hadn't sent me more calculations about my pile of boxes.

I had no idea what would unfold when I got back to Giverny. But when I arrived at the Paris airport, I saw a glimmer of hope. Henri was waiting for me with a bouquet of roses.

When we got back to his place, it was about noon. I was ravenously hungry and made myself an omelet. I then fell into bed and a deep jet-lag induced sleep. I awoke at 6 that evening, with Henri standing over me. The room was dark, so I couldn't see his face.

"You are so lazy," he said. "Do you know what time it is?"

I felt like I was dreaming. My body ached from the fatigue of a travel day across nine time zones without sleep.

"You have no idea how tired I am," I said to him as I sat up slowly. "I feel like I could sleep for days."

The word "lazy" rang in my ears and I could feel a surge of anger welling up inside me.

Chapter 19

It was a horrible argument, one of the worst Henri and I had ever had.

I hadn't seen much of him the day after I returned to Giverny. Late in the afternoon, after I had gotten up from a nap, I found him in his workshop with one of the young mechanics on his team. It was a Saturday.

Wiping grease off his hands, Henri came out into the museum hall to greet me. He turned to the young man and said, "I'll see you at dinner."

"Dinner?" I asked Henri. "You've made plans for dinner?"

Henri shrugged. "Is there a problem?"

"Actually, yes. I've been away for six weeks, Henri. I thought we might spend an evening alone together."

I could see Henri's jaw harden. "I want to wash my hands. I'll come upstairs in a few minutes."

When Henri returned to the apartment a short while later, the anger between us exploded. Everything we had ever argued about seemed to be in the mix. But that night our future together was at stake.

He abandoned whatever dinner plans he had made. We raged at each other all evening. At the end of it, we were on opposite sides of the butcher's table in the kitchen, with Henri's welcome-home bouquet of roses in a vase between us.

"Are you finished?" he asked me.

"Are we finished?" I replied. "Can you see a way forward?"

"Finding a new place to live, with room for your things?"

"Yes. I don't think that's asking too much if you want a life together."

"I can't give you an answer now."

"Henri, I have a shipping container arriving here in six weeks. I need an answer."

"There's a lot to think about."

"If you don't want to do this, I'll find my own place."

"I will tell you tomorrow."

I could feel my legs wobble from exhaustion. "I need to sleep."

I went into in my bedroom and stood in the dark, slowly unbuttoning my shirt.

In a moment, I felt Henri's presence behind me. He slipped his hands around my waist, pressing himself against me.

Our anger quickly turned to passion. I'll never forget the heat between us that night that could either fuse us together or destroy us.

~

The next day passed without a word from Henri about the decision he promised to make. When he came to say good-night, I was sitting at the end of my bed.

I reached for his hand. "Come, sit with me."

I couldn't read his mood as he sat down. But then he squeezed my hand and said, "*Oui, chérie.*"

"*Oui?*"

"I want to find a place for us in Giverny. It won't be easy. But we'll try."

We decided to do a message blitz to everyone we knew in the village, telling them of our hope to find a small house to rent.

We were turning a page together – or so I thought. Our story suddenly took on wonderful new possibilities. I wanted to make a life with Henri. Our lovemaking that night felt like a celebration of what was meant to be.

Looking back on the weeks that followed, I now clearly see the beginnings of the rupture that happened.

A few days after I returned from California, I was in Henri's kitchen and tripped over the corner of the open dishwasher door. It caught the outer bone of my right ankle, and as I fell, the inside of my left ankle smashed into the other corner of the door. The pain left me breathless. By the next morning, both ankles were badly swollen. An ugly bruise had formed on the inside of the left ankle, which had taken a hard hit.

I made an appointment to see Jose, the therapist who ran the pain clinic. He was gentle during the examination and seemed to sense my apprehension.

"You mustn't worry, Rebecca. I won't do anything that hurts you."

He was concerned about the tissue damage to the left ankle and prescribed a course of treatment. During the exam, he asked about Henri and I told him about our plan to find a bigger place. He suggested I contact the real estate agency that handled housing rentals on the campus where the clinic was located.

The campus had been the location of a military rocket-manufacturing facility, built after World War II. The engineers who worked there – many of them German – lived in a housing development on site. The houses, mostly duplexes, were of various styles. Some were elegant-looking manor houses that must have been the homes of senior staff. Many were bungalow-style with Tudor touches. Over the years, the houses had been abandoned. The City of Vernon had made a deal with the French military to rehabilitate the property and turn it into a model for a technology park with residential, retail and recreation components.

That evening, I told Henri about Jose's suggestion. Henri knew the campus well. He contacted the real estate agency handling the housing rentals. The first hurdle was submitting the required paperwork to the agency, which then recommended applicants to a board of engineers who made the final decision.

We met with an agent who showed us two houses that were available, both of them one-story duplexes. They were freshly painted, but the landscaping needed attention. Several houses on the street had already been renovated and rented. But a number of them were in a ramshackle state, overgrown with vegetation.

I knew a drawback for Henri was that we wouldn't be in Giverny. The campus was only several miles away, but we wouldn't have village life at our doorstep.

Henri had put out the word to his Giverny friends about our search. But as he had predicted, there were no immediate prospects. The embroidery ladies had come up with a few leads – mostly in Vernon and beyond – but nothing in Giverny.

Henri submitted our application to the agency and within a few days we received word that it had been approved for the board to review. The next board meeting was the following week.

With Henri's credentials as an engineer and a museum owner, I felt we had an excellent chance. I emailed a message to close friends, with photos of the house we were hoping to rent, asking them to hold a good thought.

I was hobbling around on still-swollen ankles when one evening, during a visit at the moulin with Olivier and Maxine, I stumbled in their bathroom and fell onto the back of the toilet, cracking the water tank. Strangely, the toilet sat on a platform, which had caught the toe of my shoe. The bathroom was upstairs, above the dining room where dinner would be served, a bit later than expected because of the mopping up that followed my fall.

"I can't take you anywhere," Henri teased me when I came back downstairs. "Are you okay?"

A huge bruise was forming on my right forearm where I had landed on the toilet tank, but I said nothing about that. "I'm so embarrassed," I said. "And I haven't even had a drink yet."

Maxine poured me a glass. "In all the years we've owned this place, *that* has never happened."

The next day I went to see my chiropractor, Jean-Raymond. The fall had torqued my shoulder, which he gently manipulated back into place. When he saw the bruise on my forearm, he looked at me with concern. He also knew about my recent ankle injuries.

"Is everything okay with you and Henri?"

I laughed. "We're fine. I've just been clumsy lately."

"I sometimes see women who are beaten by their husbands. The women make up stories. But you have the best stories. Like falling into a toilet!"

I knew he believed me, yet I appreciated that he was concerned for my well-being.

The worst blow came about a week later. I was standing in the doorway of the downstairs kitchen, looking out at the view, when suddenly Bernadette screamed my name. I turned to see Facel running toward me, eager to make a mad dash out the door. He hadn't been allowed to run freely outdoors ever since he had killed the baby goat.

I foolishly planted myself in his path, squatting slightly to catch him between my legs and grab hold of his collar.

He didn't break his stride and slammed into my left leg, his shoulder bone against my shin bone.

I had successfully prevented his escape, but with considerable damage to my leg. The hematoma that formed on my shin was about eight inches long and several inches wide.

I was still getting treatments for my ankles from Jose, who was alarmed by Facel's aggressive behavior. Jean-Raymond was incensed. "That dog should be put away," he said. "He attacked you, a member of the family. You say me, I call the authorities."

The hematoma slowed the healing of my left ankle, where necrosis had set in. Jose worked his magic, using electric stimulation and massage to help relieve the inflammation.

Jose usually ended our sessions with a relaxing massage of my scalp, neck and shoulders. We had wonderful conversations during those massages. He told me about the advanced degree he was getting that took him to various conferences throughout Europe. I learned a lot about Jose's specialty – lymphatic drainage – during those massages. He knew I was a writer and wanted to know more about my books. I gave him copies of my Giverny novels, which I inscribed, and he proudly displayed them on the bookcase in his office.

I regaled with him with stories of the recipe book project. When I told him I'm not a cook, he couldn't stop laughing.

"Should you put a warning in the book about that?" he asked.

"I'll write the number for poison control in your copy, okay?"

He liked that idea.

On the morning of the board meeting, Henri received a call that our application had been approved.

I was ecstatic. "Henri, isn't this wonderful?"

"I will celebrate when everything is final."

I sent out another email blast, telling friends our good news.

The lease signing was set for the following week. We asked for another walk-through, but the agency said we could do that on the day of the signing.

A couple of nights before the signing, Henri and I had dinner at the boulangerie with Bernadette and our friend Martin, who was visiting for a few days. Henri hadn't told anyone about the house and I wondered if he was afraid Bernadette might react badly. During our meal that evening, I loved that I was holding a wonderful secret.

The next morning, I was up early to get ready for an all-day work-shop with some of the embroidery ladies where we'd be learning how to make lampshades. I was going through my checklist of supplies when Henri came into the bedroom and sat down next to my desk.

"I need to talk to you," he said.

"What is it, love?"

What I remember most about that moment, oddly enough, was the tightness of his T-shirt. It hugged his chest, making his shoulders look more muscular.

"I can't do this," he said.

"Do what?"

"I can't sign the lease."

For a minute, I couldn't comprehend what he was saying. "Why not?"

"I want to stay here. This is my home."

"Henri, we made this decision more than three weeks ago."

"I'm sorry. I should have told you sooner."

"Sooner? When did you start having doubts?"

"From the beginning."

"So you've been leading me along all this time?" I looked at the calendar on my desk. "The container is due to arrive in a few weeks, Henri. What then?"

"We will go to the signing tomorrow as we planned. I will co-sign the lease."

"But I'll be living there alone?"

Henri couldn't look at me. "*Oui.*"

I stared out the window at a view I had come to love. My flower-bed was coming into bloom. The cherry tree beyond the corral had started to bud. It was a time for new beginnings.

My heart hurt. Henri's chair scraped the floor. He left the room without another word.

The rest of that day was a blur. I sent a message to Sarah, telling her I wasn't feeling well and wouldn't be at the lampshade class.

I called Jose, asking if he might have an opening that afternoon. He said he could see me at two.

I'll never forget his kindness to me that day. As I told him what had happened with Henri, I sensed his anger. I could barely breathe as I lay down on the table. And then came a torrent of tears.

Jose placed his hands on my forehead and gently massaged my temples. "Rebecca, you can always count on me to be your friend," he said.

When I returned to the apartment later that afternoon, Henri was there, emptying the shelves of an antique bookcase that had belonged to American Impressionist artist Theodore Butler, who had married into the Monet family. The bookcase was Henri's most prized possession. It had been among Butler's possessions that had been given to Henri's family by Butler's son Jimmy, who had lived in Giverny for many years and had been Henri's idol as a boy.

"There, it's yours." Henri exclaimed, pushing a stack of old magazines against the wall.

"What?"

"The bookcase is yours."

"Is this a guilt gift?"

"I want you to have it," he said angrily.

"You love that bookcase. I'm not taking it." Theodore Butler had displayed an exquisite butterfly collection in that bookcase. Henri remembered seeing the collection as a child.

I hardly recognized Henri. He seemed to be coming unhinged. "Why are you doing this? Why are you doing *any* of this?" I didn't think I could possibly have more tears, but I started to cry.

I choked back a sob. "What happened to the man I fell in love with? Where did he go?"

Torn between remorse and fury, Henri shouted, "He's right here!"

Sarah called that evening. When I told her what had happened, she was stunned.

"Would you like to come spend the night at my place?" she asked.

"I'll be all right," I assured her.

"Are you going to the lease signing tomorrow?"

"Henri insists that we should meet the agent."

"Why? Surely you won't want to live there on your own."

"I keep hoping he'll change his mind. I don't know what has pushed him to the brink. I just want this to be a bad dream."

~

Henri and I took separate cars to the house the next afternoon. He wanted to get there early to walk around the property before the agent arrived.

Strangely, he was behaving like a good husband, taking charge of the details. When I arrived, he was in the living room with the agent. The house was unfurnished, so he had brought a camping table and two chairs. The agent pulled a grungy lawn chair from a utility closet. And so began what to me was an absurd charade.

Henri had asked the agent, Madame Lambert, to provide a copy of the lease in advance. But that hadn't happened, so the process was slow as Henri translated each section for me. Madame Lambert seemed annoyed by this. I think she thought we'd get through this in 20 minutes.

Henri insisted on a walk-through and dutifully made what became a long punch list. The frame of the back door was rotted and needed to be replaced. The stove's gas fitting crumbled in Henri's hand when he knelt down to inspect it. There were broken drain pipes, and Henri discovered a gaping hole in the garage roof where a tree had fallen. When I saw on a lease attachment that the energy rating for the house was an "F," I asked why. The agent shrugged. She said the windows were new. I wondered if there might be an insulation problem in the attic and asked for an inspection. Madame Lambert looked at me as if to say, *Who are you to insist on that?*

I stood in the kitchen, which had only a utility sink. As is often the case in France, installing a kitchen is the tenant's responsibility. The cost of cabinets and appliances would be several thousand euros. I mentioned this to Henri and he said, "I'm not worried about the money." I wanted to shout at him: THAT'S BECAUSE YOU'RE NOT PAYING FOR THIS!

As Henri and Madame Lambert worked on the punch list, I wandered into the backyard. I looked at the view I would see from my writing desk. There were tall trees at the back of the property where an abandoned house was barely visible through overgrown shrubs and a tangle of vines. The houses on either side of the property had been renovated, but were vacant. I imagined myself coming home to this place after dark. There was no way in hell I was going to sign the lease, but I felt panicky that I had no Plan B.

Henri opened the living room window and beckoned for me to come inside. "We're ready for you to sign."

I shook my head in disbelief. "No, no. You need to come here."

As I watched him walk toward me, I wondered what alternate reality he was in.

"What's wrong, *chérie*?"

"Everything is wrong, Henri. I'm alone in this now and I don't see it the same way anymore."

"Do you want to back out?" he asked. "I won't pressure you to sign."

"I don't need your permission to back out of this, Henri."

"What do I tell the agent?"

"That this has been a huge waste of her time. What about that?"

~⁀

I left Henri to wrap things up with Madame Lambert and drove back to the apartment.

A short while later, I was in the kitchen, on the phone with Sarah, when Henri's car pulled into the driveway.

"What are you going to do?" she asked me.

"I have no idea."

Sarah had been in a long relationship with a Frenchman who owned a number of rental properties in the area around Vernon.

"I'll talk to Maurice. He knows every real estate agent in the area. He might be able to help you find a place."

"Thanks, Sarah. I really appreciate that. Henri is back. I have to go."

"Do you think he'll be angry? I'm worried about you."

"I don't know what's going to happen. Everything is such a mess. I'll call you later."

When Henri walked into the kitchen, I could see he was spent. He opened a bottle of wine. "We both need this," he said. "Let's sit down."

It was a long, mostly calm conversation. Henri apologized for not telling me sooner and confessed that, when he had said yes to us finding a place together, he knew in the end he'd say no.

"Every day for the past few weeks, I've been telling myself, *I need to tell her.*"

"You let the clock run down, knowing the container was coming. What am I supposed to do now?"

"You can stay here as long as you need to. There's no rush for you to leave. We'll find room for the boxes."

I leaned back into the sofa and closed my eyes. "How did you leave things with Madame Lambert?"

"She said she'd get back to me early next week about what needs to be fixed."

"It doesn't matter. I don't want to live there on my own."

"I understand."

We sat in silence for a bit. And then he said, "*Chérie*, I still love you."

I opened my eyes, which were burning with tears. "Henri, I have no feelings of love for you. Not anymore. How can I ever trust you again?"

He looked crushed, but stoically said, "Thank you for being honest with me."

"I'm not saying these things to be unkind. But I don't see a way back from this."

"Can we still be friends?" Henri asked.

"I don't know how to answer that. It's hard for me to even look at you right now."

We talked about how we'd handle our living arrangements while I looked for a place.

Ever practical, he wanted to know if we could have occasional dinners together at the apartment. I said that would be okay. He asked if I'd still like to be in contact with his friends. Yes, of course, I said. But I told him he didn't need to include me in family gatherings.

We agreed that we should be free to plan our days independently. We didn't need to check in with each other.

Our official story going forward was that we had decided to live apart. No other details. At first, Henri said he'd tell his friends, *Rebecca wants her liberty.* I quickly nixed that, trying not to lose my temper. Even in his explanation of what had happened, he couldn't shoulder the blame. Instead, he wanted to tell people I broke up with him because I wanted my freedom – and of course their response would be AFTER ALL YOU'VE DONE FOR HER!

The conversation ended with our plans for that evening. He said he was thinking about going to the Baudy for dinner and asked if I'd like to join him. I asked if Bernadette would be coming with us.

"No, I will go alone – or with you."

So in a bizarre twist, Henri and I had dinner together at the Baudy. It was the opening night of the season. We had our usual table by the bar. A constant stream of locals came by to greet us with handshakes and kisses. All seemed pretty normal.

Henri and I walked back home together under the amber glow of the street lamps. Facel trotted along beside us. Henri didn't take my hand, as was his way.

A divide between us was forming. I knew these next weeks would be difficult as we tried to find our new normal.

Back home, we followed our usual bedtime routine: We met in the kitchen in our pajamas – Henri in his red Father Christmas bathrobe – and had a cup of tea.

Our first awkward moment came when it was time to say good-night.

"*Bonne nuit, chérie,*" Henri said, as he impulsively reached out to hug me. He held back for an instant.

I stepped forward and embraced him.
As he held me close, he started to cry.

Chapter 20

The debacle with Henri wasn't the only drama in my life.

While I was in California, Roz had been emailing me with new ideas for the recipe book. She wanted to include another restaurant, owned by friends of hers, and add two more recipes, which she assured me would be translated and ready for me when I returned to Giverny.

A few days after I got back, she asked me to join her for lunch at the home of her friend Odette whose daughter Monique managed a café and gift boutique next to Monet's gardens. We hadn't considered including the café in the book because it offered mediocre buffet-style food. But during the off-season, Monique had hired a new chef, who had worked at the Baudy and was known for his inventive recipes. Roz was enthusiastic about his Salade de Fleurs made of edible blossoms – pansies, rose petals, nasturtiums and primroses – and thought it would be a perfect addition to our "garden" of recipes.

On the day of the luncheon, Roz looked lovely as she entered Odette's kitchen, wrapped in an ivory cashmere pashmina and carrying a bouquet of sunflowers. I hadn't actually seen Roz in a few months. She had spent the holidays in northern California with her family and returned to Giverny in mid-January, a few days after I left for L.A. She seemed to be in good spirits and was happy to see me.

"Oh, Rebecca, I can't wait to get started on our next book. I have some wonderful ideas."

Our *next* book. We were at least a month behind schedule with this one.

Before we sat down for lunch, she asked me to photograph Odette's garlic fried tomatoes, which was the other new dish Roz wanted to include in the book.

The meal was delicious. I felt relaxed and happy to be back in France. I mentioned to Roz that Henri and I were looking for a place. Roz was interested in hearing all the details.

"I've made a move as well," she said. "I'm back where I was last summer. In the house Monet owned, by the church."

"Was there a problem with Denis' place?"

Roz rolled her eyes. "Come by tomorrow. We have lots to catch up on. Bring your camera. I'll make the Monet fish dish for lunch."

The next day, I saw a night-and-day difference in Roz. She looked like she hadn't slept. Her hair was uncombed. She seemed to be coming down with a cold. Used tissues were strewn wherever she had dropped them, on the sofa and the floor.

There was a precarious pile of moving boxes by the front door. I noticed the box from the Monet gift shop in the stack.

"Shall I help you unpack the dishes?" I asked. "The fish should be plated on his china, don't you think?"

Roz shook her head. "We're not using the dishes. We need to return them."

"Why?"

"I don't want to talk about it. I'm so angry about that."

I didn't press her for an explanation, but I wondered if someone back home was keeping track of her spending.

"There's another matter I want to discuss with you," she said. "Please sit down." She cleared a spot for me at a small round dining table and sat opposite me. "Do you remember the day we went to Monique's café for lunch last fall?"

I nodded. "It wasn't much of a lunch. The food was awful."

"I agree with you there," she said. "Afterward, we had dessert at the pastry bar in the boutique, remember?"

"Yes, we ordered the carrot cake."

"*You* ordered the carrot cake," she said. "I paid for that and you never reimbursed me."

"I'm sorry. How much was it?"

"Three euros and fifty cents."

I suddenly realized all was not right with Roz.

"I've been upset about this," she continued. "I would like you to transfer three euros and fifty cents to my bank account."

She seemed to have no awareness of how bizarre her request was.

"That won't be necessary." I reached for my handbag and took €3.50 out of my wallet.

The woman who had boasted to me about her affluence gratefully accepted the money, which was roughly the equivalent of four U.S. dollars.

"Thank you, Rebecca. This has been bothering me for a long time."

"Do I have any other outstanding debts?" I meant to say that lightly, but I heard the edge in my voice.

I could tell something else was on her mind. "We need to draw up a contract," she said. "I'd like you to email me a list of the points you think it should cover."

"I'd be happy to. I've had a lot of experience with writers' contracts."

"Good. I'll send your list to my attorney in California."

"We're hiring an attorney?"

"I'll pay for that. He's our family attorney."

I wondered if there was going to be a problem. At the beginning of our collaboration, Roz and I had agreed to share credit and split profits and expenses. But we hadn't put anything in writing.

She quickly changed the subject and asked about Henri. "So you're looking for a place together? What brought this about?"

I laughed. "A very large shipping container that's on its way from California."

Her eyes widened. "You've decided to make a home here! How wonderful for you both. I think it will be good for you to have a little distance from his family."

"What about you?" I asked. "What are your plans?"

"My family wants me back in California," she said ruefully. "But I'm hoping I can spend at least half the year here. I have so many ideas I want to talk to you about. I've discovered some wonderful restaurants not too far from here that I want to include in our next book."

I smiled at her. "We still have a lot of work to do on this one."

We made a checklist of what still needed to be done. None of the items she had promised to work on while I was away were ready.

"I need everything in hand by the end of this week so that I can give the printer the final page count," I told her. "We can't delay."

"You'll have everything by the end of the week – and for lunch today, you'll have Monet's Fish Créole. You can check *that* off the list!"

The fish creole was a success. Roz garnished the *cabillaud* with cucumber and olives and served it with Sauce Nantua, a tomato-based fish sauce flavored with white wine and cognac.

The dinner plate she chose had an antique look, with a pale blue rim edged with silver. (I tried not to think about the Monet china by the front door, still sealed in the box.) In a stroke of *bonne chance*, I found a beautiful painter's palette tucked beside an old desk in the living room. Soft light streaming through a window facing the back garden lit the room as we placed the plate of *cabillaud* on the palette. And for a few moments, as my camera and I paid homage to the table of Monet in a house that had once been his, I felt like I was traveling back in time and sensed his presence.

~⁓

I spent the rest of the week working on the book's layout, which included the new section for Monique's café. She had helped me translate the recipes and her chef posed for a photo with his gorgeous Salade de Fleurs.

Roz signed off on the new recipes. But by the end of the week, she hadn't finished the work she had promised. I made the decision to delete the outstanding pages, which included the section she never wrote about the art of making a French baguette. I created the index and locked in the book's final layout so that I could get a price quote from the printer.

I showed Roz the book's digital files on my laptop. She loved the photos and liked the overall look of the book. I knew she wasn't happy about the deleted pages, but I could tell something else was bothering her.

"Did you receive the email I sent you about the contract terms?" I asked her.

She stiffened. "Yes, I sent it to my attorney."

"We need to have our agreement in place before we take book orders from the restaurants," I said. "How soon do you think your attorney will have something for us to sign?"

"I'll let you know, Rebecca."

A week went by. Two proof copies of the book arrived, but I decided not to give one to Roz until we had both signed the contract.

Several days later, she called to say she'd like to meet. I presumed she had a contract for me to review, so I asked her to email it to me.

"It would be best if we did this in person. Come by tomorrow morning at 10. It won't take long." She casually added, "There will be some people here."

I will forever remember that meeting as The Attempted Ambush.

It was a cold, rainy morning. Roz was waiting for me at the front door and was bundled in a heavy sweater. The house was freezing.

"Is the heat not working?" I asked her as I peeled off my rain jacket.

She seemed distracted and kept looking out the door.

"Have you called someone to look at the boiler?"

The bell rang at the front gate.

"Oh good, they're here," Roz said.

Two women hurried across the courtyard under their umbrellas. I couldn't see their faces until they were at the door. One of them was Odette and the other was an elegantly dressed older woman with a chicly chiseled haircut. I knew instantly she was a friend Roz had told me about who had been a Chanel model in her youth. I didn't catch her name as she entered the room.

Odette and Chanel (as I've come to call her) complained about the bitter chill in the room and declined Roz's offer to take their coats.

"How long have you been without heat, Roz?" asked Chanel, who spoke excellent English. I would later learn she had been married to an American.

"There seems to be a problem with the boiler." Roz said. "I'm sorry. Please make yourselves as comfortable as you can. This won't take long."

Odette, who spoke no English, took a seat in the corner. Chanel sat next to me. Roz took a clipboard with pages of notes from the dining table and sat directly opposite me.

She opened the meeting by saying she had collapsed from shock when she read my suggestions for our contract.

"Why?" I asked. "Those are standard terms for a collaboration agreement. What do you object to?"

"I don't want to discuss it. My attorney will handle this."

Exasperated, I said, "Roz, we have to settle this soon. We've received a price quote from the printer that's going to expire in two weeks. We can't move ahead until you and I have a contract."

Roz seemed flustered and began recounting the story of the carrot cake. But in this version, there was a new twist. She looked at Chanel and said, "Rebecca took all the icing and left none for me."

Roz picked up two iPhones sitting on the table next to her. One was her U.S. phone and the other her French phone. "Imagine this is the cake," she said, holding out one of the phones. And then gesturing with the other phone, she said, "This is the icing." She put them together and then pulled them apart. "This is important to me as a cook. The icing should stay on the cake."

I was dumbfounded. "Roz, you tasted the icing. In fact, you commented that you liked the texture of it."

I turned to Chanel. "This is something new," I said. "Last time we spoke about this, she claimed I hadn't reimbursed her for the cake and asked me to transfer €3.50 to her bank account."

Roz looked puzzled. "I didn't pay for the cake."

"Seriously?" I couldn't help but laugh. "The next time you see Monique, please give her the €3.50 I gave you. We'll also owe her for the coffee and tea we apparently didn't pay for."

"Are you hard up for money, Roz?" Chanel asked.

"No." Roz was visibly shaken.

"I think you might be getting paranoid, living alone and dealing with health problems," Chanel said.

I was stunned by Chanel's candor, but grateful to be out of the crosshairs.

"Roz, this isn't about the carrot cake," I said firmly. "Do you want me to speak with your attorney about the contract?"

She scrolled through her U.S. phone and gave me his contact information.

I wrote him a lengthy email, explaining what had transpired with the book. I also shared my concerns about Roz's health and state of mind. I told him about the night she had asked me to sign the directive that would have given me the authority to withhold life support if she had been admitted to the hospital.

A reply came from her son, who thanked me for my "boots-on-the-ground" assessment of his mother's situation. In a way, I hated that I had pulled the alarm, knowing it would probably mean the end of the life she had dreamed of in Giverny. But I felt relieved that her family could now step in and help her.

Her son told me on a Skype call, "I love my mother and I want her to be around for a long time. My family really appreciates all you've done for her and all the work you've put in on the book."

Roz's son offered me all rights to the book as a gift. At first, I insisted that Roz and I share credit – the book had been her idea, after all. But that arrangement presented legal complications because, under the terms of the "gift," Roz wouldn't share the expense and responsibilities of producing and promoting the book. After several rounds of contract revisions, she asked that her name be removed from the book and gave all rights to me.

I sadly agreed to that. In the span of an afternoon, I took her name off the cover and removed all photos of her in the book. I rewrote the intro, explaining that although I'm not a cook, I wanted to share with readers the experience I'd had in Giverny of gathering round a table, in the company of friends and visitors, enjoying the dishes created by Giverny's accomplished chefs. I thanked the chefs for their patience and good humor as we translated their recipes into English. When we'd get stuck on a word, improvisation was key. With one recipe, BRING TO A BOIL became BRING TO A BLUB-BLUB-BLUB. More than anything, I wanted the book to be a souvenir of wonderful memories for those who had experienced Giverny – or a reason to visit for those who hadn't yet ventured here.

When I sent the final proof to the printer, I felt relieved of a huge burden. I was proud of the work Roz and I had done, but the stress had been enormous.

It was mid-April, six weeks after my return from California. At that point, I was dealing with the imminent arrival of a shipping container, a search for a new place to live, a failed romance, and the launch of a recipe book.

So much for the blissful life I had imagined in lovely Giverny.

Chapter 21

One morning, I woke up sobbing from a nightmare that told the story of my growing distress. In my dream, I was trapped in a dark stairwell, clinging to a wobbly hand railing. I had dropped a laundry basket full of dirty clothes, which were tangled around my painfully swollen feet as I stumbled down the steps. I felt panicky. There was an urgency to this dream, which became clear as I woke up: I desperately needed to pee.

I had spent the previous few days looking at rental properties. Steep stairs, basement laundry rooms, and toilets that were nowhere near the bedrooms clearly had added to my anxiety.

I knew I wouldn't get back to sleep, so I got up and went into the kitchen to make coffee. I looked out the window at the first hint of sunlight on the hillside beyond the corral. To my surprise, standing on a mound of dirt in the middle of the corral was Dou-Dou, the ram. He looked a bit like Mufasa, the Lion King, striking a regal pose as he gazed at his world. I wondered what he was thinking about at the crack of dawn. Was he planning his day? Contemplating his breakfast options?

A thought occurred to me as I poured coffee that morning, wiping away my tears. I needed to start writing again – and more than anything, I needed to laugh again.

So with my coffee mug in hand, I sat down in the early hours that morning and set up a public Facebook page called "A Day with Doo-Doo: the life of a ram in Giverny, France." I changed the spelling of his name so that American readers would pronounce it correctly.

My introduction to the Doo-Doo page:

My name is Rebecca Bricker and I've been asked by Doo-Doo to chronicle his daily life and musings as he surveys his world from his hillock in Giverny, France. Our hope is to amuse and entertain you and give you a ram's-eye glimpse of the pastoral life of Giverny. Literally.

Doo-Doo got 50 likes on the first day. Not bad for a ram.

~⌐

Sarah had taken me to meet her former boyfriend, Maurice. He was a lawyer and a real estate investor – in his late fifties, several years younger than Sarah. He lived in the village of St. Marcel, not far from Vernon, in a beautifully restored moulin, which had been Sarah's home for several years until they split up a few months before I met her. She had moved to an apartment in Vernon, but kept in touch with Maurice, who very much wanted her back with him at the moulin.

I wasn't sure how much Sarah had told Maurice about my situation. It was difficult for me to tell the story of what had happened with Henri, especially to a stranger. But I could see the pain and empathy in Maurice's eyes when I said, "The day before the lease signing, he backed out."

Maurice kindly offered to help me find a place, but told me I'd have a difficult time – as a woman from a foreign country – getting an apartment lease without a co-signer. He already had called every local real estate agency on my behalf without luck. The only way I'd find a place, he said, was to have a friend recommend me to a landlord.

He arranged for me to see a three-story townhouse owned by a friend from his school days. She and her husband already had a few possible tenants, but Maurice's referral had put me at the top of their list.

The townhouse was high on a hill above St. Marcel, with a sweeping view of the Seine valley. Although there were other houses on the street, the location felt remote – a world away from the life I had known in Giverny. I felt so alone, a foreign woman whose unlucky love affair had turned her life upside down.

Like many rental properties in France, the townhouse had only a sink in the kitchen. I would need to install cabinets and appliances – a big expense that made it easier for me to say no.

When I called Sarah to tell her my decision, she understood. I thanked her and Maurice for their kindness. I was putting on a brave face, but I didn't have a clue how I was going to find a way out of the mess I was in.

The next day, I received an email from the shipping company, telling me the container had arrived in Le Havre and was going through Customs clearance. I needed to submit more paperwork. If all went well, the container would be delivered to Giverny in a few days.

When I shared that news with Henri, he asked where we were going to put everything.

"What doesn't fit in the storeroom, can go in the living room," I said. "You've already done the calculation."

I think, at first, he thought I was joking. I asked him to help me take the leaves out of the dining table. We cleared a big space for the boxes in what had been the dining area and made a cozy living space at the far end of the room. I situated the downsized table next to the TV cabinet and pulled the coffee table closer to the sofa and Henri's overstuffed chair. There was barely room for Facel to curl up on the rug. I watched him circle a few times before he found his landing spot. I could see his concern as he looked up at me with his big brown eyes.

I leaned over and scratched his head. "This won't be forever."

Henri's calculation about my boxes wasn't far off the mark. They filled half the living room to a height of two meters. I made an artful arrangement of the stacks, where I positioned some of my photographs of Monet's gardens.

"I'd like to have an exhibition of my photography at some point," I said to Henri. "This will be the preview showing."

I must admit he was extremely good-natured about everything. And I also must admit I took quiet pleasure in upending his well-ordered life.

Bernadette popped by a few days after the container delivery and looked aghast at the state of things, which couldn't have delighted me more.

It became my habit to write a post for Doo-Doo's Facebook page early every morning. I liked the quiet state of the world outside my bedroom window at that hour. I had a good view of the corral from my writing desk and loved watching the daily drama unfold there.

Doo-Doo was always up before me, standing on his hillock to greet the day. Strangely, he faced west instead of east. Henri's explanation for this: "He likes the sun on his ass."

I became intrigued with Doo-Doo's often antagonistic relationship with Praline, who usually didn't put up with his bad behavior. She'd butt heads with him when he'd chase her off the hillock or try to steal flowers Henri had brought for her to nibble on. There was no end to Doo-Doo's obnoxiousness. He had a pervy habit of sniffing under her tail. I was shocked one day when I watched him mount her. There rarely were moments of affection between them.

Henri said she had suffered far worse from Chocolat, the male goat who had shared the corral with her before Doo-Doo came along. Chocolat had battered and bloodied her so badly one awful day that Praline needed a vet to stitch her forehead back together. Chocolat had broken one of her horns off at the top of her skull.

Doo-Doo was a cute, cuddly baby ram when he came to live with Praline after Chocolat died. Henri told me how Praline had mothered baby Doo-Doo, who was very docile when he first arrived. But as he grew bigger, his testosterone kicked in. Henri was concerned that Doo-Doo, like Chocolat, was starting to abuse her.

One day, after the two of them had been butting heads, Henri removed the plank to the deck of the shed so that Praline would have a safe haven. Doo-Doo had a coordination problem and couldn't climb the steps to the deck. Without the plank in place, he had to sleep in the rough, under the shed in the hay.

When I asked Henri if he planned to put back the plank, he vowed, *"Jamais!"* Never.

It was definitely a #metoo victory for Praline.

Henri himself became a character in the Doo-Doo tales, which I often read aloud to him. His name was the Lord of the Manor – or LOTM, for short. Occasionally, I made a cameo appearance as FLOTM – Fair Lady of the Manor.

~~~

Henri and I had settled into a routine as housemates during this period of limbo, as I looked for a place to live. He didn't fuss about the boxes piled up in the living room. He assured me there was no rush for me to leave.

One Sunday afternoon in late April, he came upstairs after the usual family lunch – I had stopped attending those lunches – with good news.

His elderly cousins, who owned several rental properties in Giverny, had a vacancy – a small house that was a half mile away, near the entrance to Monet's gardens.

"They'd be happy for you to see it, if you're interested," he said.

The house had been a farm grain shed in the 1880s, when Monet himself had first come to Giverny. It sat across the road from an expansive meadow called La Prairie.

It would need renovations – a new kitchen and bathroom – so I wouldn't be able to move in for another six weeks or so, Henri explained. I knew he was in no hurry for me to go.

I couldn't believe this sudden good fortune. "When can we see it?"

Henri smiled. I could see his relief. He knew he had barely a slim chance of redeeming himself for what he had done, but this new prospect gave him a glimmer of hope.

A few days later, we went to see the house. It truly was a shed – the width of the house was two-and-a-half arm spans. The upstairs had been the hay loft where there were now two small bedrooms.

We stood at one of the bedroom windows, looking out at the prairie. It was early evening, that golden hour in Giverny when the landscape takes on an ethereal glow. Our view was laced with the graceful boughs of a blooming redbud tree that shaded the front terrace.

Henri told me the story of the extensive reclamation project that had brought the prairie back from neglect. He had been part of the team of conservationists who cleared the land, which is now owned by the Monet Foundation.

We were quiet for a moment, taking in the view.

He took my hand in his. "Maybe I helped clear the prairie because I knew you would be coming someday."

"Will there be a happy ending in all this?" I asked.

"I hope so."

When we returned to his apartment a little while later, Doo-Doo was on his hillock, wailing in despair. Henri checked the corral and looked under the shed to be sure nothing was amiss. In our excitement about the house, we didn't give his cries much thought until later, when we turned on the TV.

Notre Dame was burning.

Had Doo-Doo sensed there was something terribly wrong in the universe, I wondered.

The next morning, Doo-Doo was up before daybreak, lying on his hillock in the rain. He didn't stand to greet the day. He seemed to have a heavy heart, like so many in the world that day, when mournful tears fell as drops of rain.

Chapter 22

Henri and I slowly found our way back to each other during those early days of spring.

One day, he came home from his morning walk in the woods with a bouquet of beautiful wildflowers for me. When he handed me the bouquet, I saw a flutter of gold as a gorgeous butterfly found her wings. Henri wondered, in amazement, if she had just emerged from her chrysalis. I wondered, in amazement, if she had held on tight to that flower stem all the way home, knowing she couldn't let go until he handed me the bouquet.

She flew around us and landed on the kitchen window with her colorful wings outstretched on the glass, allowing the sunlight to shine through them.

"It's as if she knew," I said. "Her timing was perfect."

"I carried those flowers for an hour."

"But she hung on, waiting for her moment."

Henri slowly cranked open the window to set her free. I had a lump in my throat as we watched her fly away.

He turned to me and whispered, "I love you."

As tears streamed down my face, he kissed me – our first kiss in a very long time.

One evening in May, we gathered with friends and family for a picnic dinner on the banks of the Seine.

We set up a long table and built a fire on a swath of sandy shore called The Beach – an historic spot in Giverny, next to the inlet where Monet docked his painting boat. Tall willow trees hug the shoreline there. On that evening, the willows "wept," their sap droplets making rings in the water. But they seemed more like tears of joy. It was one of those May days – when the bright green of spring almost hurts your eyes – that make you so happy the grey days of winter are finally over.

What I loved most about that evening was the feeling that we were time travellers in a way. We could have been in a painting from Giverny's art-colony days at the turn of the last century. *Dîner sur la Seine* would be the title. Monet would have captured the scene beautifully from his painting boat. We certainly would have invited him to share our feast. I think he would have liked my guacamole, which was a big hit that evening.

It was all so idyllic. We waved at the barges and river cruise boats passing by. The dogs in our entourage splashed around in the shallows. As the sun sank behind the hills, more logs went on the fire. More wine was uncorked. No one was in a hurry to leave. We had waited all winter for that evening.

~⁹

To celebrate my birthday at the end of May, Henri and I took a trip to Müssy-sur-Seine, a charming medieval village 130 miles southeast of Paris, where my grandfather had been based after the end of World War I.

Müssy is in the Champagne region and is surrounded by vineyards and farmland. As we drove through the beautiful countryside, I read to Henri some of my grandfather's letters to his future wife, my grandmother.

They had known each other for only a month before he was inducted into the Army in 1917. They met in a small town in western Pennsylvania, where my grandmother lived. She was just 17. My grandfather, then 22, was a dashingly handsome country boy from Tennessee who had come to work in a local steel mill. Their love affair blossomed as pen pals during wartime. They were devoted correspondents who endured a two-year separation made bearable by endearments on a page. In one of her letters, she sweetly wrote: *"I surely was glad to hear that my long letter made you love me a bushel more."*

When my grandfather arrived in France in August 1918, he was careful not to disclose details of his movements, knowing U.S. Army censors were reading over his shoulder. But after the Armistice, he told my grandmother the harrowing story of the final days of the war. He had been on the Western Front, in Verdun, where hundreds of thousands of French and German soldiers had died in some of the fiercest battles of the war.

"The first night I was up there," he wrote, *"the shells were bursting all around me and it was so dark I could not see three feet before my eyes. I began to wander in my mind what I had done to cause all this to come upon me."*

After the Armistice was signed on November 11, 1918, his division hiked 125 miles, for 14 days, from Verdun to Müssy.

He wrote how he envied her Thanksgiving dinner. His Thanksgiving ration was *"1 piece of bread, 1/4 can of pork & beans, 1 drink of water."*

I had brought with me the postcards of Müssy he had sent to his mother, who lived in a remote hollow in Tennessee's Smoky Mountains called Baker's Gap. I tried to imagine the odyssey of those postcards, through war-torn France and then by ship to America. The last leg – up Mudslick Mountain – was by no means the easiest part of their journey.

One of the postcards showed the main street of the village. I stood exactly where the photograph had been taken, on a little bridge that crossed the Seine, which was more of a stream than a river at that point as it meandered to its source. Except for a car parked on the street, the scene looked remarkably the same.

I laughed when I read my grandfather's description of Müssy in a letter to my grandmother: *"You wanted to know how every little thing in France was. It is just about like it was a hundred years ago. If there has been any changes made I haven't noticed them."*

Even in 1918, Müssy seemed to have been frozen in time.

The village had been a rest station for American troops during and after the war. My grandfather appreciated Müssy's hospitality: *"This is a very nice little town. We have the Y.M.C.A, the Knights of Columbus and the Red Cross to furnish entertainment for us. We have movies at the "Y" most every night. A couple of nights ago we had a concert given by some French musicians from Paris. It sure was fine."*

The Müssy public library had a collection of photos from that era of some of the American soldiers who had stayed there. I showed the librarian the postcards, which had been mailed from Müssy in December 1918, and she happily made copies of them to add to the archives.

Before Henri and I left the village that day, we visited the War Memorial. I could feel my grandfather smiling down on me.

He had brought home a silk handkerchief from France as a gift for my grandmother, embroidered with the year "1918" next to a delicately stitched bouquet of flowers encircling the French flag. Over the years, many of the young women in our family have carried the handkerchief on their wedding day in honor of a love born during that war. My grandparents were married for 54 years.

Henri and I celebrated my birthday at a lovely restaurant recommended by the owners of the property where we were staying. The meal was superb. I have a wonderful photo of Henri filling my wine glass, standing at my side in sommelier mode, with a linen *serviette* draped over his arm.

I could feel myself slipping back into the romance of our early days together. Maybe it was the wine or the thought of my grandfather, as a soldier, writing love letters by candlelight.

I let myself savor the moment. It was the perfect ending to an extraordinary day.

Chapter 23

The reality of our new life – as a couple uncoupling – set in soon after Henri and I returned from Müssy.

He co-signed the lease with me for the Little House by the Prairie because his cousins wanted him on the contract as a guarantor. But he and I agreed that we would live apart.

"Will you leave a plank out for me?" Henri asked on our way home from the signing.

I smiled at him. "I don't recall anything about a plank in the lease." The night before, he had spent an hour translating the 10-page contract for me.

"Maybe I skipped that page," he said with a laugh.

We had each been given a set of house keys by the real estate agent, but it was my intention to change the locks after the renovations were finished. There were too many keys in circulation, between the former tenants and the contractors. Henri agreed with that.

Although we were co-signers, Henri and I weren't coming to this arrangement as equal partners. He had paid the agent's fee (half a month's rent) and I had paid the deposit (a full month's rent). The monthly payments would be my responsibility, along with the cost of appliances that needed to be installed – a refrigerator, oven, dishwasher and washer-dryer.

I was still recovering from the shock and anger of what had happened between us. I knew I needed to move on. I was delighted to have a place of my own, even with the unexpected expenses. The house was small, but charming. It had a living room that opened onto the terrace, an eat-in kitchen, two bathrooms, a downstairs bedroom, and the two small bedrooms upstairs. I planned to use one of the upstairs rooms for guests and the other would be my sewing room. I couldn't wait to unpack my quilting books and fabrics.

It would be a few more weeks before I could move in. The renovations were extensive. I stopped by the house one afternoon to take some measurements and introduced myself to the head contractor, who seemed like a nice guy. I was upstairs when suddenly I heard a familiar woman's voice. She spoke to the contractor for a few minutes and then I heard her coming up the steps.

It was Bernadette.

She seemed surprised to see me. We eyed each other for a moment, determining who was the trespasser. She made a quick retreat and fussed about the dust in the stairwell as she left.

I squinted at the freshly painted walls, which were a pale shade of green. I had asked that all the interior walls be painted white. It had been my only request. But clearly my preference had been ignored.

I was fuming on the drive back to Henri's apartment. He was outside, watering the flowerbed, when I arrived.

When I told him what had just happened, he shrugged.

"Why is Bernadette at the house, Henri?"

"The cousins want her to keep an eye on things for them."

"Is she there every day, making decisions about the décor? Did she choose the ugly tile they've put in the bathroom?"

"No, she doesn't like the tile either. The contractor chose that."

"So you've known all this time that she's over there, making decisions about the house I'm going to live in?"

"*Chérie*, she's just choosing the paint colors. That's all, I think."

"I asked you to tell the cousins I'd like the walls to be white."

"I know, *chérie*."

"They're not white."

"I don't see why all this is such a problem for you."

"I resent that there's no end to Bernadette's reach. You let her choose the sheets for *our* bed – those horrible gray sheets – and you see nothing wrong with that either."

"We'll get new sheets if you hate them so much."

"That's not the point, Henri! There are three of us in this relationship – you, me and your sister-wife."

"I'm not married to my sister."

"Emotionally, you are, Henri. The two of you are more of a couple than we are."

I looked at the flowerbed I had painstakingly tended. My David Austin roses were bursting with buds. I decided I would dig them up in the fall and plant them at the Little House. I knew it was petty of me, but I didn't want Bernadette taking possession of them, too.

~~

Giverny sits at the 49th parallel, which runs along much of the border between the U.S. and Canada. The climate is tempered by the Gulf Stream, so it's not unusual to see tropical plants in Normandy. Henri had an enormous, thriving yucca plant in our flower bed.

Because of its northern position, Giverny's summer nights are long. In early summer, the sky is still light at 10:30.

I especially loved the nights of June. I would sit out on the front steps listening to the sheep bells. An itinerant flock came to Giverny to "mow" the pastures in early summer, an eco-service provided by the prefecture. The sheep had a big job to do on the hillside above Doo-Doo Land. I thought about Henri's grandfather who used to roam the hills with his flock.

Those June days were the calm before a storm for me. I knew I'd be buried in boxes for weeks once the house renovations were finished. I began organizing and packing what I had brought from Florence.

The big June social event was once again Megan's garden party. A few days before, Henri asked if I was planning to go.

"I wasn't invited," I said.

"That must be a mistake," he said. "You can come with me. It's no problem."

"I think it is," I said. "Did your invitation also have my name on it?

"No."

"I'm not going, Henri. I have lots to do."

Henri went to the party alone. About 20 minutes after he left the apartment, I got a text message from Yuka, wanting to know if I'd like to meet her for coffee later that afternoon.

I laughed. I knew she was at the party and had just seen Henri arrive alone. She was hungry for gossip.

The gossip mill was the downside of village life.

Henri and I had stopped by for coffee one morning at the *boulangerie*. One of Henri's friends, who was sitting at the next table, had heard that I was moving to the house. When word got out that the house was coming onto the rental market, there was keen local interest. Long-term rentals are much in demand in Giverny.

The man wanted to know if Henri would be moving with me. Henri said he'd be keeping his apartment and made some joke about having an apartment in the "city" and a house in the country.

That didn't satisfy the man's curiosity. "Where will you be sleeping?" he asked.

I could tell Henri wanted to tell the guy where to stick it.

Charmingly, I interjected, "You know Henri. He likes to sleep around."

When the house was finally ready, Henri arranged for a local moving company to deliver my boxes and furnishings, at his expense. I asked Sarah to help me deal with the crew on moving day as my translator. She was a godsend. Henri made himself scarce that day.

He and I were arguing a lot in the days before the move. In what turned out to be my last night at his place, we had a horrible argument during dinner.

At one point, he railed at me for being "possessive." I had never thrown our 10-year age difference at him, but I didn't hold back. "I think there are probably a few 75-year-old men in this village who would love to be possessed by me."

I could see the depth of his pain as we lashed out at each other. "Is that it?" he finally asked. "Or do you have more?"

I regret what I said next. "It seems I'm not the only woman you've had a problem with, Henri." I knew I should stop, but I pressed on. "Yuka says Camille felt she wasn't more important to you than your steam engines and your dogs."

He looked stunned. "Yuka," he murmured. Curiously, he didn't deny it was true. But I wished more than anything I hadn't let my anger get the better of me.

I was alone at Henri's apartment the next morning and decided my exit day had come. I stripped my bed and stuffed my pillows and comforter into the back seat of my car. I quickly gathered my clothes and toiletries. I couldn't wait another minute for this to be over.

Later that afternoon, Henri came to see me. I was sitting in my living room surrounded by boxes. He said that Sofie, the housekeeper, had told him my bed had been stripped.

"It was time for me to go, Henri."

For better or worse, I had begun my new life in Giverny.

Chapter 24

When I woke up on my first morning at the Little House, the prairie across the road looked like it was buried under a foot of snow. It was actually a thick blanket of fog that had rolled in from the Seine.

It was 6 a.m. My neighbor's rooster wasn't even awake yet. I put on a caftan over my nightgown and slipped on a pair of black strappy sandals, which looked a bit odd with my pink-and-white sleep socks. I didn't care. No one would see me at that hour. I quickly ran a comb through my tousled hair, grabbed my camera and headed out the door.

I crossed the road unseen and was photographing the drifts of fog when I heard a truck approaching. I hid behind a bush. The truck passed and things got quiet again. But just as I emerged from my hiding spot, I could see the headlights of several cars coming my way. Morning rush hour had begun.

I wasn't able to get back across the road unnoticed. I laughed at my *comedienne* moment – also enjoyed from above. I heard a whoosh and looked up to see a hot-air balloon passing over my Little House.

I waved.

~⁀

The Prairie is immortalized in many Impressionist paintings of Giverny. Monet and his stepdaughter (who also became his daughter-in-law) Blanche Hoschedé Monet often painted there. The beautiful landscape is infused with vaporous light, created by the mist of the

Seine and Epte rivers that form the Prairie's natural boundary.

The property borders Monet's lily pond and provides a lovely vista of the Giverny countryside from the pathway that encircles the water garden.

Henri and his brother Olivier were involved in a project to restore the landscape as it was in Monet's era. Impressionist paintings of the Prairie, along with old postcards of the area, were serving as a planting guide. During my time at the Little House, I would often see Olivier on his tractor, inspecting the young willow trees and Italian poplars he had planted, according to their placement in the paintings and on the postcards. As a precaution, he had built sturdy wooden barriers around the young saplings.

"He lost a few trees from the first planting," Henri told me, laughing. "The cows like to use them as butt scratchers."

~⁓

One day, Henri suggested I come with him to meet some of the neighbors. This surprised me since he wasn't big on introductions. I was also surprised that we were going on this expedition by car.

Henri, at the wheel of his SUV, veered off the main road, just a few hundred yards from my driveway, and drove along a dirt road through a thicket of trees. He opened a gate hidden from view and within moments, I was on Toad's Wild Ride with Mr. Toad himself.

We bounced across the Prairie and plowed through an enormous puddle of cow poop. Mr. Toad came to a skidding stop in the middle of a herd of Charolais cattle.

"Meet your new neighbors," he said with a grin.

I got out of the car, carefully watching my step (I was wearing sandals) – those Charolais poop puddles are HUGE – and introduced myself. The cows looked at me curiously. They were so sweet and calm. I was amazed by the enormity of them. The biggest ones are the size of a car and weigh more than a ton. But despite their size, there is such gentleness about them.

They're known by the numbers written on their ear tags, which became standard accessories during the Mad Cow era, to help identify the source of contaminated meat. I wondered if, in time, I should give them proper names, befitting their personalities.

After wiping a bit of poop off my sandals, I hopped back in with Mr. Toad and off we went, in four-wheel drive, across the Prairie and into a little stream that flows from Monet's lily pond. (I'm sure my human neighbors heard me shrieking.) At one point, Mr. Toad drove alongside the fence that separates Monet's water garden from the Prairie. Tourists looked at us in amazement, as if to say "Where do we get a ticket for THAT?!"

It all ended well. We drove back to my Little House with cow poop flying off the chassis of Mr. Toad's Wild SUV. I had to pinch myself to make sure I wasn't in a wonderfully weird dream.

I actually enjoyed the process of unpacking my 150 boxes. I looked at it as a month of Christmas mornings. Each night before I went to bed, I'd stack a few boxes by the living-room coffee table to open the next morning. I'd set my alarm for 7 a.m. and was never tempted to oversleep. I'd bound out of bed and make a French-press full of coffee. Still in my pajamas, I'd sit down on the sofa, with a steaming mug in hand, wondering what would be in the first box. Some of the boxes that had come from the back of my Pasadena storage unit hadn't been opened in a decade.

One day while I was unpacking some beautiful heirloom linens and afghans that had come from my mother's cedar chest, I had some unexpected visitors who shared my love of fine needlework and were very pleased to be on hand for the unwrapping of these treasures.

Some of the pieces I took from the box instantly brought back memories: A Christmas tablecloth embroidered with cross-stitch poinsettias, made by Grammy Stout (my mother's mother, the recipient of those love letters from France), that graced the family dining table during the holidays. A crocheted Granny-Square afghan, made by my Grammy Bricker of heavy wool yarn that was wonderful to curl up under on a chilly night. A knitted afghan made by my mother that was her "masterwork," a patchwork of blocks, each made with a different intricate pattern.

In a packet of delicate doilies and beautifully embroidered linen hand towels, I discovered a note from my mother that read: "From mother's Hope Chest. Embroidered by her before she got married." The towels looked as fresh as when Grammy Stout made them 100 years earlier.

And then I found a note from Grammy Stout herself, tucked inside the folds of an exquisite piece of cloth: "Hand-woven by great grandma Ruth for her daughter Sara Ruth married to James McDowell Nov. 7, 1867 (parents of Jennie Alice Oppelt)."

There was another note from my mother telling me that one particular doily had been made by "mother's cousin, Beulah's mother." Aunt Beulah. I always loved her name.

The note that made me laugh was written by Grammy Stout and pinned to a crocheted tablecloth: "Don't put in washer & dryer. Jennie didn't make her knots tight enough & it will come apart."

I have fond memories of Aunt Jennie, my Papa Stout's sister who lived on Mudslick Mountain. She cooked on a wood-fired stove and regulated the oven temperature with a corncob she'd prop in the oven door. Her sister Hattie made blue-ribbon quilts. Hattie showed me how to hand-piece a Grandmother's Flower Garden block when I visited her in Tennessee one summer – my love of quilting comes from Hattie. A quilt she made for my mother is now mine to cherish, along with Jennie's tablecloth (which will be hand-washed and used gently, per the care instructions).

My visitors that day – my mom, Grammy Stout, Grammy Bricker, Ruth, Beulah's mother, Jennie and Hattie – sat on my bed with me as I gently ran my fingers over their stitches. I could hear their voices as I read their words. I could imagine them at a table, sharing stories and recipes over glasses of iced tea on a hot summer's day. I could smell the cornbread in Jennie's oven. I remembered the night my dad spilled red wine on that poinsettia tablecloth as he gave an exuberant Christmas toast (emergency blotting measures and a good stain remover saved the day).

My callers left as quietly as they arrived. I was sad to see them go. But the essence of them lingered in Giverny, at my Little House by the Prairie.

As I put away these keepsakes, I wrote a note and tucked it in the folds for someone I'll "visit" someday, adding a thread to this wonderful hand-me-down story.

Chapter 25

A few weeks after I had moved to the Little House, Giverny's *mairie* (town hall) issued a warning about a roving group of Roma that were in the area. They had set up camp in the woods along a road that led to the neighboring village of Limmetz and had been seen in Giverny casing properties. Our neighbor Léo, the security guard at the museum, had caught a man in the driveway in front of our apartments checking out Henri's truck.

One day, my doorbell rang at the gate to my driveway at the Little House. The man waved a business card. I thought he was from the electric company, coming to read the meter. I motioned for him to come to the door. He presented me with a card advertising his services as a handyman.

When I told Henri about this, he cautioned me. "That probably was one of the gypsies. They come onto properties offering to do work. But they're really just looking around to see what they can come back for later and steal."

That was unsettling. My driveway gate didn't lock. The front yard was concealed by tall hedges that cast long shadows at night. The steps leading up to the front terrace were not lit.

At 10:30 that same night, my doorbell rang. I couldn't see anyone at the gate in the glow of the street lamp from across the road.

I called Henri and told him I was concerned. He was getting ready for bed and clearly didn't want to come out at that hour.

He arrived about 10 minutes later, not in a good mood. He saw no one on the street and looked around the property. "It was probably just tourists walking by," he said.

"Why would they do that?"

"Maybe they were drunk." He pulled down the brim of his cap. "Can I go now?"

"Henri, I'm a woman living alone now. I'd like to know I have some backup if I feel uneasy."

Two days later, in the middle of a Saturday afternoon, there was a loud knock at the front door. I had been taking a nap. It was a hot afternoon and I was wearing only a nightgown. I saw a man I didn't recognize on the steps to the terrace. I panicked and called Henri. He didn't answer. I was standing in the hallway, where I couldn't be seen, near the front door. I was leaving Henri a frantic message when I heard pounding on the French doors in the living room. A few minutes later, the front door opened. I wasn't in the habit of locking the door when I was home during the day.

My heart was in my throat. To my surprise, the man coming through the door was the contractor who had done the house renovations. The man I had seen on the front steps was a plumber who had come to fix the stopped-up toilet.

Standing in my flimsy nightgown, I felt vulnerable, but mostly angry. The men had barged into my home uninvited. The construction was over and if they needed to return, they should make an appointment and wait for me to answer the door.

I couldn't express that with my limited French, but I made it clear I wanted them to leave.

"*Allez!*" I shouted. Go!

The plumber retreated to the terrace, apologizing. But the contractor, who was a big burly guy, didn't budge. He stood blocking the front door, so that I couldn't pass.

"*Allez! Allez!*" I shouted again.

Grabbing the door handle, I pushed the door toward him. He stumbled onto the terrace and then turned, jamming his boot in the doorway to prevent the door from closing.

"*Allez!*" I yelled, loud enough for anyone passing by to hear. He withdrew his foot. I slammed the door closed and bolted it shut.

A few days later, I made a complaint, in person, to the property manager and vowed if the contractor ever returned to the house, I would call the police.

Henri didn't make excuses for him, but I could tell he wasn't terribly upset by what had happened. "You know how things are here. People knock and walk in. That's normal."

"That's not normal where I come from," I said. "You knock and wait for someone to answer. And if that doesn't happen, you leave."

"Why are you so nervous?"

"Your dear sister Bernadette lives on the third floor of an apartment building in Vernon. She told me herself that she would never live on the ground floor of a building – or in a house by herself – because she's afraid," I said. "Sarah owns a house that she rents out. She won't live there alone because she's afraid. I'm here alone, with vagrants nosing around and a belligerent contractor shoving his boot against the door. Yes, okay, that makes me nervous. I don't need to apologize for that."

When Sarah heard what had happened with the contractor, she urged me to change the locks, which had been my intention anyway. This now became urgent because it was possible the contractor still had a key.

She called a handyman named Robert who worked for Maurice at the moulin. Robert said he could change the lock in an afternoon. He and Sarah came over to the house the next day. He removed the old lock and took it to a hardware store to get a replacement.

I hadn't told Henri I had arranged to do this, though he knew it was my plan. A few minutes after Robert returned with a new lock, Henri showed up out of the blue with a solar-powered security light mounted on a post that he had made that afternoon in his workshop.

He eyed Robert. "Who's he?"

"He's a friend of Sarah's who's looking at the lock. I'd like to change it, given all the problems I've had here."

Henri said nothing more and hammered the wooden post into the ground near the gate. And then he left.

The lock replacement had turned into a clandestine operation because I had decided I wasn't going to give Henri a spare key. I knew that would anger him, but I didn't like his attitude that the house was as much his as it was mine, even though he wasn't paying rent.

Robert handed me five keys to the new lock. I gave Sarah one. I hid another one in a metal pipe that formed the crosspiece of a clothesline in the garden. I tucked one into my handbag and slipped the other two into an envelope that I stuffed into a zippered compartment designed for a cushion in the back of my IKEA office chair.

I dreaded the likely showdown with Henri about this. I would be leaving in a few weeks for a trip to California and he was already talking about spending nights at the house to make it look like someone was home. I imagined him inviting friends over to show off the place. I cringed at the thought of Bernadette sniffing around.

But I put all that out of my mind. At least, I could get a good night's sleep knowing I was the keeper of the keys.

The day before I was set to fly to California, Henri asked me for a spare key.

I said I needed to think about that.

"What do you mean? You're leaving tomorrow. Who's going to take care of things?"

"I've made arrangements," I said.

He stormed outside and suddenly morphed into a child, stomping his feet on the flowerbed at the edge of the terrace.

Then he started crying hysterically – wailing like an out-of-control toddler.

"Henri, come back inside," I said in a calm voice. I wondered if the neighbors could hear him.

"Are we enemies now?" he cried.

"No, Henri. We're not enemies." I gently took his arm. "Come inside and sit down."

He sat at my desk in the living room and sobbed.

"Take a deep breath," I said to him. "Okay, good. Now another." I was baffled by his behavior. I had never seen this side of him.

After a few minutes, he calmed down. And then he got angry. "Why won't you give me a key?" he shouted.

"I don't want you here, bringing people over. This is *my* home. You made the decision for us to live apart. I don't understand why you feel entitled to stay here."

He got up to leave.

"Can I still count on you to take me to the airport tomorrow?"

He glared at me. "No, you can't."

I quickly called Sarah and told her what had happened. She knew of a reliable taxi service in Vernon and booked a ride for me for the next morning.

After I had finished packing, Sarah came over and we went to lunch at a little restaurant down the road that was little more than a partially covered deck on the banks of the Ru. We sat at a table by the railing, with a view of the ducks swimming by.

As our meals were served, it started to sprinkle. Our waiter asked if we'd like to move under the overhang. We said no – it was a hot August day and the drizzle was cooling. He put up an umbrella to give us some protection. By the time we paid the bill, we were both damp, but refreshed.

I shook the raindrops out of my hair, feeling like I had been cleansed.

Early the next morning, my taxi arrived on time. As the driver loaded my bags into the trunk, I took a bicycle cable lock out of my handbag and wrapped it around the driveway gate, and then clicked the lock closed.

Chapter 26

I awoke one August night, just before my trip to California, to the sound of cows crying on the Prairie. The cries came from females whose calves had been taken from them that day. Many of the young had gone to the slaughterhouse.

The cows cried all night and the crying continued for a few days. I wanted to cover my ears. My heart hurt. I was glad, in a way, that I hadn't named those sweet calves and grown fond of them.

Henri says the mothers have no memory of their young after a few days. I'd like to see some proof of that. Do we humans make up these theories to ease our conscience, I wondered.

～

I had been looking forward to spending several days with Kyle and Julia, who were meeting me in Del Mar, just north of San Diego. I had arranged for us to stay at the condo of a friend, who was out of town and had generously offered us her place, which was just two blocks from the beach.

I hoped this would be a relaxing visit for Julia. She had lost her mother only a month earlier. While jogging around a local reservoir, her mom had collapsed when her heart went out of rhythm. She had been unconscious for about a half hour before someone found her. She passed away a few days later, at the age of 52.

When Kyle sent me the news, I wept. I had never met this woman, but from what I knew of her, I wished I'd known her. I called Kyle on Skype that day and could barely say the words. "No mother should die so young and miss her children's weddings and the birth of her grandbabies. This is just so wrong."

Julia put on a brave face for most of our time in Del Mar, but Kyle told me she was struggling. One night while we were having dinner at the condo, she seemed to drift away, staring into space. Kyle and I exchanged glances. I knew he was worried about her.

He was out running one afternoon when I came back from the grocery store and found Julia at the dining room table, reading a book. She's a voracious reader, a habit I think she picked up from her mom.

I hadn't yet said anything to her about her mother's passing. So I sat down at the table with her and took a deep breath. "I'm so sorry about your mom," I said.

She nodded.

"There's no rhyme or reason. I know you're trying to understand why." I could feel a lump forming in my throat. "But if your mom were here in this room with us right now – and I have a feeling she's near – she would understand your sadness, but she wouldn't want you to curl up in a ball. She'd want you to put your feet on the floor and carry on with your life."

Julia nodded again. I could see the tears in her eyes.

"Sometimes when you feel sad or depressed, it's important to turn toward the light. When you put your feet on the floor in the morning, find a patch of sunlight on the floor. Step into it and stand there for a minute. Feel the beam of it passing through you.

"I don't know if you're a spiritual person, but I believe the people we've loved and lost in this life are never far away. Let yourself be open to that. You'll feel her presence, maybe you'll hear her whisper in your ear. She might be in the next room or sitting right beside you. Leave an empty chair for her."

Kyle returned at that moment, and I knew he sensed we had been talking about her mom. He asked Julia if she'd like to go down to the beach. He had his hand at her back as they walked out the door.

When I dropped them off at the airport a few days later, I gave Julia a big hug and whispered, "Step into the light."

She nodded and smiled a little.

As they headed toward the terminal, I felt the heartache I always feel when I watch my son walk away. I now felt that times two.

~

I always took comfort in the thought that family and friends who have left this world are near. They look out for me when I travel. When I'm lost or at loose ends, I send up distress calls and they help me find my way.

In turn, I send up hellos and words of thanks. I light candles for them at churches I visit. I've lit many candles during my travels.

I put them in the acknowledgments of my second book, which I wrote during my time in Florence. It was a beautiful summer night when I finished writing that novel. At two in the morning, I went out on my rooftop terrace. The sky was full of stars. I imagined those stars as angels, some of them "mine," looking down on all the loved ones they had left behind.

I shared the news with my angels that I had finished my book, though I think they already knew that. (Angels know everything.)

I thanked them for loving me and guiding me through my some-times-messy life on Earth.

I sat on a chaise on the terrace for an hour, watching the Big and Little Dipper slowly travel across the sky. I fell asleep, feeling the softness of wings around me.

It was one of the most magical nights of my life.

Chapter 27

Henri and I had exchanged a few emails while I was away. He wrote to say that the cousins, who owned the Little House, had decided to replace the front terrace.

I had told the property agent that there were several stones that had been loosened by weeds growing around them. One of my movers tripped on one and nearly fell. Henri, himself, had nearly lost his balance, when one stone had lifted as he stepped on it. The agent, an arrogant woman named Fanny, had assured me the cousins had insurance to pay for injuries.

Incensed, I said, "Visitors to my house aren't going to end up on crutches."

After that meeting, I sent her an email with a photo of my foot lifting one of the stones as I stepped on it. I wrote: *No insurance company is going to pay for injuries when the owners have been informed of a possible risk. If the terrace is not repaired, this now becomes NEGLIGENCE and you'll have more than hospital bills to pay for.*

Henri had cut off the bicycle lock from the front gate to give the workers access, but the crew wanted to move my car to make room for their equipment. Henri needed a key to the house so he could get the spare key to the car. I said that wouldn't be possible. I honestly couldn't remember where I had put the spare car key and didn't want him tearing the house apart looking for it.

A few days before I returned, Henri informed me that he wouldn't be able to pick me up at the airport. I was arriving on a Wednesday and his annual engine show was that weekend. He was very busy with final preparations, he wrote, and couldn't meet my flight.

I arranged for a taxi. I hadn't slept much on the plane. As the taxi left the airport, I closed my eyes, trying to relax. My stomach churned and I suddenly felt nauseated with dread.

When the taxi pulled through the front gate, I was amazed by the transformation that had occurred while I was away. The old terrace was gone, replaced by large slabs of sandstone that had been secured with a concrete border – a vast improvement.

I made a mental note: Never underestimate the power of the word NEGLIGENCE.

On the front stoop was a pot of red begonias. I wondered if it was a welcome-back gift from Sarah, who had been coming by to water my flowerbed. There was no card. I didn't think they had come from Henri.

I took a nap and then headed to the grocery store. A half hour later, my doorbell rang.

It was Henri. He looked at me in amazement as I opened the door. I must admit, I looked pretty fabulous. The California sun had given me a golden tan and had streaked my hair with lovely highlights. In fact, as I had been loading my groceries in the car a short while earlier, a good-looking guy had pulled up next to me and said, *"Qui etes-vous?"* Who are you? When I told him I didn't speak much French, he sadly said, *"C'est dommage!"* Too bad!

Henri stepped over the threshold and embraced me. He pulled back, cupping my face in his rough hands, "Look at you. There's such a change in you."

"I've been with family and friends and have had a wonderful, relaxing trip," I said. The unspoken part of that thought: *I've been away from all the crap you fling at me.*

I didn't stir the pot. He asked me to join him for dinner that evening. "We're expecting 15 people for dinner tonight at the kitchen. There won't be room for us at the table."

I thought that was a curious twist. Henri, the master of ceremonies, was bowing out of the opening event of the weekend.

We went to the little restaurant on the Ru where Sarah and I had had lunch the day before I left.

Henri seemed genuinely happy to see me. He asked if I liked the begonias (mystery solved). There was no mention of the key incident or how the construction crew managed to work around my car in the driveway. Of course, he was feeling the excitement of the weekend to come, so that lifted his spirits. He told me he had made a reservation for me at the Saturday night dinner for the exhibitors at the Baudy. I remembered the previous year when I had stood in the middle of the dining room, feeling conspicuous with no place to sit until Anne-Marie rescued me.

I knew there would be another big dinner at the kitchen on Friday evening, but he didn't mention that.

I didn't see Henri the next day. He stopped by on Friday to say hello, but didn't invite me to dinner that evening. He asked if I would be coming to the Baudy.

"I'll see how I feel," I said. "I'm still pretty jet-lagged."

I didn't go to the Baudy dinner. I knew that probably didn't go unnoticed by some. The next day, Sunday, I went to the showground after I'd had lunch. I arrived at a side gate. One of the museum volunteers, a nice guy named Nicolas, came running toward me and moved the barricade for me to enter. At least, *he* was happy to see me.

In fact, many people were happy to see me and greeted me warmly. Henri rushed toward me and kissed my cheek. I took his arm and asked him to give me a tour of the exhibits.

Nicolas' wife later pulled me aside and asked why I hadn't been at the Baudy.

"I'm just back from a trip to California and am still recovering from jet lag," I said. But I could tell she suspected something was amiss.

Later in the afternoon, as exhibitors were packing up their engines, I went into the food tent where the wives were laying the tables for the farewell dinner. Bernadette was in the thick of it. I waved at her and walked toward her to say hello. When I was within a few feet of her, she looked at me with a sour face and said, "*Bonjour*, Rebecca." And then she turned her back to me and walked away.

I enjoyed the picnic supper and sat with Anne-Marie. Her dear husband sat with us. He was in the throes of cancer treatment. He didn't look well, but Anne-Marie was optimistic.

I didn't stay till the end. I needed sleep. I said good-night to Henri. He said he'd stop by the next day. His son Paul would be staying on for a few days, so I knew I wouldn't be seeing much of Henri.

In fact, I wasn't invited to join the dinners for friends and family in the coming days during the dismantling of the show. One night, Henri brought me a pizza he had gotten at a local shop.

After all the hoopla had died down and life returned to normal, I asked Henri why I had been excluded from the dinners at the kitchen.

"There wasn't room for you," he said.

"Do you not hear yourself when you say things like that?" I asked him. I told him how Bernadette had snubbed me. "What was that about?"

He just shrugged.

Chapter 28

I was delighted to find out that a friend of mine, a talented Ukrainian artist named Nataliya Petrenko-Litvinova from Kyiv, had returned to Giverny for a month-long exhibition at a local gallery, which was just down the road from the Little House.

I had met Nataliya the previous fall when she'd had an exhibition at another gallery in the village, a short distance from Henri's place. I would see her sitting outside the gallery at a little table, sketching and doing watercolors. I loved her work and purchased a beautiful painting of a vase of vibrant red poppies set against a gold background reminiscent of Russian iconic art I had studied in a college art-appreciation class.

When I first met Nataliya, she spoke little English. On that first visit, she was traveling with a lovely Ukrainian woman named Olena, who was acting as her translator.

I enjoyed sitting with them outside the gallery. One day, I shared the story of the place where we were sitting, which was the location of a famous painting by Theodore Robinson called *The Wedding March*, commemorating the wedding day of fellow American artist Theodore Butler and Monet's stepdaughter Suzanne Hoschedé.

I pointed to a print of the painting that was on an easel outside the gallery. I was telling Nataliya and Olena about an ethereal connection I felt with Robinson when a white butterfly landed on one of Nataliya's oil paintings that hung above us on the gallery's stone facade. It was a beautiful scene of Monet's lily pond. The butterfly landed on a profusion of flowers at the edge of the pond, as if it belonged in the painting.

Suddenly, the butterfly flew over to me and sat for a minute on my head.

Nataliya gasped and Olena grabbed her phone to take a photo, but she wasn't quick enough. The butterfly flitted away.

In the year since I had last seen Nataliya, her English had improved dramatically. On this visit, she had brought her 13-year-old son, Gosha, with her as her translator.

Gosha spoke English well and had a marvelous sense of humor.

"I am the manager," he told me with a big grin.

Gosha was tall and lanky, with a wavy mop of dark hair, and looked very scholarly with his horn-rimmed glasses. He was extremely bright and took accelerated courses at school in mathematics and physics. He was also an accomplished pianist, music composer and chess player. He loved tennis. He dreamed about going to Harvard or Stanford someday. He was any university's dream package.

He worried about the expense of a U.S. education. "I think pencils and pens in America will cost a lot in Ukrainian money," he said.

I promised to buy his pencils and pens for four years. I also offered to help him with his college essays.

"I would be very thankful for that," he said.

Nataliya's new exhibition featured landscapes, portraits and pen-and-ink drawings that showed the range of her impressive talent.

I stepped closer to inspect a compelling self-portrait. Nataliya told me she was 28 years old when she painted it. I wouldn't have guessed that. At 49, Nataliya had an ageless, sensual beauty. In the portrait, her dark hair is loosely pulled back, with strands falling around her face. She gazes out from the canvas, projecting inner strength and resolve.

"What were you thinking about when you painted this?" I asked her.

"I thought about the strength of character that a woman needs to be an artist. At that time, I worked in advertising," she said. "I consider myself lucky. I now earn my living as an artist."

In the painting, Nataliya, wearing an artist's smock, is at an easel in a cramped studio space. Backlit by sunlight streaming through an open window, she stands in front of an old spinning wheel.

"When I was a teenager, I found this spinning wheel in the attic of my grandfather's sister's house, in the village of Shishaki, in central Ukraine," Nataliya told me. "My relatives wanted to burn her, but I took her with me to Kyiv. She stood in my room for a very long time."

I loved that Nataliya gave the spinning wheel a feminine identity.

"On this spinning wheel, my ancestors spun, made threads," Nataliya explained. "The spinning wheel is the ancestors, the past. An open window is also important – it is the future."

~૭

A few days later, Nataliya asked me to sit for a portrait. This was a new experience for me that required sitting still for two and a half hours. Although I was able to flex my feet and stretch my legs a bit, I couldn't turn my head very far or shift my position. I suddenly could empathize with painters' models. My thoughts wandered to Marie, Robinson's model who posed for him on Giverny's hillsides and on that little bridge by the moulin. I wondered how she would have coped on a badly sagging sofa.

I needed a focal point that would distract me.

Across the room, within my line of sight, was a painting Nataliya had done of Gosha as a young boy. He's sitting at a dining table in front of a window that looks out onto a garden. It's a luminous painting, with a blue cloth on the table along with a pitcher of flowers, a jar of something creamy looking, a plate with pastries and cheese, and a bowl of strawberries. I noticed three strawberries had escaped from the bowl and, in my fertile imagination, they morphed into two eyeballs and a nose...and below them, a shadow at the edge of the table turned into a mouth. And then I saw two yellow eyeballs in the flowers dangling from the pitcher.

This is how artists' models cope, I thought – they start hallucinating.

With each of Nataliya's brush strokes, I could feel a gentle surge of energy rise up my spine that made my scalp tingle. It was a breezy day and wind chimes at a shop down the street were the perfect background music for my dreamy state. Gosha sat at his laptop out of my view, listening to a Ukrainian news report on YouTube about the Trump-Ukraine scandal. We all laughed at the commentator's Russian pronunciation of "Monica Lewinsky" as he recounted what led to Bill Clinton's impeachment.

Gosha and I talked a lot about politics. Even at 13, he was developing a world view. He wanted to find U.S. political blogs on YouTube. I told him about Rachel Maddow's show and the outstanding journalists she had as guests. I cautioned him about the misinformation we all need to sift through. He laughed at the propaganda-laced news that comes from Russia.

I closed my eyes for a bit as Nataliya painted and thought about where Gosha's journey in life will take him. I had no doubt he had a brilliant future, as long as the world didn't turn upside down.

I had a little dream about where my life has taken me. I've had extraordinary experiences that have carved a deep well for me as a writer, a traveler, a mother, a lover, a friend. What I've seen and known sometimes brings tears – both from sadness and joy.

When I opened my eyes, Nataliya took the finished portrait off the easel for me to see. I was struck by the wistful look she had captured. She had caught a glimpse of my soul and rendered it beautifully.

During Nataliya's stay that September, I organized an exhibition of my Giverny photographs and staged it at the Lodge. I had arranged with Henri to give him a percentage of the profits in exchange for use of the space. He said he appreciated the gesture. We didn't fix the percentage.

I had printed gorgeous posters designed by a graphic artist who had done a couple of my book covers. I called the show "Reflections: on the beauty of Giverny." The designer had created a reflection of the word "reflection" in what appeared to be the shimmering, color-infused surface of a pond. I had taken that photo on a fall day on the banks of the Epte, just down the road from Monet's lily pond.

I'd had a number of the posters laminated and mounted on sticks to position around the village. Henri had printed up arrows, which he also laminated, to attach to the signs, pointing the way to the Lodge.

On the first morning of the exhibition, as I was taping a big poster on the front gate, I asked Henri if he had attached the arrows to the signs he had placed in the village.

"Yes, it's all done," he assured me.

I was hopeful there would be a good turnout. It was the weekend of Patrimony Days and Giverny's annual *vide-grenier* sale – a hugely popular flea market where residents display their treasures and discards on tables, set up around the village, that are loaded with dishes and glassware, old books and toys, linens, paintings, tools, furnishings, and collectible French ephemera. It's like walking through Yesteryear. On one of my early visits to Giverny, I experienced my first *vide grenier* and bought vintage postcards of Giverny scenes that had been postmarked during Monet's time. Little did I know then that they would set the scene for a book I would write one day.

The morning was slow, which surprised me. From the terrace of the Lodge, I could see streams of people in the streets below.

By the end of the afternoon, I'd had very few visitors and hadn't sold a single photograph.

I went down the street to collect the signs and was stunned to see that none of them had arrows.

Henri stopped by to see how the day had gone.

"Why did you lie to me?" I asked

"What are you talking about?"

"You told me you had put arrows on the signs. You didn't." I held up one of the signs that still had a clump of dirt attached to its stick. "There's no arrow on this."

"I was too busy," he said dismissively.

"You place signs all over this village during your show. All of them have arrows, pointing the way to the showgrounds. You know the importance of this. How were people supposed to find me today?"

"I'll put the arrows on tomorrow," he said unapologetically.

I wouldn't let it drop. "Henri, you *lied* to me."

He raised his hands in the air as he does when he's had enough.

I went out to the main gate to take down the big poster, only to discover that it had been stolen.

The next day, Henri put arrows on the signs and within the first hour, I had more visitors than I'd had the entire day before. I sold two photographs – one to Sarah and another to a friend of Henri's.

Nataliya and Gosha stopped by. I have some wonderful photos of them in the Lodge's living room, where I had set up a table with drinks and a tray of cookies. Nataliya gave me an insightful artist's critique of the exhibition, suggesting I experiment with printing the images on aluminum panels. It would give them a more contemporary look, she said. All of the images in the exhibition had been printed on canvas and wrapped on conventional wooden stretchers. "The textured surface of aluminum will give the images another dimension," she said. I appreciated her advice.

I felt a bit deflated as I packed up after the show. Henri came by to help.

He flipped through the pages of the guest book I had put out for visitors.

"How did it go today?" he asked.

"Not well." I turned to him, making no attempt to hide my disappointment. "I went in the hole. A big hole. I have no profit to share with you."

On the night before Nataliya and Gosha were to return to Kyiv, Madame Red Shoes organized a dinner in Nataliya's honor at her lovely home in Vernon.

We gathered at the big round table in her large kitchen whose blue-and-white decorative tiles reminded me of Monet's famous kitchen. Madame Red Shoes' kitchen, with its checkerboard red-and-ivory floor and its big cast-iron stove, often appeared in her pastel drawings. I had purchased one of them and hung it in my kitchen at the Little House.

Nataliya was exuberant that evening. Her husband Andriy had flown in from Kyiv to drive her and Gosha back home. A month earlier, he had driven them to Giverny and left the car with them to use, returning to Kyiv by plane. I could tell he was a supportive, caring husband. He wasn't Gosha's father, but he treated him like a son. Andriy was pleased to meet me and gave me a box of Ukrainian chocolates. "These are the best," he told me proudly. "These are made in Kyiv!"

I had stopped by the gallery before dinner to help them with the packing. Gosha was taping up a box containing a large painting. "I want to be postal worker someday," he said, pretending to be serious.

"Not if I have anything to do with it!" I exclaimed.

I looked around at the paintings that still had to be packed.

My heart skipped a beat when I saw the oil Nataliya had painted of Monet's lily pond that had attracted the butterfly that landed on my head.

I turned to her and said, "You don't have to pack that one. It's coming home with me."

Nataliya gave me a hug. "I'm very happy it will be with you."

As we sat at Madame Red Shoes' table that chilly autumn night, we talked about Nataliya's upcoming show at a prestigious gallery in Vienna. I had a feeling her career was about to explode. She had just won an award for a set of stained-glass windows she had designed that recently had been installed at a chapel in the mountains above Linz, Austria. There seemed to be no bounds to her creative energy and talent.

Nataliya had told me stories of her childhood and adolescence, growing up in Soviet-controlled Ukraine. She was 16 years old, living in Kyiv, when the Chernobyl meltdown happened in 1986.

"On the day of the accident, my classmates and I were in Kyiv in the open air, painting landscapes in the park," she told me. "The radiation level was already very high."

"My parents reacted quickly. My mother gathered the basic things, and that same evening, my brother, who was 11, and I went to stay with relatives in Lubny. We spent the night there, and the next day, he and I went by train to Poltava, in central Ukraine, to visit my mother's friends. The ride was not long, two hours. We lived in Poltava for a month, in a wonderful family. Meanwhile, schools began to officially evacuate children from Kyiv. My brother, with his school, and I went to a pioneer summer camp in the Crimea, and we lived there for three months. My parents, along with others, stayed in Kyiv. My mother told me that it was very strange to be in a city where there were no children on the streets.

"A couple of years after the accident, I had an enlarged thyroid gland and I had to be treated for several years. Perhaps it was from the day that I painted in the park, or maybe a completely different reason."

I marveled at the changes Nataliya had seen in her life. She had emerged from the oppressive Soviet era, after Ukraine's liberation from the U.S.S.R. in 1991, into a world where she enjoyed unbridled artistic freedom and the ability to travel. There would be no stopping her, I thought.

As we stood outside on that starry September night, I gave her a big hug.

"I'll see you in Vienna," I said with a wink.

"You will come to Vienna to see my show?" she asked incredulously.

"I wouldn't miss it for the world."

Giverny had grown quieter with the coming of fall. There were fewer tourists, which made it possible to have a leisurely lunch at the *boulangerie*.

Henri and I took a seat at our favorite corner table on the patio. It was a beautiful crisp day. Golden leaves swirled at our feet. The roosters next door provided their usual background music, as we studied the chalkboard of the chef's creations *du jour*.

That day, a dollop of juicy gossip accompanied the meal. In the hills above Giverny, a pack of wild boars had dug up a 40-year-old car that contained evidence linked to the burglary of a castle that had happened years earlier. Details were sketchy. Police were investigating.

I had many questions: Was there loot in the car? A body in the trunk? Were the boars in protective custody?

We could hear the pop of hunting rifles as we lunched.

Thankfully, boar was not on the menu. The *filet d'eglefin* (haddock) was excellent and so was the featured dessert – figs roasted in butter and served with frothy goat cheese topped with walnuts.

I thought of Roz and could imagine her savoring the taste of the buttery figs. She had disappeared from Giverny shortly after the recipe book was published, early that summer. Antoine told me she had sent her driver in to buy a copy one day. "I saw her sitting in the car," he said.

That made me sad. I wished she and I could have had fun with that project. It was such a good idea and had turned out so well, despite all the headaches. Monique's boutique had sold out their copies within a few weeks. I wasn't inclined to do a sequel. I had played the role of imposter to the limit. Jose, at the pain clinic, still teased me. As promised, I had written the number for the poison-control hotline in his autographed copy.

All year I had been saving an invitation I had received, as a local resident, from the head of the Monet Foundation to visit the gardens, with free admission for two. I had been to the gardens many times that season, but I had saved the pass for a special occasion. In the final days, I had decided that my special guest should be Henri. Who better to see the gardens with than a man who used to play there as a boy.

After World War II, when the last of Monet's descendants abandoned the property, the kids in the village had the run of the grounds. Henri loved fishing in the lily pond.

"When we needed a fishing pole, we broke off a piece of bamboo," he told me. The bamboo thicket Monet planted still stands by the Japanese bridge.

It was the first time I had visited the gardens with Henri. He himself hadn't been there for several years.

Monet's house and gardens had been blighted with neglect in the years after his death in 1926 and then damaged by Allied bombings during World War II. The restoration of the property began in the late 1970s when the former curator of Versailles, Gérald Van Der Kemp, and his American wife, Florence, raised millions of dollars – mostly from generous American donors – to return the gardens to what Monet called his "best masterpiece." The house and gardens opened to the public in 1980.

I loved that Henri, true to his roots, had contributed immensely to Giverny's revival. In 1994, he and Camille had reopened the bar and part of the terrace at the long-abandoned Hôtel Baudy. One evening while he and I were having a drink at a little table outside the Baudy entrance, Henri pointed to a junction box he had installed on a light pole across the street. "I hung that there so we could run a string of lights over the terrace. Free electricity," he said, smiling.

It gave me chills to think about the "phantoms" of the Baudy. I could easily imagine those who had gathered round the tables there: French artists Paul Cezanne, Pierre-Auguste Renoir, Alfred Sisley, Auguste Rodin, along with American painters Mary Cassatt, John Singer Sargent, Theodore Butler, John Leslie Breck, Lilla Cabot Perry, Willard Metcalf, Kenyon Cox, Henri Fitch Taylor, Theodore Wendell, Will Hicok Low, Mary Fairchild and Frederick MacMonnies, Frederick Carl Frieseke, Richard E. Miller, Lawton Parker, Louis Ritman, Guy Rose – and, of course, the artist who had enchanted me, Theodore Robinson.

One evening, as Henri and I were entertaining visitors in the Baudy's dining room, I recalled seeing a vintage postcard of the room and realized that a Robinson portrait of Marie had hung on the wall next to me, directly above our table. Robinson and Marie used to dine in this room with Madame Baudy. He was one of her favorite artists.

Between 1885 and 1915, more than 350 artists from 18 countries came to paint in Giverny. Most were from the United States. Along with artists from England, Scotland, Ireland, Canada and Australia, they created an Anglo-Saxon culture in the village.

Monet led a reclusive life behind his garden walls, annoyed by the intrusion of those who had followed him to Giverny. He befriended very few of the young bohemians. Robinson was an exception, most likely because he was older and artistically more accomplished than his cohorts. Monet critiqued Robinson's work and invited him to family gatherings, which Robinson sometimes photographed. A well-known photograph of Monet in his gardening attire, leaning on a walking stick, was taken by Robinson.

In a letter to Robinson in February 1891, Monet wrote: *In Giverny all is quiet and the life is slow-paced. The youngsters enjoyed the opportunity of skating which was offered to them. Sometimes we see some carefree and colorful people, your compatriots "checking" on the start of spring. Spring is indeed on its way and I'm sure it won't be long until you come back to your little house here.*

Henri laughed when I read aloud Monet's comment about the "carefree and colorful people" – the Americans who come "checking" on things. I thought of myself wandering the village, peering over the garden walls to find the tree with the bent limb.

Robinson did return for one more season, in 1892, a prolific summer for him when he produced several of his seminal Giverny paintings – including the one of Marie sitting on the bridge by the moulin, called *La Debacle*. The painting's title comes from the book she holds on her lap of the same name – a novel by Emile Zola about the collapse of France's Second Empire during the Franco-Prussian war, published the same year.

Robinson likely would have become America's preeminent Impressionist artist if his poor health hadn't cut his life short. He died of a severe asthma attack while in New York City in 1896, at the age of 43.

Giverny's thriving art-colony ended with the start of World War I. After the war, some artists, including Monet's stepson-in-law Theodore Butler, returned to Giverny. Butler is buried in Giverny's churchyard near Monet's grave.

The art-colony spirit of Giverny has been irrepressible. Monet's discovery of this hamlet on the Seine, bathed in its beautiful light, has continued to draw artists from around the world. But unlike in Monet's time, present-day visitors have the delight of seeing his inner sanctum.

As Henri and I walked around the perimeter of the pond on that autumn afternoon, he showed me his favorite place to fish and where Monet's famous poplar trees once stood.

The boy still lived in the man. As I photographed the dazzling last light of the season's last day, Henri stood on the little bridge at the far end of the pond, looking down at the water, and exclaimed, "Look at that bass!"

I thought he might take out his pocketknife and make himself a bamboo fishing pole.

When I told Henri that I was planning to go to Vienna in November to see Nataliya's show, he liked the idea and wanted to join me.

We hadn't taken a trip together since Malta, two years earlier. He was always too busy at the museum to go away during the tourist season. We found an Airbnb apartment in Vienna and booked our flights.

A few hours before we were to meet Nataliya for her opening-night party at the gallery, Henri and I happened upon a Pierre Bonnard exhibition elsewhere in Vienna. It was the first retrospective of Bonnard's work ever to be shown in Austria and included numerous paintings that had been part of a major Bonnard exhibition earlier that year at the Tate Modern in London.

I was astounded by the collection. These were his famous works that I had only seen in books. The painting that inspired the cover of my novel about the Bonnard forgery was on display in the main foyer.

But the one painting that caught my breath was of Bonnard's balcony view of the Seine from his studio at his house in Vernonnet, where I had met Nataliya a year earlier. She had bought a copy of my book, which I signed for her, and had shown me how an app on her phone could translate the text into Russian.

I said to Henri, "It's amazing to see this painting today. We're here because of Nataliya. I met her in that very room, at Bonnard's house. Isn't that incredible?"

He took my hand and kissed it. "*C'est incroyable.*" It's incredible.

Nataliya's opening was a big success. The gallery was located in Vienna's chic art district. The clientele was well-heeled.

The show was entitled "Universum," which explored Nataliya's fascination with the wonders of the universe. I especially loved her interpretation of the exploding energy of the cosmos that she depicted in the form of an angel.

The next day, Nataliya invited us to visit her at a secluded conference center in the breathtaking countryside of Stollhof, outside of Vienna, where she was the guest of its owner, a wealthy Russian businessman who was one of Nataliya's generous sponsors and patrons. He had commissioned a number of her paintings, which were installed at the compound.

Henri and I were guests for lunch at his villa on the property. Nataliya had prepared delicious Ukrainian dishes. Gosha joined us and was eager to talk politics. He was concerned about the situation in eastern Ukraine, where the rebel fighting against the Russians had escalated.

After lunch and a tour of the complex, it was time to say good-bye. Nataliya slipped her arm through mine, marveling how our "chance" encounter at Bonnard's house a year earlier had led to a growing friendship.

She said, "We are like stars meeting in the cosmos."

"You're so right," I said.

It all seemed like a wink and a nod from the "universum."

But neither of us could have imagined then there was unthinkable tragedy fomenting in the cosmos.

Chapter 29

An American friend whom I had met during my time in Florence was spending a few weeks in the Cotswolds of England and had invited me to come stay with her for a weekend in a lovely cottage she had rented.

We set the dates for early December. I had checked with Henri to see if there was anything on his calendar – all clear, he said. He wouldn't be going with me, but I knew he wanted me to attend his annual year-end dinner for his museum volunteers. A few weeks after I booked my trip, he found out the restaurant was nearly fully booked for the holidays and could accommodate Henri's group only on the weekend I would be away. I could tell Henri was disappointed I wouldn't be attending, but I wasn't going to pass up a weekend in the Cotswolds and a Christmastime visit to London.

I arrived in London via Eurostar mid-afternoon and checked in at a charming townhouse hotel in Bayswater, near Hyde Park. I walked around the quiet lanes of the residential neighborhood and then grabbed a cab. My destination – a pilgrimage I made on every visit to London – was Liberty's, a venerable department store since 1875, where I always emerged, after an hour or two in the fabric department, with a bulging bag of Liberty's signature Tana lawn cotton. I already had an enormous stash of Liberty cotton. But as any quilter will say, you can't ever have too much fabric – especially when it comes from Liberty.

I restrained myself and purchased a few half-meter cuts that I could tuck into my handbag. I had a dinner scheduled that evening at the posh Royal Automobile Club and I didn't want to look like a tacky American tourist who shows up for an elegant dinner with her day's shopping.

I was glad I was unencumbered when I stepped out onto bustling Regent Street. It was about 6 p.m., the start of rush hour. The traffic was gridlocked. There wasn't a taxi in sight. I asked a man standing next to me, who was also trying to hail a cab, what was going on. There was some big summit meeting of world leaders, he said. He wished me luck and headed down the steps into a Tube station.

My dinner date was with Angie, the Texas lawyer I had met at Mean Girl's garden party the summer of my arrival in Giverny. Angie and I had stayed in touch. She was delighted to hear I was coming to London.

Angie was a member of the Royal Automobile Club and later that evening I would learn they had named a cocktail after her.

I still had an hour before we were to meet, but I started getting worried after a half hour had passed with no prospects of a taxi. I saw a tricycle rickshaw coming down Regent Street and weighed my options: arrive late or arrive in a vehicle that has never shown up at the entrance of the RAC.

I swallowed my pride and hailed the rickshaw.

I don't think my screams could be heard above the din of traffic. But when a double-decker bus nearly side-swiped us, I truly thought my time of death had come.

I'll never forget the moment when the RAC doorman offered his arm as I stepped out of my carriage. He stifled a laugh as he said "Madam!" with a hint of shock and awe.

I hastily headed for a ladies' room to recover my composure and tamp down my wildly wind-blown hair.

I met Angie in front of the RAC's towering and stunningly decorated Christmas tree. We had a delicious dinner along with a few rounds of the yummy champagne cocktail that bore her name.

I managed to get a taxi back to my hotel. Though, I must say, traveling by rickshaw is something I would do again, but maybe not down the busiest street of London.

The next day, I paid a visit to Buckingham Palace, as you do when you're in town. I've taken the palace tour many times and never tire of walking the red carpet into the Throne Room as if I'm a debutante at her royal presentation.

I especially loved the Queen's gift shops. After the big fire at Windsor Castle in 1992, she got wise to the income stream high-end souvenirs could bring to pay for the renovations and hired a team of savvy tchotchke marketers.

Back in the day when the Queen was still with us, her flagship gift shop, adjacent to the gates of the palace, bore her mark. She gave prominent shelf space to exquisite china tea sets, tins of biscuits and teas, an assortment of sweets and treats, tea towels (tea is a recurring theme), GOD SAVE THE QUEEN aprons, toiletries, and an array of liquor-and-bar items. There was an eye-catching display case with knock-offs of her priceless statement jewelry along with a few affordably priced tiaras. The tiaras tie in to the featured storybook in the children's section: "Does the Queen Wear Her Crown in Bed?" And to make sure you don't mess up your royal do, there are Buckingham Palace shower caps.

Among the most bizarre gift items were the Harry-and-Meghan pillboxes – perhaps a portent of the headaches to come with their defection to California?

At the core of the Queen's souvenir collection were her pet Corgis. Corgi plush toys abound, along with Corgi Christmas ornaments, Corgi jewelry charms, even Corgi silk pajamas at $300 a pair, along with a companion teddy bear in matching jammies ($260).

I loved Her Majesty's sense of humor. I bought her "Handbag Shortbread" – a regally wrapped tube of mini "original" Scottish shortbread biscuits, which, per the label, are meant "for emergencies."

I showed my purchase to the taxi driver who picked me up at the Palace gates. He laughed and shook his head. "The Queen knows how to make a quid."

I enjoyed my weekend in the Cotswolds. I had visited there years ago on a business trip to a nearby coal-mining operation, of all things. I was in my early 20s, a newly minted journalist just out of J-school. I was working for an energy newsletter company in Washington, D.C., during the energy crisis of the mid-1970s. The publisher had money to burn and had sent me off to England to do an article about a company that was pioneering something called "long-wall" mining, a technique that sheared coal from the walls of the mine, which was a lot safer than the old-school method of blowing up a mine shaft with dynamite and hoping for the best.

The company president had arranged an extensive tour of the Cotswolds for me. I fell in love with the area, especially its storybook stone cottages and the charming names of the villages: Chipping Camden, Stow-on-the-Wold, and Upper and Lower Slaughter.

My friend Gail met me at the station in Morton-on-the-Marsh and took me to lunch at a village pub decked out for Christmas. We sat by a roaring fire and spent much of the afternoon catching up. I hadn't seen her since our farewell lunch in Florence. Gail was the friend who advised me to pack a magic carpet in case I needed to escape my life in Giverny.

I told her I'd had a rough start. She wasn't surprised.

"You need to make friends with the Sister-Wife," Gail advised. "You'll never have an easy life there if she's against you."

My return trip to Giverny unraveled with the news of a French rail strike that had caused the cancellations of many Eurostar trains from London.

I was scheduled to travel on the biggest day of the strike, which was a Monday. Even if I could get to Paris, the scene there was a nightmare. The Metro wasn't running and taxis were scarce because drivers were striking in sympathy with the rail union.

It turned out that my Eurostar train to Paris was still running, but I knew for certain that the train I had booked from Paris to Vernon-Giverny had been cancelled. Henri called early that Monday morning to say the French rail line had added a few early-evening trains to the schedule, to help stranded passengers.

Within an hour, I boarded a London-bound train from the Cotswolds, feeling like I had been shot out of a cannon, for what would be a nine-hour travel day.

Even without a rail strike to deal with, there was an added complication. I had left a credit card at the Buckingham Palace gift shop during my visit there a few days earlier. I discovered it was missing on my last night in London and called the main number for the Palace the next morning as I was leaving for the Cotswolds. I couldn't believe a real person answered the phone (on the second ring, no less). She kindly put me through to the gift shop and a woman named Vienna confirmed my credit card was there. "We'll keep it in our safe, Madam, until you come on Monday to pick it up."

If ever you lose a credit card, it's reassuring to know it's waiting for you in a safe at Buckingham Palace.

Time was tight that Monday. I jumped in a taxi at London's Paddington Station and told the driver I needed to go to the Palace.

"Do you have something for the Queen?" he asked. "Like DNA results showing you're part of the Royal Family?"

I love London cabbies.

"Actually, she has something for me – my Mastercard."

I think I gave him the biggest laugh of his morning. Despite midday traffic, he got me to the Palace in no time at all and even gave me instructions to pass on to my next cab driver to avoid Tottenham Court Road en route to St. Pancras Station, where I needed to catch the Eurostar. Precious minutes were ticking away.

I had called the gift shop from the taxi and miraculously, Vienna answered the phone. "Yes, Madam, we'll get your card from the safe as soon as you arrive. Just bring some identification."

Vienna spotted me the moment I rolled my bag through the gift shop door and made quick work of retrieving my card. Minutes later, I was back on the curb, hailing my next taxi. The driver already knew that Tottenham Court Road was a mess and managed to deliver me to the station entrance 20 minutes before boarding closed for my Eurostar train.

But I was only halfway home.

The French woman sitting next to me on the train warned that Paris was in chaos – no Metro and very few taxis. She said we must prepare ourselves for a difficult evening. She was planning to walk two hours to her home, rolling her suitcase.

I immediately called Henri. He was contemplating a Plan B, if I got stranded in Paris. But I called just as he was about to take his afternoon nap and I sensed he hadn't yet fleshed out the details of Plan B. He told me to keep in touch.

KEEP IN TOUCH??!!

I bounded off the Eurostar at Gare du Nord in Paris and waited 10 minutes in the taxi queue. I needed to get across town to Gare St. Lazare. My driver looked at the rail app on his phone and said, "There's only one more train and it leaves in 20 minutes."

Nooooooo!

He kindly scribbled his name and phone number on a slip of paper in case I needed a ride later. I raced through St. Lazare station and went to three ticket offices before I found one that could issue me a new boarding pass. A man in line ahead of me assured me the queue was moving quickly. We were both hoping to get on the same train.

When I got to the counter, the agent looked at the clock. "The train leaves in five minutes." He fumbled with the boarding pass as it came out of the printer. He was almost as flustered as I was.

Train stations in Paris have barriers that require you to scan your ticket before you go onto the platform. I nervously swiped the boarding pass on the glass screen. The gate didn't open. I looked around in a panic and suddenly a hand reached over from the other side of the barrier and held my pass in the scanner beam.

It was the man who had been in line ahead of me. He smiled as the gate opened and off we ran together, down the platform. Just as the whistle blew, he grabbed my bag and helped me up the steps. We tumbled into seats opposite each other, winded and laughing. We had made it – with barely a minute to spare.

He spoke little English and my little French wasn't enough to express my heart-felt appreciation. He had saved me from a long night alone in Paris, waiting for Henri to implement his sketchy Plan B.

I took out my phone and wrote a message, with a translation app, to my Travel Angel: *I am very grateful today for the kindness of strangers. Merci beaucoup.*

He smiled at the message and pressed his hand to his chest. In French, he said, "Destiny. Humanity."

Chapter 30

On the day before an estate sale was to begin at the house that had been my family's home for 47 years in Naperville, Illinois, I was on my last walk through the rooms when an open box of Christmas ornaments caught my eye.

A sweet familiar face smiled up at me. She was one of my favorite ornaments from childhood – a pretty girl with blonde curls tucked beneath a pale-blue scarf embellished with flowers. She had come from a distant land called Austria, a gift from an uncle who had been stationed there after World War II. She always had pride of place on a prominent branch of our Christmas tree each year.

I couldn't possibly leave her behind. I tucked her in my pocket – and then, of course, a few more followed.

There's something about Christmas ornaments that tell the story of our lives – our loved ones, our travels, our favorite things, our memories of childhood and Christmases past. Many of my ornaments are handmade, by my grandmothers, quilting friends, and some by me. I made a quilted rocking horse embroidered with my son's name the year he was born. He gave me an ornament he made when he was about six. As I unwrapped his little package, he said, "I made you a quilt, Mom." A quilt, indeed – perhaps the only one ever made of pipe cleaners.

I hung my colorful pipe-cleaner quilt and the lovely Austrian girl on my little Christmas tree at the Little House, along with the rocking horse, a Scottie dog (in memory of my family's beloved pet named Kilty), two birds a-nesting in a coiled-brass pot scrubber (from my Girl Scout days), and tiny mittens that clamp onto branches with the assist of spring-loaded pin-curl clips – Grammy Stout's ingenuity. (In the off-season, the mittens were useful as bookmarks.) Atop the tree, I placed an embroidered angel I had made for my first Christmas in a home of my own. And my favorite: a photo ornament of my newborn son in his Santa jammies. All of these ornaments had been in storage for the past 10 years. It was wonderful seeing them on a tree again.

The notable new additions to my Christmas decorations joined the friendly beasts by the manger. Henri and I had found a little ram and a goat, who looked like Doo-Doo and Praline, at a Christmas market in Salzburg during our recent trip to Austria.

Christmas dinner that year took place in Henri's apartment. As I walked in the front door, I flashed back to the year before, when I had entertained the family at my Christmas open house. This year I was a guest in what had been my home. Bernadette was the hostess, overseeing the preparations in the kitchen. I tried to let it all roll off my back. I sat toward the end of the table next to a woman in her 40s, the daughter of Henri's relatives who owned the Little House. She was pleasant and we chatted about this and that. And then she asked a question that pierced my heart.

"Do you feel homesick at Christmas?"

I held back tears. I resented her insensitivity, but I knew she didn't realize her stupidity.

"Yes," I said. "My heart aches today."

～♪

A few weeks later, Henri and I were headed to Ibiza – at last. We had booked the same house, where Henri had taken himself to the year before while I was in California.

We covered every square mile of that island during our week's stay. Henri knew all the side roads, some of them barely roads at all. One day, he drove down a nearly washed-out track that cut through a grove of centuries-old gnarled olive trees and stopped at the end of a rutted driveway, blocked off by a swag of heavy chain. Henri parked the car.

"This is where Camille and I used to live," he said quietly.

"Would you like to take a stroll down memory lane?" I asked. "I'll wait here."

He sat in silence for a moment and then shook his head. We continued on our way.

Henri gave me an amazing tour of Ibiza. We traveled its rugged coastline, dotted with pirate watchtowers, lighthouses and beach clubs. The almond trees, which were blooming during our visit, looked like they were dusted with snow. We had paella to die for at Henri's favorite restaurant, perched on a cliff with a view of the Ses Margalides Islands that seemed to float like giant sun loungers in the sea.

On our last day, we went to a restaurant on the beach, where waiters adroitly balanced trays with immense pitchers of sangria. After a delicious seafood lunch, Henri and I settled into a cushioned settee, soaking up the last sun of the afternoon. I was mesmerized by the gentle waves lapping the shoreline of the cove where we sat, with its postcard view of a lighthouse on a promontory that jutted into the sea.

Our waiter took a photo of us – it's my favorite of Henri and me. We're leaning against each other, beaming with happiness. We truly look like we don't have a care in the world.

I would often remember that carefree day, yearning to relive it. Like so many life-changing events that were looming on the horizon, we had no idea of what was coming.

Chapter 31

In the weeks after our return from Ibiza, we heard news almost daily about a virus that was spreading in China.

We were used to seeing masked Chinese tourists in Giverny. They looked like alien creatures, often moving through the village in large groups, all wearing white surgical masks. I understood their caution, given the viruses that had been a concern in Asia. But it always seemed unnecessary in the bucolic hamlet of Giverny.

The first Covid case in France was a Chinese tourist, who had been admitted to a Paris hospital in late January and died a few weeks later. It was the first Covid death outside of Asia.

As more cases began popping up around Europe, I said to Henri, "We could be dealing with this for months. Do you think it's going to be bad?

I'll never forget Henri's reply. "I think this is going to change our lives."

~

The first Covid lockdown in France was announced by President Macron during a live address to the nation on March 14, at 8 p.m. It was a Saturday. He instructed all restaurants, cafes, bars, clubs, and cinemas in France to close at midnight – in just four hours. Schools, theaters, museums and non-essential businesses were to close as well. The only places allowed to remain open were food stores, pharmacies, banks, petrol stations and "tabac" shops, which sell cigarettes, newspapers and lotto tickets.

By Tuesday, March 17, the entire population of France would begin confinement in their homes. Valid reasons for leaving home: food shopping, trips to the pharmacy, medical appointments, caring for vulnerable people, childcare needs, pet care and personal exercise (no group sports).

The rules, to be enforced by the police, were strict: We couldn't go out without a government-issued document called an *attestation*, stating our name, address, date and place of birth, and the reason for leaving our quarantine location. We even had to indicate the time of our departure and weren't allowed to be out for more than an hour. For exercise outings, we had to stay within one kilometer (about a half mile) from our quarantine address.

Fines for violators started at 135 euros ($150). Repeat offenders faced much stiffer penalties.

Curfews went into place in some parts of France, including the French Riviera where the nightlife and beach scene are so enticing. In Giverny, the local gendarmes set up road blocks to intercept Parisians who had slipped out of the city for a play day *en plein air*.

For me, the police surveillance added a huge layer of stress. I was staying in France on a long-term "visiteur" visa and feared I could run into big trouble if I got stopped.

During the first week of confinement, I needed to get some cash. Giverny shut down its only ATM machine during the off-season, so I would have to go to my bank in Vernon, several miles away. Henri wrote out what I should say if I got stopped.

The thought of having to explain myself to the police in a language I don't speak well was overwhelming. I asked him to come with me.

The police didn't like seeing more than one person in a vehicle, but we took a chance. Henri stayed in the car while I went to the ATM machine. We decided not to stop for groceries on the way back lest we be seen getting out of the car together. It was an uneasy ride home. But fortunately, there were no police on patrol that day.

I hated going to the grocery store. I'd mentally hold my breath as I walked through the door. We didn't have masks during the first lockdown. The stores ran out of hand sanitizer and disinfectant wipes during the early weeks and those items weren't restocked for months. Even liquid hand soap disappeared from the shelves.

On the day before the first lockdown began, there was panic buying at the store where we always shopped. Henri loaded a cart with toilet paper, much to my embarrassment. When we approached the checkout counter with our separate carts, I told him I wasn't going to stand in the same line with him. "You're acting like an American," I teased him. But unlike the U.S., France never ran out of toilet paper.

~

The situation in Italy was far worse. Initially, the hardest hit areas were Lombardy and Veneto. But the virus spread rapidly and by early March, all of Italy – 60 million people – were in lockdown. So many people were dying. I cried when I saw a photo of a nurse slumped over a desk, sobbing from grief and exhaustion. By the end of 2020, Italy's Covid death toll reached 100,000.

A dear friend named Rachel, who lived in Florence, had started a donation box at her neighborhood grocery store, for food and supplies for healthcare workers at the local hospitals.

"I put a bottle of brandy in the box," Rachel told me on Skype one day. "And I bought one for myself as well."

Suddenly, she said, "I hear music!" She carried her laptop to the living room window so I could share the moment. Neighbors shouted out greetings from their open apartment windows as the music played.

It became a daily noontime ritual in much of Italy: Everyone singing to each other from their windows and balconies. My former neighbor, an Englishwoman named Beth, wrote on Facebook: "We all sang out the windows, waved and called out to neighbors, and well, cried our eyes out. We'll be doing it again tomorrow at 12.00. We're all alone, but nobody's alone!"

~~

In the early weeks of the first lockdown, the French government allowed people to change their quarantine locations. This was mainly for Parisians, who had properties in the countryside or at the seaside and wanted to escape the city.

Bernadette, who lived across the river in Vernon, informed Henri that she was going to move her son Jérémy, who also had an apartment in Vernon, to the apartment next to Henri's museum, where a guest room and bathroom – along with Henri's office – adjoined the family kitchen. Her son had been furloughed from his job as a groundskeeper at a mental-health facility. He wasn't coping well being home alone, so Bernadette decided he should move to the apartment. He could be outdoors and help Henri in his workshop. Jérémy had a mental impairment, which would entitle Bernadette to come to the property to "care" for him, which I suspected was a big part of why she wanted to make this change.

When Henri told me about this, I said, "Surely, you're not going to agree to this. You're in your office every day. Adding two more people to the mix downstairs is going to increase your risk of exposure and mine."

He assured me he wouldn't let that happen. But the next day, while Henri was sitting with me in my living room at the Little House, Bernadette called and told him she would be moving Jérémy to the apartment later that afternoon.

Henri had her on speaker, but the volume wasn't loud enough for me to hear her clearly. He told her he didn't want that – it was too dangerous. I could hear the anger in her voice. She apparently hung up on him.

"What's happening?" I asked.

"She's bringing Jérémy to the apartment today, to stay."

"But you told her it wasn't safe."

I could see Henri wasn't making this decision. Bernadette had taken charge.

"You need to call her back. This isn't safe for any of us."

I worried about Henri. He had been a smoker for 60 years and was prone to debilitating bouts of bronchitis every winter. I'd read stories about people with pre-existing respiratory problems dying of Covid.

He called her back and the conversation didn't go any better. She hung up on him again. After the third try, with another hang-up, he said, "I need to go speak with her in person."

Later that evening, I joined him for dinner at his apartment. We were bending the rules, traveling back and forth to see each other. I carried my attestation form, checking the box saying that I was helping someone in need.

He told me that evening he had been adamant with Bernadette. He didn't elaborate, but assured me once again that Jérémy and Bernadette wouldn't be on the scene.

~⁀

The quarantine period in France had been extended to mid-April, but it would likely go longer. Monet's Gardens announced it hoped to open May 1, with government approval, a month later than usual. But that sounded unrealistically optimistic to me.

I had driven by the front gate of the gardens on a rare outing. Surprisingly, the gate was open. A work crew was grooming the *Grande Allée*. Daffodils and tulips were blooming right on time. They knew nothing about Covid.

On my way home from the grocery store one day, I took the back road. Just beyond the Tree Tunnel, I stopped the car at the side of the road and put down the window. It was late afternoon, when the light is lovely. I turned off the engine and just sat for a bit, listening to the sounds of the woods around me. Birds were chirping, not all in the same language. I'm not an expert on bird chatter, but I don't think they were talking about a deadly virus that was reshaping the human world. But then, who was I to know.

Not another car passed as I sat soaking up the serenity around me. I just needed a few minutes to decompress from the dire news that had been pounding us day after day.

This, too, will pass, I kept telling myself. But the loss was already enormous. How will the world heal from this, I wondered.

I wept on Easter (April 12, 2020) as I watched the "Music for Hope" concert with Andrea Bocelli that showed major cities around the world in lockdown, with haunting images of the nearly deserted streets of Florence, Venice, Rome, Madrid, Warsaw, Paris, London, New York, Mexico City, Cape Town, São Paulo, Buenos Aires, Los Angeles and Beijing. I couldn't control my sobs as Andrea Bocelli sang "Amazing Grace" on the steps of the cathedral in Milan, to an empty piazza.

Sometimes Henri and I talked about different scenarios that started with "if you get sick" or "if I get sick." But those sentences usually ended with a reassuring squeeze of hands (despite warnings about no hand contact). It was a small gesture of love in the Time of Corona.

And then came the tragic news that Henri's Camille had died. Henri didn't tell me whether it was Covid that took her, only that she was gone. He said they would postpone a memorial gathering for her until the restrictions were lifted. My heart ached for him.

Chapter 32

Finally, after two months of confinement, the Covid case numbers started coming down in France.

The government eased some of the restrictions, allowing travel 100 kilometers (60 miles) from home – *"à vol d'oiseau"* (as a bird flies) was the exact wording of the new decree. With a straight-line radius forming our outer limit, we didn't have to worry about losing precious kilometers with every bend in the road.

But actually, distance didn't matter to Henri and me. We were content just having a day out and the freedom to wander.

We drove through the Normandy countryside on a beautiful May day. The weather was gorgeous – sunny skies, nice breezes.

We ended up in Gerberoy, the village where I had slit a tire on my first visit there two years earlier. We chose to leave Henri's car in a parking area to avoid a repeat of our previous mishap.

Restaurants and cafes in France weren't open yet, so we stopped at a boulangerie to get sandwiches. We ate our picnic lunch on a bench under a chestnut tree in the heart of the village.

Gerberoy's famous roses were in bloom. As we walked the cobbled streets, we stopped often to take a whiff.

Our next stop was the nearby resort town of Forges-les-Eaux, but the park we had hoped to see was still closed. Instead, we sat by a sparkling pond and enjoyed watching the ducks. One seemed to fall from the sky as he came in for a long graceful landing, using his webbed feet as water skis. There was a lone Canadian goose among them. A fellow foreigner, an ocean away from home.

As we sat in the sun, I was transfixed by the pinpoints of light dancing on the ripples of the water.

I hadn't felt so relaxed in weeks. It was a day of simple pleasures, *"à vol d'oiseau."*

~⁀〜

That summer, Henri's son Paul, his wife Leisha and their 12-year-old daughter Sareena came to Giverny for a visit. The opportunity to travel again was such a boost. We gathered at our favorite little restaurant on the Ru.

Paul and Leisha were planning to go to the seaside the next day and asked Henri and me to join them.

Henri said, "No, no."

That surprised me. *"Pourquoi pas?* Why not?"

"I don't like the beach," Henri said.

"Henri, this isn't about the beach. It's about being with your family," I said, squeezing his hand. "What I wouldn't do to have a day with my son." I hadn't seen Kyle in almost a year.

I looked over at Paul and gave him a little nod.

The next morning, seven of us piled into Paul's big SUV. Henri's other son Alex and his son Luc had joined the party.

We had a relaxing day in Dieppe, on the shore of the English Channel, lounging on the pebbly beach. Sareena and Luc played in the surf. We ended the day with rosy cheeks from sun exposure we hadn't experienced in months.

The next day, after a family dinner at Henri's apartment, he informed me that we had been invited to a dinner party the following evening at Yuka's. He and I were alone at his dining table when this conversation started. Paul, Leisha and Alex were in the kitchen, cleaning up.

I quietly asked him, "Will Bernadette be there?" I hadn't seen her since his big blowup with her during the early weeks of confinement.

"Yes, I think she'll be there," he said.

"Henri, this is very awkward for me."

Leisha appeared and sat down at the table across from me. She apparently had overheard the start of our conversation. Paul and Alex joined us.

I didn't know what more to say, now that we had an audience.

I looked at the assembled group and said, "There's a problem with Bernadette."

"We know," Leisha said. "What she wanted to do wasn't safe."

They knew. I later learned that Bernadette had told them what had happened during the lockdown, but I had the feeling that, in her version of the story, I was the one who had prevented Jérémy from moving to the downstairs apartment.

"I agree," Alex said. "It was very risky."

I was grateful that they saw the danger in Bernadette's plan. But there was now an open wound between Bernadette and Henri – and me – that was on public display.

~⌇

I always felt like I was picking my way through a labyrinth of trip wires with Henri's family. There were times when I truly felt it wasn't my place to be present.

One evening, Henri announced that Camille's memorial gathering would be in a few days and that he'd like me to attend. It was going to be held at the home he and Camille had shared in Giverny, just behind her parents' house.

I didn't say anything at first, but the next day, I told Henri I wanted him to have this time of remembrance without me. I knew it was going to be a large gathering of her family and friends. I didn't want to feel conspicuous as the woman who had replaced her. More than anything, I wanted Henri to freely experience the memory of her and find some closure.

I had gone out for a long walk with Sarah that afternoon. When I came home, it was early evening. Henri was sitting on a bar stool in the kitchen making a salad for our dinner.

He looked up at me. His eyes were red. "We used to live there, at that house…"

I could see he was overwhelmed. "Oh, my love," I said as I went to him.

I cradled him in my arms as he wept.

~

By the fall of 2020, the Covid numbers were rising as people returned to offices and children went back to school.

The government did nothing until the daily cases topped 25,000. On October 30, the curtain came crashing down with another lockdown that would last at least a month. Under the new restrictions, friends and families weren't allowed to gather. There were already concerns about Christmas.

We barely had 24 hours to prepare. The day before the lockdown began, a Thursday, people flocked to grocery stores and hair salons. Traffic out of Paris was a gridlock of headlights as those with somewhere else to go headed out of the city.

Earlier in the week, I had suspected another lockdown was coming and had stocked up on toilet paper, masks and hand soap, along with a backup supply of the basics. I got cash and gas and refilled prescriptions.

So on the last day of freedom, I wasn't in a panic. I went to the hair salon (a guilty pleasure) and afterward, sat in my car for a few minutes taking in the scene. It felt a little like Christmas Eve with last-minute shoppers scurrying about. I noticed the bookstore was doing a brisk business. Sadly, it would close at midnight along with all "non-essential" businesses. (I would argue books are absolutely essential in a pandemic.)

I also noticed a lot of people buying flowers, especially pots of chrysanthemums. It seemed a bit odd, but later I learned that it's a French tradition to take flowers to the graves of loved ones, in celebration of All Saints' Day, on November 1. Confinement restrictions had been eased to allow people to visit cemeteries.

As I sat in my car, I thought about items that might not be easy to get in the next weeks and possibly months. During the last lockdown, online shopping wasn't a sure bet because the postal service was so slow. In fact, in Giverny, mail delivery was cut back to a few days a week.

I was parked in front of a wonderful bakery with tempting pastries in the window. My first purchase of the afternoon: 2 freshly baked chocolate fondant cupcakes, for dessert that evening.

Within the next hour or so, I had loaded my car with little treasures:

~ 2 Christmas cactuses, to brighten my kitchen window

~ 1 flat of pansies for the window box

~ 1 bucket of birdseed for my feathered friends who had roosted at my place the previous winter

~ 1 ream of printer paper and an ink cartridge to print those horrible forms we had to carry, stating our reason for leaving home

~ 1 roll of cheerful Christmas wrapping paper and matching ribbon (an impulse purchase as I was waiting in line to pay for the paper and ink)

I felt a little better, especially after dessert that evening. I saved part of my cupcake to have with a cup of tea the next day. Henri devoured his.

The next day, French news reported that the two items in high demand during Thursday's shopping frenzy were ink cartridges and yoga mats.

~~~

As the November lockdown dragged on, there was a public outcry about the government's ban on the sale of "non-essential" items.

As of October 30, the government had forced all "non-essential" businesses in France to close. Grocery stores, including large super-markets, remained open, with many offering a wide range of merchandise beyond food and basic household supplies. Non-essential businesses cried foul, complaining that supermarkets shouldn't be allowed to sell non-essential goods. After a few days of protests, with some small shops defying closure orders, the government ordered supermarkets to stop selling non-essential items and issued a list of banned merchandise.

As a result, for most of November, no store in France was allowed to sell books, toys, DVDs, CDs, clothing, jewelry, textiles, large household appliances, home-decor items and flowers. (The decree didn't apply to online shopping, which caused another uproar along with a petition to boycott Amazon during the holiday season.)

At our local supermarket, white shrouds covered shelves of black-listed items. Books disappeared entirely from the racks. I saw a child crying at the end of an aisle of toys, that were in plain view, but that had been taped off as contraband. One day, I noticed a cloth strip concealing a shelf above the paper napkins: I peeked underneath to see...CANDLES.

No candles to be had in the darkness of a pandemic? I suddenly felt inspired to write a dystopian tale.

When Henri and I sat down to our Frenchified Thanksgiving dinner, we lit the last candle from our pre-Covid stock. Henri cut the last flower in the garden for our centerpiece. The sad-looking hollyhock, drooping in its vase, perfectly captured the mood of 2020.

There was a collective sigh of national relief when the government finally backed down and allowed non-essential businesses to re-open in time for holiday shopping. In a surprising show of unity, big box stores, small shops and Amazon France agreed to postpone Black Friday sales for a week, until December 4. I took little comfort in seeing the restoration of "Black Friday." What a horrible custom America had exported to Europe. But at least it was bolstering a collapsing economy that had become a worrying side effect of Covid.

Penalties for disobeying Covid rules had escalated: Three-peat offenders could face fines of $9,000 and six months in prison.

A black man in Paris was brutalized by police for not wearing a mask, which was caught on video. The French government was pushing for a new law to restrict the filming of police.

Henri's 93-year-old cousin remarked wryly about the heavy-handedness of the French police during the pandemic. "Life was easier when the Germans were here."

In a surprise shift, the government ended the lockdown on December 15 and implemented a national curfew from 8 p.m. till 6 a.m. The prime minister cautioned, "It will be strictly controlled with limited possibilities for exemption." The curfew would be lifted on Christmas Eve, but gatherings would be limited to six people. There would be no curfew exemption on New Year's Eve.

There was no longer a need to carry an attestation during the day, but one would be required for any nighttime outings. Valid reasons for going out at night were limited to travel between home and work, health issues, compelling family matters, and taking a pet for a walk.

Police surveillance would increase. Since the beginning of the second lockdown, the Ministry of the Interior reported there had been 2,924,775 police checks.

It was a lonely Christmas. Henri and I had brunch at my place and then we took a long drive in the countryside.

We came upon a spot that I remembered from a day trip I had taken with the artists' group that had stayed at the moulin.

It had been a stunning fall day, with the shadows of billowy white clouds shapeshifting on the fields. An ancient stone cross stood by the road, marking the way for soldiers during the Crusades.

"Henri, stop the car," I said when I saw the cross. Ever since our outing that day, I had never been able to find this spot.

I stood at the side of the road, watching the sun dip beneath the distant ridge, and could hear the chatter and laughter of our painting group that day. I ached for life as we had known it.

I longed for the day when friends and family could come visit me in my little corner of paradise and I could bring them to see this gorgeous view from a road that dated back to the Crusades.

THAT was my Christmas wish and my hope for the new year.

~⁀

On the day before New Year's Eve, Henri brought home a crate of English Channel oysters. I had seen the crates stacked outside the fish shop in Vernon, which was doing a brisk business.

We savored our treat. The oysters were juicy and plump, fresh from briny waters. We drank champagne and toasted what we hoped would be a much better year to come.

It was past 8 p.m. when Henri and I got in his SUV for the quick drive back to my place, just a half mile down the road. We were in the habit of taking a track road, not far from Henri's front gate that went above the village and dropped down near the front gate of the Little House.

We used to laugh on these clandestine expeditions, with the head-lights off, feeling like we were a couple of teenagers out after curfew. We never worried too much. Police didn't patrol sleepy Giverny.

Henri had thrown a bag of oyster shells into the back of his SUV. There would be garbage pickup the next day.

He stopped at the end of the driveway and had lifted the lid off the garbage can when headlights appeared, coming down the road from the end of the Tree Tunnel. I wondered who else was out at this hour. Apparently, we weren't the only renegades in the neighborhood.

A van stopped at the gate. I assumed it was a neighbor. But then I saw GENDARMERIE on the door.

What transpired in the next few minutes felt like a scene in a war movie to me.

A female officer got out of the police van on the passenger side and shone a flashlight in Henri's face. She asked what he was doing and he said something about *poubelle,* the French word for "trash."

I bit my lip, stifling a giggle. I thought, who drives to the end of their driveway to take out the trash?

The female officer noticed me in the front seat and asked Henri who I was.

"*Ma femme,*" he said.

Oh, Henri, what a stupid thing to say, I thought. In French, *femme* means "woman" or "wife." I clearly was a woman, but I wasn't his wife.

The driver got out of the van and was in attack mode. He shone a flashlight on Henri and asked if he had been drinking. Henri said no, but I knew he couldn't worm his way out of that lie. The officer told him he was going perform a breath test.

At that point, I felt more outraged than intimidated. We hadn't yet driven onto the street. We were still in the driveway, on Henri's private property. The pit bull had no authority to do anything to us.

He turned his flashlight on me and asked Henri who I was. Henri changed his story and identified me as his *copine* (girlfriend).

The female officer upbraided Henri for changing his story. In French, she said, a girlfriend is not a wife. *Damn straight,* I said to myself, but I knew this wasn't the moment to link arms with a like-minded French soul sister.

Pitt Bull said something to me in French. I couldn't hear him because of the engine noise from both Henri's SUV and the police van.

When I didn't answer, he barked, "*Parlez-vous français?*"

"*Un petit peu,*" I said with a hint of a Southern Belle accent that sounded a bit like Scarlett O'Hara in *Gone with the Wind.*

For added emphasis, Henri told him I didn't speak much French.

With the flashlight in my eyes, he asked in English, "Where are you from?"

"The United States," I said, squinting. This guy was pissing me off.

"Where do you live?" he shouted.

"Rue de Falaise." I didn't give the house number.

He didn't seem to know where that was. Still shouting, he ordered us to go back to the house where he said we had to stay until 6 a.m.

Henri got in the SUV and turned around.

We didn't speak until we were back inside. Henri poured shots of calvados for us both. We sat in the living room that was lit only by the Christmas tree.

I could see Henri was shaken.

"He had nothing on us," I said. "We were on your property. The car wheels were in your driveway. You can't breathalyze someone when they're taking out the trash."

He lay his head against the back of his overstuffed armchair. "That's the American in you talking, *chérie*." He sipped the calvados and let it roll on his tongue. Then he said, "He could have done anything he wanted."

~~

I didn't sleep a wink that night. I finally got out of bed at 4 a.m. and sat in the living room in the glow of the tree.

At 6, I woke Henri and asked him to take me home.

It was that day, on the last day of 2020, that I made my decision to move back to the U.S. I couldn't – wouldn't–live in a police state that had become drunk with its authority.

Chapter 33

My life with Henri changed after the curfew went into place. The screw tightened when the start time moved from 8 p.m. to 6 p.m., after the holidays.

Henri and I no longer had dinners together. We could have seen each other in the evenings, with me arriving at his place before 6 p.m. and then spending the night. But I didn't sleep well at Henri's. He often got up at night and had a snack in the kitchen, which was next to my bedroom. I'd hear a bar stool scrape across the floor or the sound of the fridge or a cupboard opening and closing. Sometimes, it took a while for me to get back to sleep.

In our new routine, the only time I saw Henri was in the morning when he'd stop by for coffee. He'd stay for a half hour and then head out to run errands or meet friends. We were allowed to be out during the day.

I was reluctant to leave home because of Covid. When the vaccine rollout began, I took heart. I watched with envy as my friends in the U.S. starting posting on Facebook that they had gotten their first dose as early as January.

Other than healthcare workers, only those over 75 or with compromised immune systems were eligible for the vaccine in France. Henri, then 77, signed up for his appointment in the first days after the Pfizer vaccine was available, in mid-January. But within several weeks, Pfizer temporarily halted its European operation in order to gear up for expanded production. France kept aside enough vaccine for its initial recipients, like Henri, to get a second dose. But the rest of the country had to wait another couple of months for more vaccine.

Later in January, Kyle and Julia called me to announce their engagement. I was thrilled and loved hearing the story of how he proposed. He had written a poem that sent her on a scavenger hunt. I found out later that he had hoped to plant the last clue somewhere at Disneyland Paris. But Covid scuttled that idea.

They were planning a November wedding in northern California, near Walnut Creek where they lived. Julia's grandmother was a member of a country club in nearby Danville and had helped them book a date – not an easy task with so many couples looking for wedding venues because of postponements during Covid.

A week later, France announced a travel ban that prevented people living in France from leaving the European Union without proof of an urgent reason to travel – weddings didn't make the list. Non-French residents were allowed to return to their home countries, but France made no guarantee that we'd be allowed back in.

That absolutely was the last straw.

I began planning my exit. I decided I wouldn't travel until I got both doses of the vaccine, so that was the first hurdle. The rollout hadn't resumed yet in France, but there were reports that appointments would become available again in March.

I checked the appointment website daily. One night at midnight, a few dozen time slots appeared at the hospital in Vernon. I was able to schedule both doses. The second would be March 31.

Henri, who had already gotten his second dose, was delighted for me. I was under the age requirement of 75, but I had an underlying condition that made it possible for me to jump the queue.

He knew I was at wit's end and understood my anxiety when the travel ban went into place.

"I need to have a home base in my home country," I told him. "Never in my life, in all the traveling I've done, have I ever experienced the panic of not being able to return home."

During the first two days after the ban was announced, there was a notice on the website of the U.S. Embassy in Paris saying they were seeking "clarification" from the French government. Finally, the embassy confirmed Americans could return to the U.S. for any reason. But if the purpose wasn't urgent, France could refuse re-entry.

"How can I go to Kyle and Julia's wedding, not knowing if I can return to France?"

"*Chérie,* the ban is going to be over by summer," he assured me. "France wants to bring tourists back."

"I can't wait until summer to see what happens. If I'm going to move back to the States, I have to start planning now."

I asked Henri if he wanted to be part of the new life I was contemplating. "I know you would never consider moving to the States with me," I said, testing the water. "Your life is here."

He nodded.

"Could we figure out a way to split our time between California and Giverny?" I asked.

He thought about that for a moment and then said, "My answer is no answer."

I tried not to let that land as a gut punch. "Then that's a no," I said matter-of-factly. "I will make all the decisions for this move on my own."

"I want you to be happy, *chérie,*" he said. "I won't get in your way."

~

I began to think seriously of where I would go. My friend who had been renting the condo in Del Mar, where I had stayed with Kyle and Julia, told me that she and her husband had decided to retire and move to Spain and would likely be leaving in May.

It was mid-March at that point. I spoke with her landlady who was delighted to take me as a tenant.

I started contacting shipping companies. A container ship had run aground in the Suez Canal, creating an impasse that had left 400 ships in a bottleneck. The ripple effect had disrupted shipping schedules globally. Containers were waiting to be loaded on ships and piling up at ports.

After days of futile searching, a U.K. shipping company found a container that could be loaded in Giverny within two weeks, but I had to make the payment by the close of business that day – within two hours. The cost: $18,000. I charged it to two credit cards and circled the pick-up date on my kitchen calendar. The ship would sail for California from the Normandy port of Le Havre on May 1.

Those days were a blur of bubble wrap coming off a giant roll that I had propped next to my kitchen table at the Little House. The movers would wrap and pack everything, but I wanted to give extra attention to my Limoges wedding china and Waterford champagne flutes. I enthusiastically had unpacked most of it when I moved to the Little House in 2019, thinking I would be having dinner parties. I never imagined I'd be alone, with only a half hour of human contact each day.

As I wrapped my fragile treasures, I felt remarkably calm. From my kitchen table, I had a view of the Prairie in all its spring glory.

Chapter 34

The Seine had flooded the Prairie and other low-lying pastures in Giverny that spring.

An historic property named Le Vivier (The Fish Pond), just down the road from the moulin, had taken a direct hit. The owner, who had a herd of goats, brought them to Doo-Doo Land, the name I had given the corral in my Facebook posts about Doo-Doo and Praline.

Because the corral sat on high ground – and also because Henri was an animal lover – Doo-Doo Land had become Giverny's animal refuge in times of flooding. A few years earlier, during another flood, Maxine and Olivier's menagerie of wallabies, kangaroos, an alpaca and two emus along with their flock of dark-colored Ouessant sheep (Doo-Doo's breed) were evacuated to Doo-Doo Land. Henri sprayed a red X on Doo-Doo's back so he wouldn't get lost in the crowd when it was time for the flock to return home.

The goat evacuees caused a disturbance in Doo-Doo Land. The boss of the herd was a Billy Goat Gruff, who had big horns, an impressively long goatee and plenty of attitude. He liked pushing Doo-Doo off the hillock. Surprisingly, Doo-Doo didn't push back. He seemed to know he was sorely outnumbered.

The hillock, which had been reduced in size after Henri had plowed under an invasive patch of nettles, had become a popular spot for group gatherings and sunbathing. I had noticed there was no social distancing and wondered about "herd immunity," a concept that had emerged in the Covid age.

The darling of the herd was a baby goat with severely bowed legs. I called her Baby Girl. She was bullied by Billy Goat Gruff, who used to toss her in the air like a rag doll. But she'd always clamber back to her feet and carry on. Strangely, she was alone in the herd. There was never a mama close by. She ate constantly and devoured the tender grass that grew along the corral fence. With her bowed legs, she was low to the ground and could reach where the bigger goats couldn't.

Henri took her to his museum workshop, where he and his team of mechanics designed splints to straighten her legs. For two months, they fashioned new splints as she grew. On the day they finally removed them for good, I nearly cried watching her run and jump around the corral. It was as if Henri and his team had put springs in her legs.

When the flood waters receded, the owner of the herd gave Baby Girl to Henri as a gift, along with another goat in the herd that he identified as her mother. He told us she was a young mom, barely more than a year old herself when she gave birth.

Henri had told him I had a written a book about Giverny's Impressionist era and asked if we could visit Le Vivier. I was delighted when the owner invited us to come by for drinks one afternoon.

Le Vivier, with a two-story cottage situated on the banks of the Ru, is a secluded property barely visible from the main road. Its high walls surround a fish pond and a garden where, in Monet's time, artists painted nudes. Although nude models were common in the studios of Paris, it pushed the limits of decorum to have nudity on display in a garden, no matter how secluded. The models luxuriated on sun-dappled linens or were depicted shedding their clothes before taking a dip in the pond. Ironically, the pond had a somewhat sacred past. It was where the monks of ancient Giverny used to breed fish. During Giverny's art-colony days, Le Vivier became known as the "nymph pasture." The fish had strayed from their divine origins, devouring mosquitoes that threatened to blemish the pearly skin of the naked ladies.

An arched stone bridge crossed one end of the pond. A painted white pergola sat on top of the bridge, its pillars supported by stone blocks carved with the bearded faces of kingly men.

Henri and I had a lovely afternoon at Le Vivier. The owner and his wife were very grateful for Henri's kindness during the flood. I gave them a signed copy of *The Secret of Marie*, with a page marker at Chapter Four. The love affair between the main characters in the story blossoms in Le Vivier's garden.

In that scene, Gérard, the Frenchman who owns the moulin where the story takes place, and Kate, the visiting American writer who's a guest at the moulin, are looking at a book of nude studies that had been painted in the garden by Frederick Carl Frieseke, a well-known American artist in Giverny who was from Owosso, Michigan. In a letter to a friend, Frieseke had written: *I am more free in France. There are not the Puritanical restrictions which prevail in America – here I can paint the nude out of doors.* It seemed Frieseke had a streak of mischief. On his first visit back home to Owosso in 1902, he told a friend, "I get much pleasure in shocking the good Church people with the nudes."

That evening at my place, Henri and I enjoyed looking through a beautiful Frieseke book I had purchased on a visit to the Metropolitan Museum in New York a few years earlier. The book had added a couple of pounds to my suitcase, but it was too beautiful to pass up.

Much like the scene that unfolds in Chapter Four of *Marie*, Henri and I, aroused by the erotic beauty of the paintings, found ourselves enjoying pleasures of the flesh that Giverny's hedonistic American rebels painted so well.

Later, as we lay satiated on damp bedsheets, Henri ran a finger along the curve of my back and smiled. "My father and his friends, who were teenagers then, used to prop a ladder against the garden wall at Le Vivier and spy on the naked women."

What I didn't realize during our visit to Le Vivier was that Henri was keeping a secret from me.

Early that morning, he had found Praline dead under the shed.

Praline belonged to Bernadette, who took responsibility for her and Doo-Doo's care.

Henri had called Bernadette immediately to tell her. While he and I had been enjoying our afternoon at Le Vivier, Bernadette had buried Praline – digging her grave next to the hillock and dragged her carcass across the corral. She later told Henri that Doo-Doo had stood by, watching.

When Henri broke the news to me later that night, I had a vision of this as a movie scene: Bernadette alone, sweating and shoveling dirt into the grave, with operatic death-scene music – *The Godfather* soundtrack came to mind – playing in the background, with inter-cuts to Henri and me, in the throes of passion.

The week before Praline died, I had noticed a big change in her. Her udders had turned black and were so swollen they dragged on the ground as she walked.

I asked Henri if a vet should come.

"She's very old," he said. "It's her time."

I sat with her a few days before she died. She was half asleep, sunning herself by the corral gate. She looked serene.

I thought about the day she bent the gate out of shape with her hefty hips and made a run for it. Doo-Doo wasn't far behind. Henri and Facel chased them down. Henri was a skilled sheriff and deftly steered them back into the corral with a long pole.

Praline staged a couple of jailbreaks, in fact. I always wondered what she was yearning for – was it the roses in my flower bed or did she want to see Paris and climb the Eiffel Tower? Goats are good at climbing.

When I wrote about her death on Facebook, a dear high school friend, who had called me often during Covid to help keep me sane, saw the parallel in my journey and hers. He had known from the early days of my Doo-Doo posts that I was telling an allegorical tale that reflected my own life in Giverny.

He worried about the head-butting. I assured him Henri and I weren't engaged in physical combat. But he saw the toll my life here had taken on me during our Covid Zoom calls.

For all her suffering, sweet Praline was finally free. "And so are you," he said to me.

About a week after Praline's death, I was sitting on the end of my bed, looking at my lovely view of Doo-Doo Land. I had just taken a shower and was drying my hair.

Out the window, I noticed a little white animal nibbling the grass along the driveway, halfway between the corral and the street.

I jumped up. It was Baby Girl.

I grabbed my phone and called Henri, who was down at the moulin having a morning coffee with Olivier and Maxine.

I had been telling Henri for a few weeks that he should fix the bottom of the corral gate where Praline had bent the metal frame. Baby Girl was tiny enough to squeeze through the gap.

I heard his SUV roaring up the road. The moulin was only a few blocks away.

I was standing guard over her, still in my bathrobe, in case she decided to head for Paris.

He scooped her up in his arms and hugged her. She put her little head against his chest. She clearly was in love.

Even though I would soon be leaving him, I still had moments when I loved Henri, too.

As I walked back to the apartment after all the excitement of yet another jailbreak, I looked over at a pile of stones beside the hillock where Praline was buried. Doo-Doo was napping beside her grave.

Henri pounded a block of wood against the bottom of the gate to straighten it, so that he could lash it to the fence post.

Baby Girl was watching him from inside the corral.

I smiled, knowing the spirit of Praline lived on.

~

On May 1, all my belongings were in a 40-foot container heading to the Port of Los Angeles. The container size had doubled from two years earlier because of the furniture I had purchased in France. They were high-end pieces. The sofa, made in Italy, was the most comfortable sofa I had ever owned. Its back, footrests and headrests could be adjusted with the push of a button. It had become my favorite place to write. If I were to have bought something similar in the States, the price would have been exorbitant. Despite the cost of international shipping, I had learned that if you have expensive furnishings and household goods, it's cheaper in the long run to ship them than to buy them again.

Henri's cousins had allowed me to end my three-year lease early, without penalty, which I appreciated. We met with one of the minions from Fanny's agency for the final inspection. The house was immaculate. The walk-through should have taken no more than 20 minutes. After an hour and a half, I went to sit in the car. Henri was listed as the primary tenant on the lease – even though he never contributed a cent toward the rent – so I felt justified in letting him assume his role. I thought back to the first rent payment I made, sitting with Henri in Fanny's office. I wrote the check and Fanny handed him the receipt.

The inspector general, as I called her, tried to ding me for weeds in the front flowerbed by the terrace. When I moved in, the flowerbed was nothing but weeds. I had a photo of that on my phone, which I showed her. She pulled up a tender green sprout at the edge of the terrace, claiming it was a weed. In English, I said, "That's a prize-winning geranium." I googled a photo of it. "It won the Royal Horticultural Society's Plant of the Centenary at the 100th Chelsea Flower Show." She didn't understand a word I said, but she heard the disdain in my voice and moved on.

I moved back to Henri's apartment for the final weeks before my departure. I had booked a flight for June 10, but the shipping agent said I would need to be in California for the container's arrival, which was scheduled for June 3, in case Customs needed to do an inspection. I rebooked my flight for June 1.

At first, Henri and I amicably settled back into our old routine, from the early days when we were new together. We had breakfast in our pajamas and bedtime tea in our pajamas. The cozy hours, I called them.

It wasn't long before the friction started. As stoic as Henri had been through all my preparations for the move, he was feeling the burn of my departure as the date drew near.

One night, we had an argument after I'd had a Skype call with Angie, the woman from Texas whom I had seen in London. I reminded Henri of the incident, soon after my arrival in 2018, when Bernadette wanted to tell their sister Lucile that I had invited Angie to stay at the Lodge.

"It was pretty clear to me then that I was going to have trouble with Bernadette," I said to him.

I had poked the bear with that comment. Bernadette and Henri still had a strained relationship after their blowup during Covid. "I don't want to talk about this," he said.

"How do you propose that I say good-bye to your family?" I asked.

"We'll have a family dinner," he said.

"Surely, you don't expect Bernadette to attend."

Henri angrily pushed back his chair from the table. "I told you, I don't want to talk about this," he said.

The next morning, he was in a mood. I had many loose ends I

needed to tie up and needed Henri's help. His car mechanic was interested in buying the Lego-mobile, but we hadn't had a meeting with him yet.

When I mentioned this, I could see it was all becoming too much for Henri. "You don't appreciate all I do for you," he shouted at me. "You always need more and more."

He stormed out of the apartment, slamming the door.

I opened my laptop and rebooked my return flight for May 7, just a week away. There was no point prolonging the agony of this good-bye.

~~~

Some Covid restrictions were still in place in France. Henri and I had planned to take a trip through Brittany before I left. It was a part of France I had never seen. But restaurants hadn't opened yet. Many parks and museums were still closed.

"We'll go to Brittany next time you're here," Henri told me. I thought it was interesting that he was imagining a *next time.*

I wanted to say good-bye to special friends before I left. I booked one last appointment with Jose. Despite our rough start, he truly had been a friend to me and had relieved much of the physical and emotional pain I had endured.

He was holding back tears as we said good-bye. "In these times, we don't know if we will ever see each other again." I cried all the way home.

Jean-Raymond, my chiropractor, was eager to come to see me in California. "You say me, I come," he said. He was delighted to know he would be a character in this book. "Will it be a movie?" he asked, wanting to know what kind of tuxedo he should get for the Oscars.

I had tea with Madame Red Shoes. She happily accepted my invitation to come to Del Mar for a visit. She loved to travel and often escaped Normandy winters by flying off to tropical locations.

She asked how I was leaving things with the Sister-Wife. I told her what had happened during the pandemic and how she had blamed me for not allowing her son to quarantine at the Lodge property.

"That's what Henri told her," she said. In that moment, I didn't think to ask if that was her supposition or whether, in fact, she knew that to be true.

I remember asking Henri if Bernadette was telling people that I had prevented Jérémy from moving to the property. He shrugged and said, "*Je ne sais pas.*" But the expression on his face told another story. It was the first time I suspected Henri had laid the blame with me.

A wonderful friend of ours named Jean-Michel invited me to come see him before I left. He was the same age as Henri and had lived with his wife in a beautiful house in the village for many years. Even though he was not from Giverny, he became fascinated with the village's history and over the years, had developed an archive of old Giverny postcards and photographs, historical documents as well as letters and memorabilia from local families, which he digitally preserved and shared on a website of the village's olden days called *Giverny Autrefois.*

Jean-Michel was an excellent photographer and had ventured into the amazing world of drone photography. His aerial footage of Giverny was stunningly beautiful – truly, a bird's eye view of the forests, fields and streams that made up the patchwork of Giverny's gorgeous landscape that hadn't changed much since Monet's time.

I was sitting next to Jean-Michel on the sofa in his living room when he said, in his excellent English, "I have a present for you." He took a memory stick out of his pocket and put it into his laptop, then cued up the video on his big-screen TV.

The title appeared: "The Last Good-bye." He had set to music a video of his aerial photography of Giverny.

"So that you won't forget this beautiful place," he said, smiling at me.

"How could I ever forget?" I tried to smile, too, but I felt the tears coming.

The video ran for about 20 minutes. I wept the entire time. Jean-Michel patted my hand as I tried to control my sobs.

After it was over, he put the memory stick in my hand.

His wife, Christine, sat down on the sofa, on the other side of me. "Will Henri take you to the airport?" I knew there must be some curiosity in the village about why I was leaving and on what terms with Henri.

I shook my head. "No, it will be too sad."

She nodded.

Sarah and I had made that decision. I was afraid Henri would be distraught on the drive to and from the airport. "I especially don't want him dealing with the horrible drive home," I told her.

She arranged for her son, a professional limo driver who often did airport runs, to take me to Charles de Gaulle. Sam would pick me up at Henri's place on the morning of my departure.

Sarah was at a tea Madeleine kindly had organized for me at her home with a few of the embroidery ladies. I received a couple of lovely cross-stitch gifts that I'll cherish forever.

When I said good-bye to Sarah, I thought of Dorothy in *The Wizard of Oz*, saying her good-byes to the Lion, the Tin Man and the Scarecrow, before she headed back to Kansas. Dorothy whispers to the Scarecrow, "I'll miss you most of all." That's how I felt about Sarah.

I left Sarah with a stack of my quilting fabric and Madame Souliman's needlepoint canvas. "Maybe you're meant to be the one to finish this," I told her. I also gave her many of my potted roses to add to her garden. "When these bloom, think of me."

Henri had been angry when I told him I had moved up my departure date. I tried to diffuse the tension by telling him I had much to do when I returned to California. I was hearing news about a car shortage. A friend had warned me it may take weeks for me to find a car to lease, which was my plan.

I told Henri, "My to-do list when I get to California is now longer than my to-do list here. It's time for me to go."

On the day before my departure, Henri prepared a nice lunch for the two of us at the apartment. He opened a box of very ripe cheese and put an oozing hunk of Neuchatel on the cutting board. Soft French cheeses can be very erotic.

He casually said, "I've been thinking about that Ray Charles song today: If you ever find someone new who means more than me to you...I'll never stand in your way."

"That's sad," I said.

"It's the way I feel," he said. "I won't stand in your way. I want you to be happy."

I thought about that for a minute and replied, "I want the same for you, Henri."

After lunch, we made love. He brought me to an incredible climax. Our passion brought on a long, languorous nap.

Later that day, Henri and I took the Lego-mobile to his mechanic, who paid a fair price for it, considering it was a piece of crap. I was glad to be rid of it. The car's faulty transmission had given me many heart-stopping moments as it lurched into traffic circles.

On the way home, we stopped at the moulin to say good-bye to Olivier and Maxine.

My gift to Olivier, who didn't speak English, was a one-of-a-kind copy of the French edition of *The Secret of Marie*, which had been published during the early months of the pandemic – an event I celebrated alone when my author copy arrived. I had found a photo I had taken of Olivier during my first visit to the moulin in 2004. He was 46 then. He looked youthful, with a bit more hair. I had glued the photo inside the front cover of the book and inscribed a dedication to him.

I told Olivier about a book talk I had done in the U.S. a few years earlier and how all the women in the group wanted to know if the character Gérard was inspired by a real person.

"Yes," I said. "But his real name is Olivier."

They immediately wanted to organize a trip to Giverny to meet Olivier.

Henri told Olivier that, in the story, Gérard was an architect. Olivier was pleased to hear that.

As an author, I had a soft spot in my heart for Gérard. When I started writing *The Secret of Marie*, I imagined him as more of a "prop" character, the moulin owner who introduces Kate, an American magazine writer, to the world of Giverny. But on the day I started writing the book, as I moved into an early scene where Gérard makes his first appearance carrying Kate's breakfast tray of coffee and croissants, he seemed to look at me from out of my laptop screen and say, "I'm not a minor character." I smiled and told him, "Okay, let's see what you've got." By the next chapter, I knew he would be Kate's lover and a major character in the story.

I remembered on my first visit to the moulin in 2004 how Olivier would bring me delicious warm croissants from the *boulangerie*. He'd put out yogurt, fruit, hard-boiled eggs, muesli and a pitcher of freshly brewed coffee – a lavish spread considering I was his only guest. Each morning, he'd join me for coffee. Even though he didn't speak English, I had enough high-school French to have conversations with him. I was amazed when he told me how his mother had worked in the Monet household when she was a young woman, before she married his father and started raising a large family of her own.

In the moulin dining room, there was a poster on an easel of a Robinson painting called *Père Trognan*, who is on a horse crossing the Ru, which powers the moulin's water wheel. Next to him in the picture is the bridge where Marie posed for the painting that would years later become the cover of *The Secret of Marie*.

Olivier told me that Robinson may have used my room, with the big arched window, as a studio. I didn't say anything, but I thought of my phantom whom I had been singing to every night and couldn't help but wonder.

I remember apologizing to Olivier for my limited French. He pointed to a photo on the dining room of his infant daughter and told me I was like her, just learning to talk. He promised if I stayed in France for a while, my French would quickly improve.

I thought it was so fitting that on my last night in Giverny, I was saying my last good-bye at the moulin. It was where *my* Giverny story had begun.

We were all gathered in the moulin kitchen as Henri uncorked a bottle of wine. That "baby" daughter, who had recently turned 18, joined us. She squealed with laughter when she opened the book and saw the photo of her much younger dad.

~~⁓~~

That evening, after dinner, I gave Henri his own inscribed copy of the French edition of *Marie*. I wrote:

Henri ~

As I wrote this Giverny love story, I found one of my own. You will always be in my heart, no matter the miles between us. Je t'aime, my darling.

~Rebecca

May 7, 2021

~~⁓~~

Henri and I fell asleep in each other's arms that night. He was up the next morning before I was. I could hear him making breakfast, as I stepped out of the shower.

He had soft-boiled a few eggs – in his electric kettle, of course. There was a toasted, buttered baguette, a fruit salad of banana, kiwi and orange slices, and a steaming mug of coffee waiting for me.

"You need a good breakfast. You have a long journey," Henri said.

Facel lay under the table with his head on my feet.

Henri wanted me to have a second egg.

"I can't," I said, with my hand on my tummy that felt tied in knots.

Sarah's son Sam was about 10 minutes early. He parked in the driveway. I texted him to say I'd be ready at 7, as we had agreed.

Henri helped me roll my suitcases to the front door. He was so brave and kept smiling at me, until I kissed his cheek and whispered, "Take good care of yourself." I held his face in my hands. "You still belong to me."

He caught his breath as his eyes filled with tears. We held each other close for a few minutes.

Facel stood at our feet, with such a sad look in his eyes. He knew. I remembered one night when Henri and I were slow-dancing to Dean Martin's *You Belong to Me*, Facel wanted to join us. He jumped up, putting his front paws on our shoulders and the three of us teetered to the music.

Sam loaded the luggage in the trunk. Henri stood in the doorway with Facel at his side.

As Sam drove toward the front gate, I rolled down my window and waved. Henri waved back. The man who didn't like good-byes didn't turn away. He stood waving until I was out of sight.

Chapter 35

When Sam pulled into Charles de Gaulle Airport, I was stunned. "I don't believe this," I murmured.

"It's unreal, isn't it?"

All of the terminals were closed except for one. The buildings looked post-apocalyptic, as if they had been blasted with a radioactive shockwave. The windows and facades of the terminals were filthy. Weeds had grown through the cracks in the vast empty parking areas that filled the central area of the airport.

"There are only 38 flights a day leaving from here," Sam said. Before the pandemic, Charles de Gaulle had been one of the busiest airports in the world.

I was so grateful to Sam for his good company that morning. I told him what a wonderful friend his mom had been to me and how much I was going to miss her.

When I walked into the terminal, I felt like I had entered an alternate universe. Most of the travelers were African. By the looks of the departure/arrival boards, it seemed that Air Ethiopia was running most of the flights that day. Some passengers were in business attire with briefcases. Many wore colorful garments made from bold African fabrics. Many women carried large baskets, looking like they had just come from the market. I wondered how they were allowed to travel under the current ban. What were their urgent reasons? Most looked like they were on business trips or holidays.

It was chaos at security check-in. As I put my laptop and toiletries on the conveyor belt, someone got pulled out of line at the body scanner. I nervously watched my laptop go into the X-ray tunnel. I usually tried to avoid letting my laptop and carry-on go ahead of me.

When I got through the scanner, I quickly collected the laptop, but discovered my toiletries bag filled with Covid essentials – a going-away gift from a local pharmacist – was missing. When I reported this to a security agent – a French woman with a nasty temperament – she insinuated that I was making a false claim and demanded that I unpack my carry-on for her to inspect. She didn't find my toiletries bag and then accused me of lying.

She had no English, so I took secret delight in saying, "You should be fired for allowing a theft in the security line."

Just then, there was another disruption at the scanner. She lost interest in me and my stolen toiletries bag and went off to share her charms with someone else.

There were only 25 people on my flight, an American Airlines wide-body. I had booked a seat in First/Business Class with surprisingly few airmiles – 57,000 miles plus a fee of $60 for a one-way ticket. There were 30 seats and five passengers in First/Business Class. The remaining 20 passengers in Economy were at the back of the plane. An empty middle section was in total darkness, except for the running lights on the floor.

The flight crew was American, based in Dallas. I asked one of the attendants how American Airlines was staying in business. "We don't make money off passengers and luggage anymore," she said. "It's all about cargo."

She came back a while later with a snack basket. I didn't recognize any of them – not the snacks themselves or the brands. She looked puzzled when I asked her to tell me what they were. "I've been away for seven years," I told her.

"Oh, honey," she said, with great empathy. "You need to get yourself to Costco."

That was the beginning of my reverse culture shock. I had to ask about things – like what's Instacart? And Postmates and Uber Eats? I saw a Prime truck for the first time, a few days after my return. In

France, Amazon Prime was a joke – it meant your package might be delivered within a week.

I quickly adapted to online shopping and getting groceries delivered in an hour. One day, a Prime truck and a FedEx truck pulled up, almost nose-to-nose with each other, at the end of my driveway. They both were delivering packages for me. "It's like Christmas," I said to the drivers. "I love this country!"

I fumbled a lot when I tried to pay for things in stores. Do I swipe or scan? Which way does the card go into the reader? To simplify things, I tried to pay with cash one day and the guy at the register freaked out. "We don't take cash," he said, looking at me like maybe I was from another planet.

"I'm sorry. I just moved from France. I'm still learning about things."

"France! You speak English really well."

"There's a reason for that," I said. I didn't explain. I just wanted to pay for my coffee and muffin.

That afternoon, a Best Buy delivery guy came to set up my new TV (my French TV got smashed on its ocean voyage). I asked him how to switch on the broadcast networks. He informed me that TVs don't work that way anymore. I started taking notes about apps and services I had never heard of.

"I just arrived from France, " I explained and then told him what the guy at the coffee shop had said, thinking he'd get the joke.

Mr. Best Buy concurred. "You really do speak English well. And you've got a great American accent."

~

I still had loose ends to tie up back in France as I waited for accounts to settle. Henri had gone quiet and was ignoring my requests for updates.

I finally emailed him a list of questions. We agreed on a time to talk on WhatsApp, but the connection was bad. He called me back on his landline, which turned out to be an expensive call. It took a good half hour to get through my list. He had let a bill go unpaid and it had been turned over to a collection agency.

"Henri, please take care of this and tell me what I owe you. I'll transfer funds to your account to reimburse you. But I want to close my account soon."

He paid the bill, but complained about how much that phone call had cost him. "All we talked about was money."

"Please just answer my emails so I can be done with all this," I said. I could tell by his anger that he most likely wanted to be done with me as well.

~⁓

I had heartbreaking news from Sarah about a month after I returned to California. Her six-month-old grandson had died of what doctors believed was crib death – Sudden Infant Death Syndrome.

Sarah was distraught as she described his funeral. "His coffin was so tiny," she said. "You can't imagine…" She couldn't finish the sentence. The family buried him in a children's section of a Paris cemetery. Sarah told me she had laced fresh flowers through Madame Souliman's tapestry and they placed it on his grave.

I felt some comfort knowing that Madame Souliman, herself on High, was looking after this baby boy.

~⁓

My French visa expired on July 19. I didn't even take note of that. I had decided I would never again live as an expat abroad. I felt euphoric about being HOME.

I turned my attention to launching a new business venture as a writing coach for book authors. I spent many hours and more than a little money creating a website and a business plan. I hired a graphic artist to create a logo for my new company, which I registered with the city of San Diego. I filed a trademark application for the logo and the company name. I rewrote my LinkedIn profile and joined a couple of networking groups. I was serious about making this new venture a success. The income I hoped to generate from coaching was critical to funding my new life in Del Mar. Rents there were exorbitantly expensive.

My social life revolved around two close friends, Cindy and Norm, who had lived in San Diego for 20 years. Norm's sister, Nancy, and I had been best friends since our college days when we spent a year in Britain as part of our studies. She lived in London then and attended the Guildhall School of Music. I was at the University of Edinburgh in Scotland. We both marvel how that year abroad changed our lives. The world opened to us in so many wonderful ways. Nancy became an opera singer and eventually made her home in Berlin.

Cindy and Norm had lived in New York City for many years before moving to San Diego. Cindy, a cytologist, was still in love with New York and missed it constantly. Norm, a former actor, had settled into life in southern California and worked as a paralegal. He was a shorts-and-flip-flop kind of guy, who loved the mild climate of San Diego. He enjoyed bird-watching and could identify a bird by its song. He loved hanging out on the patio of my condo near the beach, watching the birds (not the ones in bikinis who often passed by on their way to the beach). I, too, began to appreciate the calls of the birds in the 'hood. I learned to identify the raspy caw of egrets as they soared on updrafts from their protected lagoon habitat along the local beach road. Sometimes during my swims in the neighborhood pool, I would hear the piercing *kak-kak-kak* of cooper hawks who perched in the treetops watching for possible prey.

Both in their early 70s, Cindy and Norm had left their jobs during the pandemic and were ambivalent about returning to work. The Delta strain of Covid was surging that summer and infecting even those who had been vaccinated.

The three of us were like-minded about Covid precautions and formed our own bubble. We didn't go anywhere indoors without wearing masks, which meant that when we went out to dinner, which was often, we always sat outdoors. When winter arrived, we'd do take out and have dinner at my place.

Norm loved to drive and enjoyed taking Cindy and me up the coast to the clifftop overlooks in Encinitas at sunset. We'd wait patiently for the moment when the sun dipped below the horizon, hoping to see the Green Flash, an optical phenomenon that happens under certain conditions when a burst of green light appears as the rays of the setting sun refract through the atmosphere. The flash usually lasts just a second or two. One evening, as I was driving down the hill from my condo, I saw a green glow that lasted a full four or five seconds.

I saw dozens of green flashes during my time in Del Mar. They are supposed to be portents of good luck.

Nineteenth-century French novelist Jules Verne waxed rhapsodic about the Green Flash:

...it will be 'green,' but a most wonderful green, a green which no artist could ever obtain on his palette, a green which neither the varied tints of vegetation nor the shades of the most limpid sea could ever produce the like! If there be green in Paradise, it cannot but be of this shade, which most surely is the true green of Hope!

After an acrimonious couple of months, Henri and I had found our equilibrium with each other. We had long talks by phone, which surprised me. Henri hates talking on the phone. Our WhatsApp connection wasn't always great, so sometimes our chats ended in mid-sentence.

But sometimes our conversations would go more than an hour.

We typically spoke around noon my time, 9 p.m. for him – or later, if he'd been out in the evening. He sent me photos almost every day, from his morning walks or from dinner parties with friends. On our calls, he kept me current with the latest happenings in Giverny. Some days, I felt so wistful, wanting to be there again. The Covid restrictions had eased. As Henri had predicted, France had lifted the travel ban.

One day, he sent me an email with an excerpt from a letter French novelist Gustave Flaubert had written to his paramour, poet Louise Colet in 1852:

Toi, je t'aime comme je n'ai jamais aimé et comme je n'aimerai pas. Tu es et resteras seule, et sans comparison avec nulle autre. C'est quelque chose de melangé et de profound, quelque chose qui me tient par tous les bouts, qui flatte tous mes appetits et caresse tous mes vanities.

I used a translation app to read it in English:

You, I love you as I have never loved and as I will not love. You are and will remain alone, and without comparison with any other. It is something mixed and deep, something which holds me at all ends, which flatters and caresses all my vanities.

I stared out the window for a long while after reading that email. I couldn't imagine putting everything back on a boat and setting sail for France again.

But there was such a pull on my heartstrings that day.

Chapter 36

By fall, Kyle and Julia's wedding plans were in place. The guest list had grown to 114, which worried me given the Delta surge. When they had come to Del Mar for a visit during the summer, I gently suggested that they think about Plan B. A garden wedding with a dozen people could be nice, I said to them, and so much safer. "I'd hate to think of you two coming down with Covid on your honeymoon."

But this was to be a country-club affair. A significant number of the guests were over 60, in the Covid danger zone. Because of my underlying medical issue, I wore a mask whenever I was indoors and had asked Kyle if he could arrange for patio seating for those of us who felt uncomfortable eating inside. He said he'd look into it, but couldn't make any promises.

During a tense phone call with him, I said, "I'm your mother. I shouldn't have to beg for this."

He clearly was on edge tending to all the details of planning a big wedding. But I was taken back by this hard-boiled side of him I had never seen.

I had a difficult realization as we navigated the run-up to the wedding: I needed to adjust my expectations to keep from getting my feelings hurt.

When I arrived for the wedding, three days before the event, I turned on my phone as the plane's wheels hit the tarmac. Kyle had sent a message saying he'd be too busy running errands that evening to meet me for dinner.

I remembered the week of my own wedding, 36 years earlier.

My soon-to-be husband and I had planned several days of activities for our guests. But before all the festivities began, we set aside an evening to take our parents to dinner, on the day of their arrival. We were starting a wonderful chapter of family life together and wanted to celebrate that.

As I headed to the airport exit, a kind woman at the information desk directed me to the Uber pickup area across from the terminal. It was a half-hour ride to the hotel. The driver was kind, too. He rolled my bags into the lobby, which he didn't have to do.

The hotel didn't have a restaurant, so I thought I'd order in. But I saw there was a restaurant across the road, so I freshened up and took myself out to dinner. It turned out to be a sports bar, with a patio in back. The heaters on the patio weren't working and it grew chilly as the sun set, so I didn't linger over my meal.

What I'll always remember about that evening is the heartache of loneliness. This was to have been the start of a wonderful celebration and there I sat, alone at a table facing a strip-mall parking lot – the mother of the 32-year-old groom, who is my only child.

After my sports-bar-patio dinner, I went next door to Trader Joe's to get provisions. I wanted to have wine and nibbles on hand for wedding guests staying at the hotel. I had booked a suite that had a living room and small kitchen and envisioned having drop-in visitors.

The fatigue of my travel day was setting in as I rolled my grocery cart out of the store. To my surprise, there were no cart barricades, so I proceeded down the sidewalk leading back to the main road. At the crosswalk, I vowed to the universe I would return the cart by the end of the weekend (I did) and gingerly maneuvered it off the curb. There was no stop sign or light, so I waited to be sure I would be seen. It was pitch dark by then. One car stopped and soon the pathetic sight of me had stopped all traffic. With all those headlights on me, I wanted to yell, "I'm not a bag lady! I'm the mother of a very inconsiderate groom!"

It definitely was a low point. I had spent the entire year focused on getting to this wedding. My journey home had been an odyssey plagued with obstacles and duress even Homer himself couldn't have imagined.

Two days later, on the day before the wedding, I finally saw my son. We had lunch with a college friend of mine who had flown in from Tulsa.

Before the rehearsal dinner that evening, as a group of us gathered in the hotel parking lot, I turned to see a man smiling at me as he approached. It was my ex-husband, whom I hadn't seen in seven years, not since Kyle's graduation from graduate school. I had seen recent photos of him, so I wasn't surprised by how his sun wrinkles and laugh lines had aged him. I'm sure he was surprised by how my "Covid kilos," as my European girlfriends and I referred to our pandemic weight gain, had changed my silhouette. We hugged and marveled about the major life event that was about to transpire. He had remarried and his new wife and members of her family had come with him to celebrate.

At the rehearsal dinner, I gave a toast to the bride and groom. I stood – unmasked, so that I could be heard – at the entrance of the pizza parlor's party room. I told a story that drew laughter. I choked up at the end as I lifted my glass to my son and the beautiful young woman who would become my daughter-in-law the next day. I had no feeling of sadness or loss, as some moms-of-sons feel. I felt only happiness for what I hoped would be their wonderful life together.

The wedding ceremony, which took place at the edge of the country club's golf course, was beautiful beyond belief.

As Julia said her vows, birds sang in the pine trees behind her and a sunbeam bathed her in white light. She wept as she spoke of her mom. There was no doubt in my mind that her mother had something to do with that sunbeam. I looked across the aisle from where I was sitting. An empty chair, which had her name on it, held a beautiful basket of flowers.

I thought of my mom and dad and how much they would have enjoyed this day. On my left ring finger, I wore my mother's diamond wedding ring and my father's gold wedding band and knew they were with us in spirit.

The reception was a Covid nightmare. Of the 114 guests, I was the only one who wore a mask. The bride's lovely grandmother, who was a country-club member, saved the evening for me. She had graciously arranged for two tables to be set up on the balcony outside the dining room, next to a tall pyramid heater, for those who wanted to dine outdoors. My college friend and my former sister-in-law joined me there.

After dinner, we returned to the party for toasts and dancing. During the mother-son dance, I had a wonderful few minutes with my son as we reminisced about the song he had chosen – Seal's "Kiss from a Rose." We had played that song until the CD wore out one summer on our drives around town to his activities. As we danced, I told him how happy I was that he had found his life partner. For years, when he was single and glum on Valentine's Day, I had promised him, "She's out there looking for you and when you find each other, it's going to be wonderful." It's a good thing moms are usually right.

As the evening wound done, I stood at the candy table, looking at a pink plush-toy walrus my mother had given my son as a baby. He was adorably dressed in a snug-fitting, mini tux that my son had ordered for him online. He's a chubby walrus and likes to eat, so I put a few pieces of candy in front of him.

I sensed someone standing next to me. It was my ex, who had come to say good-bye. He said he wasn't feeling well and was going back to the hotel. I suggested we go to a quieter spot, away from the music.

I will always treasure that private moment. "We did a wonder-ful thing," I said to him as we embraced. There was a stoop in his shoulders that was new to me. In that moment, I let go of years of anger over why our marriage had ended. As I watched him walk out the door a few minutes later, I wondered if I'd ever see him again. Through Covid, I had learned to savor the here and now.

In the days after the wedding, I thought long and hard about love and the disappointments and heartache that often come with it. I was profoundly disappointed in my son's disregard for me. I knew I needed to let go of that, but I felt entitled to feel the pain of what had happened. There will be many happy occasions to come in our family life. We'll move on. But I knew that, going forward, I would need to better manage my expectations.

When I returned home, I sent my ex some photos I had taken during the ceremony, with a thank you for his generous underwriting of wedding expenses and for all his financial support of our son over the years.

Love, in all its messiness, had ruled the day. I saw a blessing in that, especially in a fraught time when sadness and anger can easily overshadow joy.

Chapter 37

Two days after the wedding, I was at the Oakland airport waiting for my flight back to San Diego, when a photo popped up on WhatsApp from Henri. Its caption: The Frankenstein of Giverny.

At first glance, I thought someone had introduced him to Snapchat. It looked like a photo filter had enlarged his front teeth. Actually, his real teeth were descending from his long-neglected gums.

I called him immediately and he told me the story of how the teeth had been feeling loose since summer. His dentist said they would have to be pulled sooner than later. The day had come. He had just spent a couple of hours having most of his top teeth extracted.

"I'm so sorry, *chérie*," he said. "I won't be able to come see you."

Henri was due to arrive in San Diego in a few days. He had booked the flight a few weeks earlier when the U.S. announced it would lift the Covid travel ban that had prevented Europeans from visiting the U.S.

I could hear the disappointment in his voice. His dentist thought he could make the trip in about a month.

"*Chérie*, what are you doing for Christmas?" Henri asked. "If you don't have plans with your family, I could be with you in California."

That surprised me. I never would have imagined Henri not spending Christmas with his family.

"Bernadette, Valérie and Jérémy are going to Majorca for the holidays."

I wondered if the house-with-no-heat had already been booked – or maybe it had finally lost its allure.

"Alex and Paul think it's risky to gather with this new Covid variant," Henri said.

The Omicron strain has taken hold in Europe and was threatening to be the biggest Covid surge yet.

"I'd love for you to come spend Christmas with me, Henri."

"Even if I look like Frankenstein?"

That made me laugh.

Henri had a lot of gum swelling after his surgery. He abandoned his temporary dentures, which didn't fit well. He felt better with no top teeth at all, which meant he had to change his diet to soft foods.

"I'm eating a lot of soup and mashed potatoes," he told me.

I hardly recognized him in the post-op photos he sent. With his stubble of a beard, the sunken curve of his mouth wasn't that noticeable. But the contours of his face had changed.

Henri didn't seem to mind. "The pain is gone and I'm eating again," he assured me. Henri was a warrior in the face of adversity.

He rebooked his flights and was scheduled to arrive two days before Christmas.

I got a big tree – a Noble fir about seven feet tall. I hadn't had one that size in a decade. I unpacked all my Christmas ornaments and bought new strings of lights. I placed my mother's set of Christmas caroler candles from the 1950s on the fireplace mantle and my German pyramid windmill on the dining table. I hung a fresh wreath on the door, trimmed with berries and Scottish-tartan ribbon.

Henri was traveling through London so that he could get a nonstop flight from Heathrow to San Diego. But the U.K. had changed its Covid rules and was requiring a PCR test, within 24 hours of travel, even for those transiting to a non-U.K. destination. Henri couldn't find a testing sight at Heathrow that was open on a Sunday, which was when he'd need to test.

It all became too stressful for him. He then developed a gum infection and the dentist told him he couldn't travel for at least another month.

"I'm sorry to do this again, *chérie*," he said when he called to cancel our Christmas. His voice sounded husky. I wondered if he had been crying.

It was a hard blow for me. I had been so looking forward to spending the holidays with him.

Two days before Christmas, Norm, Cindy and I went to a bird sanctuary at an oceanside lagoon up the coast from Del Mar. I sat on the balcony of the nature center, staring at the sea.

I looked at the time. Henri's flight was about to land at San Diego Airport without him.

Norm and Cindy helped cheer me up. We went for a ride around a San Diego neighborhood called Christmas Card Lane, known for its beautiful decorations and light displays. On Christmas Eve, we had takeout from a local Italian restaurant at my place, in the glow of my gorgeous Christmas tree, and watched *A Christmas Story*, which I had never seen.

I was alone Christmas morning. Henri called about noon. He'd spent Christmas Eve with our dear friend Claire, who undoubtedly took the sting out of scuppered travel plans and tender gums with a good bottle of whiskey she'd stashed somewhere.

Norm and Cindy came over later on Christmas Day and we made a feast of the ham and all the side dishes we had ordered from Whole Foods. They brought pies from a favorite bakery. None of us cook, but we're experts at ordering gourmet food.

We had a good time together, as always. But it was one of those years when I was glad Christmas Day was over.

Chapter 38

After the holidays, I began to experience symptoms of anxiety and depression. This wasn't new to me. I'd had a debilitating experience with both during the two years it took my estranged husband and me to reach a divorce settlement. Back then, I was so anxious I couldn't sleep. I was averaging two or three hours of sleep a day. I was wracked with worry about the future and whether I could handle everything that was coming at me as a single mom. I wasn't able to focus. I had trouble digesting food. I had tension headaches that felt like a vice was squeezing my skull. I eventually recovered, with the help of a good therapist and Zoloft.

This time, it was different. I had a tickle in my chest that felt a bit like a heart palpitation that my doctor diagnosed as acid reflux. Just to be sure, she sent me to cardiologist. He said my heart was fine. I took a low-dose of Ativan at bedtime to help get me through the night. But I'd often wake up at dawn, unable to get back to sleep as my worries woke up, too.

I was worried about my driftless state. I felt I had no traction with the life I had planned for myself in California. My new business had not taken off – not to the level that would sustain my monthly expenses. My rent was high, but still below market. My new neighbor, who had moved into the condo that shared a wall with mine, was paying $4,350 a month.

What worried me most was my lack of interest in anything that used to interest me. I didn't feel like reading or quilting or gardening. I had no spark of creativity or imagination that always spurred me to write. I had no stories floating around in my head.

Each day, I spent too much time reading the news, which was depressing. Sometimes, I'd go to the pool, which gave me a lift.

But most days felt empty to me. Although I saw Norm and Cindy a few times a week, I was lonely. When I had first moved to Del Mar, I looked online for quilting groups and went to a large fabric store to see if there were any quilting guilds close to me. A lot of guilds had stopped meeting during Covid. I thought about starting my own group, but then worried about having people gather at my condo. The Omicron variant was rampant.

My despair grew. I felt like I was in a canoe, rowing against the current and banging against the rocks. I needed to get the wind at my back, but I had no clue how to do that.

I revisited a manuscript I had started writing before Covid – the story of my time in Giverny. The story was mostly focused on my relationship with Henri. I had put the manuscript aside because I couldn't explain his behavior. When an author can't figure out a main character's motivation, there's a problem.

The story didn't have an arc at the point where I had left it. Covid hadn't happened yet. I hadn't yet thought about returning to California.

I sifted through my notes and revisited my outline. I couldn't see the end of the story and put it aside once more.

~

One evening as Norm, Cindy and I headed to dinner at our favorite Italian restaurant in the lovely beach town of Cardiff, I was startled to see a two-decker commuter train hurtling toward us along a track that paralleled the highway.

I had never seen a train from the perspective of someone who might be standing on a track the moment before impact. The curve of the track along the highway made it appear, from where I was sitting in the front passenger seat, that we were in the direct path of the train.

I couldn't shake the image from my mind for a few minutes.

Shortly before Covid swept Europe, I was on a train to Paris when someone threw themselves onto the tracks. I was appalled that some of my fellow passengers, including the Frenchman sitting next to me, were upset that their Sunday lunch plans had been spoiled. I looked incredulously at my seat mate and said, "The person who's dead in front of this train could have taken us all with him – or her. Don't you realize how lucky we are?"

I then started a conversation with him about what brings a person to the side of the tracks. Is it an impulse or a plan? I wondered what this person had done that morning. Did they have breakfast? Did they write a note? What were their last thoughts as they saw the train approach?

It was an existential conversation – so French, I thought. But when we parted at the station two hours later, he said good-bye in a way that happens so often on a train journey, when strangers in a compartment have bonded for a few hours and become companions in their travel experience.

I looked back at the front of the train, not wanting to see the mark of the person who ended their life in front of it. But I stopped for a moment to honor their passing.

At Paris' Gare St. Lazare, suicide trains are brought in on a separate track. The front of the train is shielded by a high opaque barrier so traces of the deceased can't be seen. Railroad staff wait on the platform to usher passengers into an office where they're offered a refund. That seemed surreal to me. You can't "unlive" the experience, but you can get your money back.

During Covid, Nancy had been sitting in traffic in Berlin and witnessed a woman jump to her death from the top floor of a building. For days afterward, she said she was haunted by what had happened. "I can't unsee her falling," she told me.

It took me several days to unsee the train, with its bright beacon of light shining from the top deck, as that blinding mass of metal streaked toward us.

My heart felt the rawness that so many of us had endured during the Covid age. We had lost loved ones and fallen out with loved ones. Friendships had fractured. Lost jobs and homes had forced some into bankruptcy and homelessness. For some, the only relief had come at the side of the tracks or at the ledge of a window.

That day, I resolved to guard my mental health, to find a way back to wellness. I wasn't sure of the path, but I was determined to find a way.

Step into the light, I had told Julia. I needed to follow my own advice.

Chapter 39

As much as I tried to avoid doomscrolling – a bad habit I had picked up during Covid – I couldn't help following the frightening news about an imminent Russian invasion of Ukraine.

I had been in touch with Nataliya since my return to California. We'd spoken on Skype a few times. She used a phone app to translate what I was saying into Ukrainian. Gosha translated what she was saying in Ukrainian into English. Sometimes the two of them got into a discussion about whatever the topic was. I loved our calls, but I think we all felt a little exhausted after they were over.

In early February, President Biden was sounding the alarm about the Russian tank buildup in Belarus along Ukraine's northern border. Kyiv was in the direct line of an invasion.

I sent Nataliya a Facebook message and asked if we could set up a time to skype. We arranged that on a Sunday evening, in early February. They had just finished dinner. Nataliya and Andriy sat on their living room sofa on either side of Gosha. They assured me they were fine. The news was overblown – life was normal in Kyiv.

I was relieved to hear that, but I wondered if they were putting on brave faces. At one point, Gosha said, translating for his mother, "She worries that war might come."

In the days that followed that call, as the prospect of an invasion seemed certain, Nataliya and I exchanged private messages on Facebook.

Nataliya: *We personally try to think only about the good and not to panic, but in the future it will be what will be. I hope God saves us.*

On the day of the invasion, Nataliya posted on Facebook that she awoke to the sound of bombs dropping on the outskirts of Kyiv.

The next day, she sent me this message: *We are going West very slowly. We left Kyiv.*

She would later tell me that she and Andriy decided to leave Kyiv the day the bombing began. They packed two cars. Andriy would not be allowed to leave the country because, with the declaration of martial law, all men under 60 were required to stay and protect the homeland. He travelled with them as they headed to the border of Poland and then stayed with a friend in a village near the city of Ivano-Frankivsk, in western Ukraine, to help with the volunteer effort. Nataliya and Gosha continued on, in the second car, to the border.

I lost contact with her for a couple of days. And then she wrote: *We have a bad network connectoin and low battery. We are saving flue and electricity. When we will get to Poland we will have a sleep and connect with you. We hope, we will cross the border in 2-3 days. Our internet is low, we can read yiur messages, but it takes a lot of time to send them. We haven't slept for 3 days. But we are alive.*

She ended with a heart emoji and praying hands.

I could tell from the typos that she was writing quickly.

That message came on February 27, three days after the invasion. Henri and I were in touch daily about her situation. He was trying to find accommodations for Nataliya and Gosha in Giverny.

That same day, I sent her an update about the situation: *I don't know how much news you're able to get...talks are scheduled tomorrow (Monday) between Ukraine and Russian delegations at the Ukraine-Belarus border. The Ukrainian army is putting up a good fight and still holds Kyiv and other major cities. Sanctions are severe and widespread now as global outrage increases.*

She sent a heart emoji as a reply.

The next day, February 28, I wrote: *I just spoke with Henri. He is following the news in France about the situation at Ukraine's western border. He says there's still food and fuel in the western part of the country, so hopefully you're able to get what you need as you wait. Poland, Hungary and Romania are welcoming Ukrainians. Airbnb is making accommodations available for as many as 100,000 people. Russia is now in an economic crisis because of the sanctions. Even neutral Switzerland has frozen Russian assets. Please let us know when you arrive in Poland. We're here to help you in any way we can. I hope Andriy is safe and well. Sending you much love.*

I hadn't received more than the heart emoji from her in two days. I kept checking my Facebook messages, even in the middle of the night.

Finally, on March 1 she wrote: *We're fine. Local residents give tea, soup, sandwiches. It snowed, -10 C. It's cold, but bearable. We save fuel. In two days, 12 out of 19 km were driven in line at the border. 7 km left. Hopefully we'll be at the border today. Hugs to you and Henri.*

She signed off with another heart emoji.

I tried to imagine being bundled up in a car in the snow, with no heat and temps at 14 degrees Fahrenheit. It had taken them two days to travel seven-and-a-half miles.

Later that day, they arrived in Poland. Andriy had booked a room for them at a nice hotel near the border so they wouldn't have to stay in the refugee-arrival camp.

After their first night in Poland, she wrote: *Hello Rebecca. We slept well and are glad that there is a peaceful sky overhead. My heart hurts for those who are in Ukraine, but we believe that our troops will win, the truth is on our side. Thank you and Henri for your support on the road, it is very important that you are not alone in this world. It takes longer to get to France. I'm very tired. But maybe in time I will be there. From the beginning I will rest in Austria.*

They drove to Stohllhof, where they stayed at the conference center, as the guests of the owner, her patron.

Before we could skype, she needed to go shopping for a computer cord. "We left so quickly, we forgot some things — like the cords to our computers," she told me when we finally spoke.

"What about your paintings?" I asked, afraid to hear the answer.

Except for a couple of small watercolors, she had left all her artwork behind. Her main concern was fitting Gosha's piano keyboard into the car. "The child's piano is more important," she told me.

Later, she wrote: *I hope my pictures will wait for me whole. I could not even choose which of the paintings is more important to me. How fragile everything is in this world. How illusory are the material values that we create. There is something to think about.*

I would have chosen the painting of Gosha as a little boy at the breakfast table – the painting that had nearly hypnotized me during my portrait sitting in Giverny, with its strawberry nose and eyeballs rolling across the table. As a mother, I couldn't have left that one behind.

A couple of weeks later, after she and Gosha had settled in Austria, Nataliya sent me a harrowing account about the day of the invasion: *Rebecca, we are very grateful that you follow our destiny. And your kind words support us. I am answering your question how much time we had for the collection. At 5:12 in the morning my friend called me and said that she saw explosions from her window, she saw how the civilian airfield in Boryspil was being bombed. I learned from her that the war had begun. The fact is that Kyiv is a very large city and is located on two banks of the Dnieper River. My friend's house is on the left bank and that's why she heard and saw the explosions. Andriy's apartment is located on the right bank at the other end of the city, and even then we had not seen all this horror. As soon as my friend called, the siren began to howl for us to go down to the bomb shelter. We didn't have a bomb shelter in our house. I walked around the apartment for 30 minutes and couldn't find the TV remote control. My body was shaking and I wanted to go back to sleep to wake up "yesterday" in a peaceful country. And the remote was lying on the table, I just didn't see it, though I looked at it. When I turned on the TV, I saw that rockets were exploding in different places in Ukraine. And even near my mother's dacha. I then realized that a full-scale war had begun and I needed to take my son abroad, not knowing exactly where, but I had to save him. And on this first day of the war, when all the people were still thinking what would happen next, I was collecting things, but rather packing them in a panic. Gosha did not want to leave. But I convinced him that as an adult he would help his country more. I collected mainly Gosha's things, a computer and an electric piano. I took quite a bit from my things. I also took my handkerchiefs with prints of my paintings. They took up little space. Unfortunately, I took only two watercolors from the paintings. Oil work remained at home. At 19.00 we left the house in two cars (Andriy in his own, and Gosha and I in my car. We came to Giverny for an exhibition in it.) and drove towards the border. From my house the first 100 km we drove in 12 hours. We didn't drive, but rather crawled in a car in a huge traffic jam. So in a half day we packed our things and left Kyiv. And no one could stop me, maternal instinct helped me and made me do something.*

As I read this, I thought of Nataliya's own mother who had hurriedly sent Nataliya and her younger brother on their escape from Kyiv after the Chernobyl disaster. Nataliya's fight-or-flight instinct was clearly part of her DNA.

I so admired Nataliya for what she wrote next:

I want Gosha to grow up, learn and then help Ukraine to recover consciously. All the way Gosha really did not want to leave Ukraine, he was very worried about his classmates. But our military advised women and children to leave the city so that civilians would not interfere with their fight. I think that when Gosha learns he will be able to contribute to the development of Ukraine. I pray that all children remain alive with living parents.

The horrific events that would follow in the weeks and months to come – at the bloodied hands of a mad man – would devastate the world.

Chapter 40

In the swirl of all this bad news and angst, Henri arrived in San Diego on a beautiful day in early May of 2022.

As I stood at the foot of an escalator at the San Diego Airport, the world seemed to spin a bit slower for a few seconds.

Henri jumped off the escalator's last step with his amazingly small carry-on bag (his only luggage) and rushed toward me. I thought of that winter's day in Florence when he had run through the snow to greet me.

We were oblivious to the airport commotion around us. We held each other tight. There were lots of kisses. We hadn't seen each other in almost a year.

～

We spent three blissful weeks together at my condo in Del Mar.

Henri loved Del Mar and took walks on the beach every morning. He chatted with the engineers about an annual dredging operation that was underway to remove excess sand from the adjacent lagoon and came home each day with a full report about their progress.

We hung out at my favorite neighborhood coffee bar called Bird Rock that overlooked the lagoon. We took drives along the coast. Henri enjoyed seeing the noisy, smelly pelicans and seals that had encamped in a cove in La Jolla. He watched in amazement as para-gliders soared over the cliffs above Torrey Pines State Beach. He liked my habit of watching the sun set.

One day, we made a pilgrimage to an antique engine museum in Vista, California, about a half hour from Del Mar. It was a huge property with an impressive collection of steam engines. Henri was astounded by the vast "graveyard" of machinery waiting to be restored. "We have 10 projects in the queue in Giverny," he remarked. At the museum in Vista, dozens of engines and machines sat in a field, rusting in the elements.

Our days at the condo were very relaxed. We made love and took long naps.

Every day, Henri sat down at the dining table with his sketchpad and colored pencils. He loved drawing the bird-of-paradise flowers that were in bloom. He was enthralled with the hummingbirds that came to the feeder by my dining room window. He had never seen a hummingbird. They don't exist in Europe.

For my birthday at the end of May, we spent a couple of days in Pasadena. I invited several friends to join Henri and me for dinner at a restaurant with a lovely garden patio. Another friend who had offered to host the party at her house had called that morning to say she had tested positive for Covid.

I was happy for Henri to meet my friends. At last, he had a glimpse of my old life and the people I missed. I gave a toast to friendship and the joy of being able to gather around a table again.

It was a wonderful birthday that included a visit to Pasadena's Norton Simon Museum. Henri was delighted to see the Impressionist collection and many landscapes from Giverny that we both recognized.

"Do you miss Giverny?" he asked.

"More than you know."

Henri and I hadn't talked much about the future, not until our last days together. We had been both testing the water, I think, wanting to see if the temperature between us felt right.

On our last night, we had dinner at a restaurant in Del Mar with an ocean view. I broached the subject of what next. Henri asked if I'd like to come back to Giverny, to make my home there again.

I wouldn't be able to renew my French visa because I had been away for more than a year. I'd have to begin again, from scratch, which seemed overwhelming.

"You would need to commit to this," Henri said. "The expense of moving is great. It's a big decision – I don't envy you."

I turned to Henri, so that I could read his eyes. "We would need to share the expense of the move," I said. "We would do this as a couple. Are you willing to do that?"

He thought about that for a moment and then said, "*Oui.*"

Such a little word to carry such a heavy load, I thought.

The sun was sinking below the horizon. I took Henri's hand. "Wait for it," I said, holding my breath. "There!" A tiny spark of green appeared and then vanished in a blink.

"A green flash is supposed to be a good omen," I said to him.

Regardless, we began planning my return to Giverny.

Chapter 41

In early September, I returned to Giverny for a seven-week visit. I wanted to immerse myself in village life again, in the post-Covid age.

I had been so distraught by the Covid scene in France when I left in 2021, I couldn't imagine wanting to return. A friend in California had asked me if I'd ever want to live in Giverny again. Emphatically, I said, "Never."

It felt strange to be back at Henri's apartment. I was surrounded by old memories – not all of them wonderful. In fact, the flashbacks to our many unhappy times together in that apartment were unsettling.

Henri and I were in agreement that we would move to a house together. Our plan was to rent, not buy. We wanted to stay in Giverny, but to my surprise, he had been looking at properties in Vernon and in some of the outlying villages. I didn't want to be isolated out in the countryside, so we focused on Vernon and Vernonnet. A Giverny real estate agent had told Henri that very few houses in the village come on the market for long-term rental because owners want to cash in on the tourist season.

But first, I had to get a new visa. Henri and I began collecting the documents I'd need. We knew the drill. Henri went to the *mairie* to get his attestation form stamped with the mayor's official seal. He provided me with a copy of his passport along with a utility bill, confirming his address, and a letter of invitation stating that he would provide my accommodation. In all the years I had lived in Italy – where I had rented three apartments – I had never needed a man to "accommodate" me.

Henri and I decided to take the trip we had postponed in 2021, to Brittany.

The weather in Brittany was changeable, as storm systems over the Atlantic came ashore. The skies were dramatic and sometimes, so were the waves that crashed on the rocky beaches.

Every day, we ate fresh oysters that had been pulled from the beds we'd see along the shore. Their aphrodisiac effect wasn't lost on Henri and me. As many storms as Henri and I had weathered, I marveled that our passion never waned. I suppose, in a way, it was what held us together. So many times in our lovemaking, I felt the release of my anger and the intensity of my underlying desire. I knew it wasn't necessarily a good thing – to build a relationship on makeup sex – but there was something addictive about it.

I was surprised that despite the intimacy we were enjoying, we weren't getting along very well. Part of it was the wear-and-tear of a car trip. Henri's hearing loss had worsened. He couldn't hear the voice of the GPS system on his phone or mine, so I had to speak the directions loudly. Even then, he wasn't getting everything. He'd miss a turn or at the last second, as we were in a traffic circle, he'd disagree with the directions and take another exit. Sometimes, his instincts were right. But many times, we'd head in the opposite direction for miles before I could convince him – pointing to the arrow indicator on Google's map – to turn around.

A long-standing problem Henri and I had had over the years was his disregard for my personal belongings. Once at the Little House, he sat down at the living-room coffee table and pushed aside my camera using a sloshing mug of coffee.

One morning on our trip, I came down to breakfast at a self-catering cottage we had rented, to find a buffet he had made with bread, cheese and ham on the kitchen table. Henri had put the ham, in its greasy plastic wrapper, on the lid of my laptop.

I could barely control my temper as I wiped off a $3,000 MacBook Pro that he had used as a serving platter.

He seemed unfazed.

Finally, on our last night, as we unwound from our 10-day journey over a bottle of wine, I brought up the touchy subject. "Henri, we've not been getting along very well on this trip. I'm wondering why. We had such a good time together in Del Mar."

He noted the strain of changing locations every couple of days and the fatigue of driving many hours a day. He had done all the driving. I agreed and suggested that in the future we choose one place as our base.

Later, as we were getting ready for bed, he turned to me and said, "I know the reason. When I'm with you, you're the boss." And then he grinned, "But when you're with me, I'm the boss."

It may have been the first introspective revelation Henri had ever had.

"It's important to be a nice boss," I said.

"Bien sûr!" he replied. Of course.

But, of course, he didn't see the irony in that.

~~~

I was happy to see my chiropractor Jean-Raymond again. He re-aligned me after my long-haul flight from California and my 10-day car trip through Brittany.

Henri had told me that Jose had left the area. I had sent him a couple of private messages on Facebook over the past year, but I had never gotten a reply.

One day, I drove to his clinic, on the campus of the old rocket factory. The property was overgrown with tall weeds and the front gate was chained shut.

I realized, when Jose had said good-bye to me the year before, that he probably knew he would be leaving. "In these times, we don't know if we will ever see each other again," he had said.

I presumed he had returned to Spain. His family was there. He went home, like I had. I felt so sad knowing I probably would never see him again.

Jose had been a hero during Covid. He had gotten permission from French authorities to go to Madrid, where Covid was raging in early 2020. He told me, "It was like being in a war zone. In one day, I saw 100 patients die."

⌒⌒

Our Giverny friends were eager to hear news of Nataliya. One of the local gallery owners had offered to host an exhibition of her work. Henri had found a few possible places for Nataliya and Gosha to stay.

Nataliya wanted to go abroad, fearful that Putin might provoke a war in Europe. By early summer, she had received a visa from Canada, which was welcoming Ukrainians with a government-subsidized resettlement program – unlike the U.S., which was putting the burden on private citizens to act as financial sponsors.

Nataliya had asked if I could write a letter of invitation so that she and Gosha could come to the U.S. She especially wanted Gosha to visit Stanford. But the entry rules were strict. I'd have to pledge to support them and submit my financial records for the government to review. I explained to her that I didn't have the required resources to be a sponsor. She understood and was positive about their prospects in Canada.

She and Gosha spent a couple of months in Vancouver, where she won first prize in an art exhibition that featured her new paintings, some with a Ukrainian theme. Gosha had enrolled in an intensive English course and was looking at colleges in Canada. By September, they had moved to Edmonton, where Gosha, at the age of 16, had been accepted for a degree program at a polytechnic institute.

It was a meteoric rise from the ashes, fueled by Nataliya's vision, determination and amazing strength.

Andriy had returned to their home in Kyiv – which, at that time, was not in the combat zone – and sent a photo of her paintings in storage, all safe and sound.

A well-known Giverny artist named Christophe Demarez had invited Henri and me to dinner one evening in late October. There was a special purpose for this dinner. Henri and Christophe were doing a painting swap.

Years earlier, Camille had given Henri a painting by a local artist who had recently passed away. When I moved in with Henri, the painting hung in the living room above the harmonium. It was a dark abstract picture – mostly brown and black with touches of deep blue. The shapes looked like toy building blocks. Christophe had been a friend of the artist, Christian Zeimert, who had lived in Vernonnet, and regretted he didn't own one of his paintings. Henri agreed to Christophe's offer to give him the painting in exchange for one of Christophe's own works.

I liked Christophe's work. His colors are bright. His canvases are large. In recent years, he had gone through a period of rendering local scenes – like the bar at the Hôtel Baudy – or Paris locations with distorted shapes and curved lines, creating the effect of a Fun House mirror.

Before dinner, Christophe invited us look around the gallery to choose a painting. Curiously, Henri was drawn to a scene of a woman's boudoir. He said the intimate setting and style reminded him of Bonnard. Soft sunlight streamed through lace curtains, casting intricate shadows on the wood floor. A creamy-white-and-gold pitcher and bowl on a washstand by the window caught the light. Potted flowers decorated the room. The bedding was in shades of pink: a long bolster pillow, in a patterned rose-colored fabric, seemed to have been tossed at the bed's footboard. A rumpled pale pink duvet, tumbling onto the floor, gave the impression that the woman who had slept there had just left the room. Bonnard often portrayed naked women luxuriating in their untidy beds.

"This is a perfect painting for a bedroom," I said to Henri. "You need a big painting on the wall above the sofa."

My favorite was a Matisse-like scene that Christophe had painted from the sitting room of his apartment on the French Riviera. Through open glass doors that opened onto a balcony, there was a sweeping view of the Mediterranean above the tops of palm trees. A painting on the wall of the sitting room in the picture continued the line of the seascape, in a clever wink from the artist. A cat was curled up on an armchair, upholstered with a boldly printed blue fabric. In the style of Matisse and Bonnard, the chair looked like it might fall off the canvas.

Henri didn't make a selection that evening. He said he wanted to "think about it in my sleep." Christophe put his new acquisition on an easel and we went up the garden steps to Christophe's lovely secluded house on the hillside above the gallery.

Yuka and Marc joined us for dinner, which was a nice surprise. I hadn't seen Yuka since before the pandemic.

Our last encounter had been uncomfortable. She and Marc had come to my photo exhibition at the Lodge. When they entered, I was sitting in the living room, having tea and a chat with Madame Red Shoes.

Yuka had barely said hello before she admonished Madame Red Shoes, "Don't speak English with her! She needs to speak French."

I couldn't believe Yuka's rudeness. How dare she come to an exhibition of my work and tell me what language I had to speak.

I reached over and gripped my fingers on the edge of the coffee table. "Yuka, when a child is finding her balance – like this – before she's able to walk, telling her she has to start walking isn't going to help her learn any faster."

Yuka seemed miffed and walked out the front door and down the front steps. She stopped partway when she realized Marc hadn't followed her. He had stayed to talk with me about my photographs. A few minutes later, Yuka returned.

After they left, I said to Madame Red Shoes, "Well, that was awkward."

"I don't want to talk with you in French," she said. "I like speaking with you in English. If we spoke in French, I would be the teacher and we wouldn't be able to have our wonderful conversations as friends."

At Christophe's dinner party, Yuka was friendly and interested to hear what had brought me back to Giverny. I wondered if she had been offended that I hadn't stopped by to say good-bye. During the pandemic, I'd occasionally see her out walking. She has a very distinctive stride that resembles a forced march.

Henri, Christophe and Yuka had been friends for more than 20 years. Henri has a wonderful photo of the three of them in a garden in Giverny. They're so young. Henri and Christophe look like a couple of jolly *bonhommes*, sitting at a café table with their cigs and coffee. Yuka stands beside them, wearing a summer frock and straw hat, smiling shyly at the photographer who, I presume, was Camille.

I was fascinated by the conversation that evening, though some of it escaped me. It was all in fast French, but I got the gist of the story Christophe told.

His grandfather had been a physician in Vernon and one of his patient's was Pierre Bonnard's wife and muse Marthe de Méligny. I quickly realized that Christophe didn't know I had written a book about Bonnard and his troubled love life. He looked surprised when he referred to the young model who had killed herself and I called her by name.

He spoke of Marthe's fragile mental state and obsession with bathing. He then revealed he owned the basin she often bathed in. It's an iconic prop in many of Bonnard's paintings. When Bonnard moved to the south of France in the 1930s, he left behind some of his belongings – including the basin – with the next owner, who, years later, sold the basin to Christophe. I imagined it would go for a small fortune at auction.

And then it was time for show-and-tell. Christophe produced a small wooden box addressed to Claude Monet that had contained paint pigments he had ordered. What came next gave me goose-bumps: Christophe unwrapped a piece of canvas painted by Monet himself that had been among the abandoned pictures found at his house, which had slipped into a derelict state in the late 1940s.

The hidden treasures of Giverny never ceased to amaze me.

~◡

A few days before I was to fly back to California, Henri suggested we take a drive. It was a gorgeous fall day: sunny, blue skies with the hint of autumn colors appearing on the wooded hillsides.

We took the road to Les Andelys, home of Chateau Gaillard, an imposing fortress built in the late 12th century by King Richard the Lionheart of England to protect the Norman frontier. The chateau, now in ruins, sits on the cliffs with a breathtaking panoramic view of the Seine Valley. The road up to the chateau is a series of hairpin turns that, from a drone's view, looks like a serpent on the side of the hill.

We had just left the town center to make our way up to the castle when Henri's phone rang. He stopped in the middle of the two-lane road to take the call.

He had actually stopped at a T-intersection. A large van was coming down the hill toward us. Henri didn't seem to care that he was blocking the road.

"Henri, pull over," I said, pointing to a place at the side of the road where he could park.

"There's a problem with Facel," he said. "I have to know what's going on."

"You can't sit here in the middle of the road and discuss it. Pull over!"

A driving-school car that was behind us, slowly pulled around Henri. I'm sure the instructor, who gave Henri a bewildered look, made a point to his pupil to never follow Henri's example. The driver of the van impatiently honked his horn for Henri to move.

Henri finally pulled over to sort out the problem: Facel had gone for a swim in the pond at Giverny's Impressionist Museum and couldn't get himself out of the water. This was the second time this had happened in a week. Over the years, the museum staff had tolerated Facel's swims, which were a regular occurrence and big hit with the tourists. But Facel, at 13, was beginning to show his age. Arthritis was slowly crippling his back legs, which made it difficult for him to push himself up steps or out of a pond.

Léo, our neighbor, had been on guard duty and rescued Facel when he had gotten into this predicament a few days earlier. The museum employee who was on the phone with Henri said it was Léo's day off. Henri reached him at home, and Léo saved the day once again.

Henri and I had had many conversations about the risks of letting Facel roam freely, given his leg problem. He often came home wet from a swim somewhere. I worried that if he got stuck in a stream or in the Seine, where he loved to cool off on hot days, he'd drown.

With the crisis *du jour* averted, we started our climb up the serpentine road to the castle. From a side road, a tour bus pulled out in front of us. Henri hated getting stuck behind trucks and buses. But on that narrow road, there was no room to pass – or so I thought – and no clear view of traffic coming down the hill because of the hairpin turns.

As we began our ascent, I sensed Henri's impatience. Suddenly, he jammed his foot on the accelerator and pulled up alongside the bus.

"Henri, what are you doing?" I shouted.

We were coming into a blind curve obscured by a thicket of trees. Just as we were even with the bus, I could see around the bend. An oncoming car was a few hundred feet from us.

"Henri!" I screamed.

He sharply turned the steering wheel and cut in front of the bus, still pushing hard on the accelerator.

I could barely breath for a few seconds. I looked at Henri in disbelief. He was laughing maniacally, like a crazed teenager.

"You could have killed us, Henri. Not only us, but everyone on the bus, in that car. What the hell is wrong with you?"

He grinned. "I could see what was coming."

"No, you couldn't. I saw what was coming a second before you did because I'm on this side of the car. It was a blind curve. You had no idea what was coming."

We didn't speak the rest of the way home. I stared at the beautiful scenery, as the sun sank low in the sky, casting long shadows over the golden fields.

The question that kept running through my mind: Did I really want a life with this man?

When we got back to the apartment, he said he'd make a dinner reservation. He then went down to his workshop.

About an hour later, he returned and asked if I was ready to leave.

"No," I said. "We need to talk.'

He sat down on a bar stool in the kitchen. I stood a few feet away, mentally cementing my feet to the floor. I wasn't going to lose my footing in this conversation.

"What you did today could have put a lot of people in hospital beds or in coffins.

"*Chérie*, I could see around that bend," he said dismissively.

"No, you couldn't." I pressed my heels into the floor. "You couldn't see through those trees. You were as surprised as I was when we came around that bend and saw that car coming at us. You had to sharply cut the wheel to avoid a collision. You narrowly missed hitting the bus. Don't reinvent what happened."

He stared at me for a few seconds. "No, I couldn't see around the bend. But I knew I could handle whatever was coming at us."

I was stunned. That was his enormous ego talking. "You could have killed a lot of people today, Henri, and you don't seem to care. You're 79 years old. Someday in the not-too-distant future, you're not going to have the reflexes of the stupid teenager who lives inside you."

Henri laughed.

"You think it's funny. The thought of apologizing to me hasn't crossed your mind, has it?"

He shrugged. "I'm sorry you were so frightened."

I exploded. "Don't pin the blame for this on me! Yes, I was frightened because your recklessness terrifies me. You need to apologize to me."

He looked out the window and was silent for a moment. Then he looked at me, without a trace of remorse in his expression, and said, "I'm sorry I took a risk."

Even if he wrote "I'm sorry I took a risk" 50 times, with two pencils taped together, I was certain he'd do it again someday.

I took a deep breath and said, "I can't make a life with a man who won't keep me safe."

On the last day of Giverny's season, we stopped by Christophe's gallery so that Henri could choose his painting. He didn't choose his favorite, the Bonnard-like painting of the bedroom scene. Christophe overheard me say to Henri, "It's pretty, but it's too feminine for the living room." Henri's living room is a manly room with its hodgepodge of massive furniture.

Instead, Henri chose the Matisse-like painting of the Mediterranean view that I liked. I took a photo of Henri and Christophe with the two paintings they had swapped.

Christophe disappeared for a moment and came back, carrying a painting that I could see only from the back. He stood in front of me, and to my surprise, he said, "For you."

He turned the canvas toward me. It was the bedroom painting.

"Christophe…" I didn't know what to say for a moment. "What a generous gift. *Merci beaucoup.*"

He smiled. "This gives me pleasure."

I glanced at Henri, who looked surprised and delighted.

After we got home, Henri hung both paintings in his living room.

That evening, Henri and I joined Bernadette and their friend Raoul at the Baudy, to celebrate the memory of our *bon amie* Claire Joyes, who had passed away unexpectedly that summer.

She had fallen ill suddenly. She was treated for fluid in her lungs at a hospital in Rouen and was convalescing at the hospital in Vernon when Henri had visited her.

For a couple of weeks, he had been trying to get in touch with her. She wasn't answering her phone and he wasn't getting a response when he rang the bell at her gate. On a hunch, he went to the hospital in Vernon and found her.

She was in a private room and breathing through an oxygen tube. Henri said she was weak, but mentally alert. They had a good conversation and talked about the care she'd need once she was back home.

Two days later, she died.

I received the news from Henri the next day. Naturally, he was devastated. They had been friends for many years. "She's gone," he said. I could hear the raw emotion in his voice.

Henri said her local friends would honor her in some way. But it seemed everyone was too grief-stricken to organize a memorial.

During my fall visit, I suggested to Henri that he and I should raise a glass to her on the Baudy's closing night of the season. I had a wonderful photo of Claire and Henri on a closing night there a few years earlier: The two of them share a dinner napkin between them – tucked into her collar and his. They're smiling and raising their wine glasses, clearly enjoying the evening.

Henri and I discussed who else we could invite to Claire's final night at the Baudy. Yuka had been a close friend, but Bernadette objected to including her. Apparently, Yuka had known Claire was seriously ill – she had been in touch with Claire's sister – but she hadn't told Bernadette and Henri about Claire's deteriorating condition. Claire's family had asked Yuka not to discuss this with anyone.

"Yuka lied to us," Henri told me. "We asked her if she had heard news of Claire."

"What if Claire's family had told you she was ill and asked you not to tell anyone?" I said. "Yuka was honoring their request."

"Bernadette will not come to the Baudy if Yuka is there."

That's so like Bernadette, I thought. Grinding her axe, even in this.

It was twilight when Henri, Bernadette, Raoul – a longtime friend of Claire's – and I sat down on the Baudy terrace. We ordered champagne, one of Claire's favorite beverages. Bernadette had brought one of Claire's books. She had written several about the history of Giverny. Her bestsellers, translated into many languages, were lavish coffee-table books inspired by recipes from the Monet household cooking journals, featuring beautiful photos of table settings that evoked the lifestyle of his era.

We shared our memories of Claire. I remembered an afternoon with her at her rambling garden cottage that had been the home of Lily Butler, the daughter of American Impressionist painter Theodore Butler whose wedding march Theodore Robinson had painted. She wanted to hear about my Robinson research and a discovery I had made in a museum vault of a misidentified photo that turned out to be the first known photo of Marie's face. Robinson had always photographed her in profile or with her head down.

She shared with me old photographs of her family's estate in southern France. Claire was a blue blood who didn't celebrate Bastille Day. I remember she actually refused to attend a dinner party at Yuka's on July 14 because she didn't support the uprising in 1789 that marked the start of the French Revolution.

Claire had been married to Jean-Marie Toulgouat, whose lineage was impressive. He was the son of Lily Butler, the grandson of Theodore Butler, and the great-grandson of Monet's second wife, Alice Hoschedé. He was born the year after Monet died and was a highly regarded artist in his own right. As a boy, he played in Monet's house, surrounded by Monet's unsold and unfinished work, along with the paintings Monet had collected by Renoir, Cezanne, Pissarro and Manet. Toulgouat passed away in 2006. His paintings were widely collected and were sold at a prestigious gallery in London that represented his estate. I took Claire to the Vernon station one Sunday morning for a trip to London for an event honoring her late husband. She was all aflutter – (then) Prince Charles would be in attendance.

As Henri and I walked back to his apartment that evening, I took his arm and said, "You received an extraordinary gift last Christmas, even though you may not have realized it at the time."

"What was that?" he asked.

"You had hoped to spend Christmas with me," I said. "But instead, you got to spend it with Claire. How lucky were you."

Chapter 42

When I returned to California in early November, I felt undone by what had happened in those seven weeks with Henri. I couldn't shake the terror I had felt on that serpent-of-a-road in Les Andelys. I had shared the story with Sarah, who was appalled. As much as she wanted me to move back to Giverny, she questioned how I could have a good life with Henri.

What stuck in my mind was a long talk I'd had with Madame Red Shoes before I left. When I told her Henri wanted me to return and had promised we'd move to a house together, she furrowed her forehead and shook her head. I knew what she was about to say came from her love and concern for me.

"Rebecca," she said firmly. "You need to have your independence, a life apart from him."

Madame Red Shoes had been such a comfort to me during the debacle with the lease signing, when Henri had pulled the rug. She had put out the word to her friends that I was looking for a place and had come with me to see properties. She had listened empathetically as I told her what had happened with Henri. When I finished, she said, "He's a selfish man."

She had made a life for herself and her three sons after her husband had left her, when she was in her late thirties, for another woman. She was determined to keep her beautiful home, an enormous house that had been a leprosy asylum in Vernon in the 15th century. Some days, we would sit in her solarium, with its two-story stained-glass windows decorated with herons and cattails. Some of her paintings were set in that room, decorated with fan-back rattan chairs and oversized floor cushions in colorful fabrics.

Her life hadn't been easy. As a single mother, she rode the train to Paris, where she worked at the famous department store Galeries Lafayette, in the china department. Every day on the hour-long train ride, she worked on a memoir about her childhood and the years before her marriage ended. She enjoyed showing me one of the copies she'd printed for family members. She had included old photos with the text.

"What a treasure this is," I said.

I took great inspiration from Madame Red Shoes. At 88, she was still traveling to far-flung places. When I saw her during my autumn visit, she was recovering from a fall that had injured her shoulder. She hadn't been able to work on her pottery or pastels. She was getting treatments that weren't helping and was hoping a scheduled cortisone shot would give her relief. She wanted to get back to her drawing class and was eager to begin planning a trip to the Yucatan in the spring.

"I want to be like you in 20 years," I told her. She was exactly 20 years older than I.

She leaned over and patted my arm. "Keep your independence."

~

After many frustrating, futile tries online, I finally got an appointment to submit my French visa application. There was a new system that required me to go to a document processing center in Los Angeles, where I would submit the paperwork, which would then be sent on to the French Embassy in Washington, D.C.

I drove to L.A. the day before my appointment, not wanting to risk getting stuck in a traffic jam on the day. I had spent hours putting my file together, making sure I had additional documents that weren't on the list, like a copy of my birth certificate. I'd had too many experiences where I'd show up at an immigration office without a document that hadn't been on the checklist.

A new item had been added to the checklist —a something called Schengen Travel Insurance. Standard medical coverage wasn't enough. The Schengen policy had coverage for Covid treatment – and coverage for the cost of shipping your coffin to your home country. The cost of the policy was 350 euros (about $375). I had purchased the insurance coverage online from a French insurance company, which processed the payment and emailed a copy of the policy to me all in the same day.

My appointment was December 1, which was a Thursday, and took about 20 minutes. Because I had already had a French visa, the woman at the counter told me that I might hear back from the embassy within a few weeks, perhaps before Christmas. I didn't expect that to happen, especially with the holidays coming. I had read on the embassy website that visa decisions could take as long as six weeks.

The application, along with my passport, was sent that day to Washington via overnight courier. I paid a FedEx fee to have the passport returned to me so that I wouldn't have to make another trip to L.A.

A week and a day later, I was astounded when a FedEx delivery guy rang my doorbell. Inside the packet was my new French visa embossed in my passport.

~

The visa would take effect January 1, 2023. The woman at the visa center said she thought I would need to arrive in France within three months of the effective date, but she wasn't sure. Dealing with the visa service had been a nightmare – most people I had spoken with there didn't have a clue.

I suddenly had to make a plan. This was really happening. I called Henri. He seemed delighted and promised to step up his housing search.

I contacted shipping companies and gulped when the quotes came in. The same U.K. company that had shipped my goods in 2021 – for a staggering $18,000 – had raised the price for a 40-foot container for the same route to $26,300. Why the huge increase, I asked the agent. There was no longer a shipping crisis. Containers were readily available. She apologized for the increase and blamed it on inflation in general and the cost of fuel in particular. I had dealt with the same woman before. She was friendly and helpful and told me she'd ask for a discount since I had been a previous customer. But she couldn't get the price below $22,600.

I finally found a company that could do it for just under $19,000. I called Henri back to give him the bad news. "Are you still willing to split the cost of this?" I asked him. He said yes and would make arrangements to transfer funds. I told him we wouldn't need to make the payment until the week of the move, which would be scheduled for late February.

I needed to give 60-day notice to my landlady, to terminate the lease early. A few days after Christmas, while I was spending the holidays with Kyle and Julia, I sent her this email, with a copy to her daughter:

I have some news: I am moving back to Giverny. I never imagined this would happen when I arrived here last year. But I left behind a Frenchman who would very much like me to return.

When I made the decision to come back to the U.S., I felt undone by the harsh Covid restrictions (especially the travel ban) that were in place in France at the time, with no relief in sight. But things are different now and I would very much like to resume the life Henri and I had together before the pandemic.

Thank you for allowing me to make your beautiful condo my home. Del Mar has been one of the loveliest places I've ever lived.

I truly had loved the beauty of Del Mar and its beaches and sunsets. Tears would come as I drove over the hill on Del Mar Heights Road toward the beach. On the downward slope, the horizon line rose to my eye level – a phenomenon of physics – which always astonished me as the ocean seemed to magically rise high in the sky.

I had seen more Green Flashes during my time in Del Mar than most people could hope to see in a lifetime.

But I felt ready to move on. Another equally beautiful place awaited my return.

Chapter 43

On the morning of January 6, 2023 – just a week after I had given notice and signed a shipping contract – I awoke at 7 and as I put my feet on the floor, mud squished between my toes. I thought surely I was dreaming.

In the middle of the night, a city water main had ruptured and spewed thousands of gallons of water at tremendous force down the hill where my condo was situated. The patio area, which was sheltered by a high wooden fence but no protective wall, took the brunt of the flow. The rushing water carved a channel under the fence and washed out the flower bed, pushing mud under the sliding patio doors.

By the time I got up – after the rupture had gone unabated for four hours – the entire condo was filled with an inch of muddy water. The carpet in the bedroom, on the opposite end of the condo from the patio, had acted as a giant sponge, pulling water from the living room down a long corridor, where I had stacked boxes of photos in preparation for the move. I could see a waterline forming on the bottom of the boxes as the cardboard soaked up the water that had flooded the hallway. My first impulse was to rescue the boxes. But there wasn't a dry place to move them.

My more immediate concern in the first moments: Was I sloshing through mud or shit?

I heard voices out on the street beyond the patio and quickly got dressed. At the top of the street, the disaster was in plain view. A 24-inch pipe, showing years of neglect, had torn apart and created a sink hole, about 10 feet across, that could have held several SUVs.

The day became a blur of engineers, contractors, cleanup crews and guys in suits with clipboards offering their business cards and apologies.

What I couldn't understand was why me? A family down the street had also sustained some damage, but I was told I had taken the full impact. My neighbor whose unit shared a wall with mine seemed unconcerned. He had noticed a puddle by his patio doors. But he didn't realize that water was seeping through the floorboards in my unit and running across the slab under his dining room floor and up into the common wall. He would be displaced, too.

At one point that day, I went outside to get some fresh air and looked down the street. It was a normal, sunny day. People were out walking their dogs, riding their bikes, heading to the beach.

I was now homeless, but no one seemed to notice. I felt targeted. It felt personal.

Most of the workers and their supervisors had left by 5. It was a Friday. The weekend had started. A man and a woman on the crew had stayed to help me empty three trunks that the rest of the crew had missed. It was nearly 7 when we finally finished. They kindly helped me carry things to my car that I would be taking to the hotel. The City of San Diego was footing the bill for me to stay at a nearby Residence Inn for the next six weeks.

I called Norm and Cindy and asked them to meet me there. I was exhausted and didn't think I had enough energy to unpack the car.

The next morning, I awoke feeling like I was coming out of a bad dream. The poofy hotel mattress felt like a cloud. I felt strangely suspended, like I was about to go over a waterfall.

I sat on the edge of bed, wondering where to begin. Fans and de-humidifiers were blowing round-the-clock at the condo. I wouldn't be able to start sorting through the mess for a couple of days, until things had dried out.

A week earlier, I had scheduled a hair appointment for that after-noon and I decided to keep it. I desperately needed a scalp massage.

Two-and-a-half weeks later, I watched a 40-foot container pull away from my driveway with all my belongings that had been salvageable. There were losses, but most of my photos – that I feared would be ruined – came through mostly unscathed. Some photo albums that had spent a week in a drying facility bore the telltale marks of the flood, with ink running down wavy pages.

I had accomplished in two-and-a-half weeks what I had planned to do in seven at a much more leisurely pace. I was walking with a cane by that point. My ankles were wobbly again, from all the hours I had spent on my feet.

I still had much to do, but the stress of the move itself was over.

In the end, I was on a plane to France only 10 days earlier than I had planned. I tried to understand the reason for all the drama. What was the urgency of it all? Did the universe want to make sure I wouldn't change my mind and stay in California?

I had been torn in this decision, I admit. I had come back to the U.S. to start a new chapter of my family life. I wanted to be close to Kyle and Julia and their children if and when that blessing arrived.

I had quickly learned during the runup to the wedding that I needed to better manage my expectations. In the year since the wedding, I had only seen Kyle and Julia for a weekend. They had busy lives, demanding jobs, and an active social life with Julia's family who lived close by. I was only an hour plane ride away, but I wasn't down the street.

I was happy to spend my last Christmas in the States with them. I had intended to return home on December 27th. But Southwest Airlines went into a scheduling meltdown and I couldn't rebook my ticket until New Year's Day.

I tried to see a gift in the extra days I spent with them. It came during a conversation I had with them about the decision I needed to make.

Kyle eased my guilt. "Mom, you need to do what will make you happy."

I knew he was blissfully happy in his new life with Julia and her family. I told them if they ever needed me, I could come back in a day. I had actually done that once, when I was living in Italy and my parents were in distress.

I imagined having grandkids visit me in France, making memories they could share with their kids someday about their Grammy who had lived in Giverny.

But once again, I reminded myself that I needed to better manage my expectations.

Chapter 44

Henri was waiting with open arms and a surprised look when I emerged from the international arrivals area at Charles de Gaulle Airport.

I had two luggage carts loaded with four suitcases and a carry-on. I had somehow managed to hook the carts together, but the exit door was the width of a single cart. A British guy coming up behind me saved the day. He threw his duffle bag on one of the carts and pushed it through the door ahead of me.

Henri seemed to be waiting for an explanation after I thanked my travel angel.

I kissed Henri on the cheek and said, "Don't worry, luv, I just met him. It probably won't last."

He then looked at the pile of bags. "How long are you staying?" There was a smile in his eyes.

I rarely travel with more than two bags. But my shipping container wasn't due to arrive for two or three months, so I needed clothes for two seasons. It was barely above freezing on my arrival day in mid-February. I pulled my puffer coat out of my carry-on before we left the terminal for the parking lot.

One suitcase was full of immigration and tax files and a stack of binders with notes for the book I had been working on (this one).

Another bag had a few packing cubes with those precious things I didn't want sinking to the bottom of the sea if the shipping container slid off the deck.

A lot had happened with Henri since I had last seen him. Just the week before, he had gotten his dental implants – more than a year after that ordeal had begun. He had sent me a photo of his new smile, which looked just like his old smile. It looked even better in person. I always loved his smile.

But Henri had not been in great shape otherwise. An old back problem had flared. He was in so much pain that he had spent the holidays in a wheel chair. Painkillers finally got him back on his feet.

His hearing loss had worsened considerably. He seemed to be totally deaf in his right ear. When I spoke to him in the car, he didn't turn his head toward me or acknowledge he had heard me.

At one point, I put my hand on his leg to get his attention. "Henri, can you not hear me?"

He shook his head. "I've become an old man since you left."

That surprised me. Henri was always the ever-youthful, invincible guy who called people much younger than he "old."

It was early evening by the time Henri and I got back to his place. He made dinner. We lingered over a bottle of wine.

I fell into bed next to him, exhausted. But I hungrily wanted him. We were like a couple of teenagers when we finally came up for air.

I kissed his cheek and whispered, "Where's the old man?"

It wasn't long before stress fractures started to show in this new life we were making. At first, they mystified me.

Henri had rented an all-electric KIA for me. Electric cars and hybrids, with their automatic transmissions, were a godsend to me. And with the fuel shortages that had hit France because of strikes at the refineries, I didn't have to deal with long lines at the pumps.

Henri enjoyed driving the KIA on an expedition we took to Paris to see the "Monet-Mitchell" exhibition, which was in its final week.

It was Henri's first trip to Paris since 2016. Henri hates Paris. Mostly, he dislikes Parisians, whom he finds to be arrogant.

But we had a wonderful day. The exhibition was at the spectacular Fondation Louis Vuitton building, a modern massive glass-and-steel structure designed by Frank Gehry, in the lovely Bois de Boulogne section of Paris.

Before visiting the galleries, we had a fabulous lunch at the Fondation restaurant Le Frank, presumably named for Gehry. The space felt like an out-of-kilter geodesic dome, constructed with glass panels that towered over us at precarious angles. Suspended from the high point of the ceiling was Gehry's "Fish Lamp," a mobile of 17 fish made of torn pieces of translucent plastic laminate and illuminated by LED lights.

I told Henri about director Sydney Pollack's 2005 film *Sketches of Frank Gehry* that explored Gehry's creative process.

I picked up my napkin, folding and twisting it into a contorted shape. "This is what he does," I said. "And then the engineers have to figure out how to build it."

Before lunch, Henri had already inspected the joints of the exterior steel beams that held the glass panels in place. "You see the wood blocks wedged between the metal plates?" he said. "That's how they allow for contraction and expansion."

The menu of Le Frank's Michelin-star chef didn't disappoint. For dessert, I had Monet's "Vert-Vert" cake. The recipe comes from his household cooking journal and is unusual for a special ingredient that gives the cake its green coloring: spinach juice.

I had noticed, in the main foyer, an enormous photo of Monet in a white hat and white jacket. I said to Henri, smiling, "I think I've seen that photo before, but where?" It is a widely disseminated photo of Monet, but Henri has the framed original that came from the Monet-Butler household, with Monet's name inscribed on a small brass plate at the bottom of the frame.

I had been a bit skeptical about the concept of the exhibition which was to create a visual "dialogue" between Monet and

American abstract expressionist Joan Mitchell, who had spent much of her adult life in France and in 1967, purchased a two-acre estate in Vetheuil, the village where Monet had lived before he moved to nearby Giverny. Mitchell was born in Chicago the year before Monet died, and took art classes in her youth at the Art Institute of Chicago, where she later earned a Bachelor of Fine Arts degree in 1947.

The Fondation Louis Vuitton had an impressive collection of her work and, for the exhibition, had juxtaposed her abstract compositions next to Monet's, to compare their palettes and renderings of the same landscapes, along the banks of the Seine.

What made the concept work was the installation. The gallery spaces were enormous, with vaulted ceilings that were a few stories high. As Henri and I entered one gallery, I turned to him and said, "Wow. Look what they've done." Straight ahead of us, on the far wall, was an immense multi-panel abstract by Mitchell. In the middle of the gallery, two large display boards had been mounted, flanking the view of her work, with two unframed Monet canvases: The one on the left showed the trunk of a willow with its delicate branches "weeping" over the banks of the lily pond. The one on the right showed a mass of water lilies seemingly suspended in the reflection on the water's surface, etched with wispy willow foliage. All three paintings – Mitchell's large panel and the two Monets – looked like they have been painted from the same palette, dominated by a rich forest green and lavender-blue.

I loved that Henri and I shared a deep interest in art. I had been a journalism major in college, but my special area of study – my "minor," as they called it – was art history. I've often thought if I were to go back to my college days and choose a different career path, I would have become an art historian.

That evening, Henri and I were still talking about the exhibition. He reminded me of the stories about Mitchell that Christophe had told us at his dinner party. Christophe knew Mitchell well and on a number of occasions had helped her get home after she'd tied on a few too many at a local bar. She was a colorful character in Vetheuil, where she lived until her death in 1992.

~~~

After our big trip to Paris that day, Henri decided to recharge the KIA. First, he plugged it into an outdoor outlet, adjacent to the driveway, by the door to the boiler room. But the power surge caused the breaker to flip. He then brought the cable into the boiler room and plugged it in there.

The green light on the charger cast a glow on the ceiling of my room, which had a window, without a curtain, that looked down on the boiler room. The green glow didn't bother me, but about 10 minutes later, the light started flashing.

Henri was already in bed. I knocked on his door and told him the charger was flashing. I wondered if there might be a problem.

What happened next astounded me. He angrily got out of bed, cursing under his breath. "You don't appreciate anything I do for you."

"What does my appreciation for you have to do with the charger? Let's unplug it for tonight and plug it back in the morning. I don't want the light flashing in my room all night."

"It wouldn't bother me," he retorted.

I lay awake that night, as I had so many times in that bed, trying to understand Henri's behavior. I hadn't been back in Giverny a week and already we were coming undone.

The next day, I asked him to sit down with me so we could talk about his outburst the night before. I pointed out that when he's unhappy with me, he often comes around to one of two complaints: I don't appreciate him or I don't trust him.

I asked him how the blinking car charger was connected to his resentment that I didn't appreciate him.

He didn't have an explanation. I could tell he was still angry.

"We've had a lot of problems in the past, you and I," I said. "I don't want us going back to our old ways. We have a chance at a new start now."

A few days later, we had a big blowup. His housekeeper, Sofie, was in the habit of showing up at his apartment once or twice a week, whenever she had free time, to clean and do the laundry. Henri didn't mind this arrangement because he wasn't at home during the day.

"I'd like to know when she's coming – at least a day in advance. No drop-ins," I said.

"Why?" Henri asked.

"I write during the day and have calls with clients. I don't want her running the vacuum when I'm on a call," I said. "She barges in here – she opens the door as she knocks. One day, I was coming out of the bathroom wrapped in a towel and there was Sofie in the hallway."

I hadn't forgotten my first encounter with Sofie several years earlier. The day before I met her, Henri had told me, "You are the woman of the house. You decide what needs to be done. But be nice to her. If she quits, we'll have a problem. It's not easy finding housekeepers."

I can still see Sofie standing next to Henri in the wide archway between the dining room and the kitchen when he introduced us. She politely said *bonjour.* She spoke no English.

Henri then said to me, "Tell Sofie what you'd like her to do today."

To Henri, I said in English, "I'd like her to change the bedsheets."

After he translated my request, she looked at me with a stony face. "It's not time," she replied in French.

I looked at Henri and asked, "What does she mean by that?"

They had a brief exchange in French. He then said to me, "She changes the sheets every other week."

I raised an eyebrow. "I'd like her to change them today and every week."

A bad start.

She changed the sheets that day, but left a load of wet towels in the dryer and a load of wet sheets in the washer. When Henri came home that evening, I asked who would be finishing the laundry.

"What do you mean?" he asked. "Sofie will be back in a few days to do the ironing."

"She left wet laundry in the washer and dryer today. Who will take care of that?"

Henri shrugged.

"It's not going to be me, Henri. You need to tell her not to start a task she can't finish."

He sighed. I could hear an "oy" under his breath.

After her next visit, I came home to find a broken vase on a small table in the dining room.

Henri appeared from the kitchen. "Sofie said she was sorry about the vase. She was trying to kill a spider on the wall with the vacuum hose and knocked it over.

It was my turn to shrug. "It wasn't my vase. It was yours."

As I walked down the corridor, I noticed a stack of neatly folded towels on top of the dryer. I wondered why she hadn't put them on the shelf where they belonged. I then realized they were soaking wet.

In disbelief, I called for Henri.

"Oui, *chérie*?" he said as he entered the bathroom.

"Look at this." I had lifted the corner of the top towel on the stack.

"I don't see the problem."

I handed him the wet stack. "What about now?"

My head-butting with Sofie turned nasty one day as I was getting ready to leave for an appointment. After the vase incident, I started putting all the breakables on the dining room table so that she could freely dust the furniture. Sofie didn't dust knickknacks, which was fine with me, given her clumsiness. It had become my job to collect, dust and put the knickknacks back in place.

The dining table hadn't been polished in years. The wood was scratched and stained with water marks. It was laughable that she suddenly wanted to polish it that particular day. From all the cleaning I had done in that apartment when I first arrived, I knew for a fact that Sofie had rarely dirtied a rag.

I pointed to the clock, indicating I needed to leave. "*Pas aujourd'hui,* Sofie." Not today.

She insisted that I clear the table.

I emphatically said again, *"Pas aujourd'hui!"*

When I told Henri that evening what had happened, he repeated what he had said before. "It won't be easy finding another house-keeper if she quits."

Sofie didn't quit. She knew better. She got a fat paycheck from Henri every month.

At Christmastime that year, I gave her a loaf of pumpkin bread I had made, and after that, she was friendlier. She worked for me when I moved to the Little House, and we didn't have any problems. She wasn't a great cleaner – she only went upstairs twice during the two years I lived there – but she was great at ironing duvet covers and linen dresses and could make a neat bed.

But there seemed to be an attitude shift with Sofie now that I was back living at the apartment with Henri. I wondered if she saw herself as his Queen Bee. Very French. I sensed she ran the show and got away with that because Henri was afraid of losing her.

She was back to her old habit of leaving behind wet laundry. One day, I discovered a wet load that had been sitting in the dryer for four days. Henri and I pulled out three big bag loads of damp, tangled sheets, towels and jeans.

"This stuff is going to mildew," I said to him. "When is she coming again?"

He didn't seem to know.

An hour later, she showed up, as usual without notice. Henri showed her the three bags we had pulled out of the dryer that we had put in his dressing room. One of them held a pile of wet towels.

Sofie set up the ironing board in the dressing room, where there was a single bed that grandkids used to sleep in when they'd come visit. After about 45 minutes, she called out, *"Au revoir,* Rebecca," and left by the back door.

I went to check on things. She hadn't finished the ironing. There was an untouched bag of damp rumpled sheets and a bag of wet towels. She had tossed one damp sheet across the bed and hung another from the end of the ironing board that she had propped against the wall.

I phoned Henri, who was down in his workshop, and asked him to come upstairs.

When he came through the back door, dressed in his coveralls, I was standing in the doorway of the dressing room.

"I thought you should see this," pointing to the wet sheet on the bed. Feel this." I picked up a corner and held it for him to take.

He turned up his greasy palms, not wanting to touch it. He glanced down at the bag of wet towels at the end of the bed. He told me he had spoken with Sofie briefly when she arrived. "She said these need to be dried."

"That's not our job, Henri. That's what you're paying her to do. When is she coming back to finish the ironing?"

"Friday."

"It's Monday. This damp stuff is going to sit in bags for another four days?"

He grabbed the bag of towels and went down the hall into the bathroom. I could hear him cursing as he jammed the towels into the dryer. He came back into the hallway and squared off with me.

"I don't want to deal with domestic matters," he shouted.

"You've had women taking care of you all your life."

"That's right!"

"I'll take care of Sofie," I said.

"If you make her mad, she'll quit."

"The problem is she's the boss and you're afraid of her. She doesn't get to come here whenever she feels like it, leaving work for us to finish that you're paying her to do."

Henri threw his arms in the air. "You make my life so difficult!"

"Really? I'm so sorry to hear that, Henri."

He stormed out and slammed the door behind him.

In the weeks before I arrived in February, Henri had had a stream of visitors, mostly his mechanic friends who had come to work on various projects. My arrival had added further disruption to Henri's routine.

He was behind with his paperwork and raced out of the apartment one morning with bills in hand that were nearly overdue. He had been skipping his morning walks. We had had some late nights, enjoying the honeymoon phase of our reunion, and he was sleeping later than usual in the mornings, which cut into the time he usually spent in his office.

Henri had also been driving me to appointments and to visits with friends, which threw a wrench in his day. We had returned the KIA to the rental agency after our trip to Paris because its electrical system went haywire the next day. I didn't want to spend money renting another car. I needed to buy a car.

That process took a month as we dealt with the complications of getting financing and insurance. Toyota's financing arm wouldn't approve a loan for me unless I had a guarantor. Our banker, whose name was Quentin, had warned me that I'd have trouble getting a car loan if I didn't have French-sourced income.

All of the back-and-forth with the dealership was an added strain for Henri. One day in exasperation, he said to me, "I want my old life back."

I felt like I had been cut by a knife. "Do you mean that, Henri?"

He looked tired and ragged. His eyes had lost their sparkle. He was often in a bad mood and was short-tempered with me.

"Henri, what do you *need*?" I asked.

He closed his eyes for a moment. "Calm. I need calm."

He turned away and stared out the kitchen window. Then I asked, "What do you *want*?"

He kept his back to me and didn't reply.

"You need to think about that," I said quietly. "Because I don't feel very wanted."

Our mood brightened one Saturday night in late March when we went to a local disco dance party organized by Giverny's social committee. It marked the end of winter hibernation. The season would officially begin in a week, on April 1.

It was nice seeing friends again, some of whom go to tropical climes in the winter. I was greeted warmly by many who were glad to hear I had moved back to Giverny.

There were new faces, too. A group of Ukrainians who had come to live in the area since the start of the war were special guests that night.

The local deejay had a great playlist – lots of sing-along French songs and exotic Moroccan tunes that got the ladies shimmying.

On my list of my proudest accomplishments in this lifetime, I added one that Saturday night – I got Henri out on the dance floor.

His moment of Saturday Night Fever didn't last long. Once he sat down, some guy in a green chipmunk costume asked me to dance. I don't know who my mystery partner was or why he was dressed as a chipmunk. But we tripped the light fantastic under the disco ball.

The next day, I found out my Chipmunk dance partner had been a woman. Twist!

A couple of nights later, Maxine and Olivier invited us for dinner at the moulin. Henri wanted to take my car, which I'd had for only a week.

"No, no'" I said. "You know how their dogs are. They'll jump up on the car and scratch it."

As we got in Henri's SUV, he said testily, "You know how to spoil an evening."

He had used that line on me a few years earlier. I had actually written it down and taped it above my desk – I thought I'd work it into a story someday.

"This spoils your evening – me wanting to keep my car from getting scratched?" I asked. "I just spent 28,000 euros on that car and would like to keep it nice for at least a few weeks."

I hadn't yet closed the door on the passenger side.

"We're late," he said impatiently. "It's not nice to keep Maxine and Olivier waiting."

"It's also not nice for us to show up in the middle of an argument. Is it going to be possible for us to have an enjoyable evening? If not, I can stay home."

We were locked in a battle of wills. It reminded me of the head-butting between Doo-Doo and Praline.

"Can we have an enjoyable evening?" I asked again. I finally reached over and closed the door. And then to have the last word, I said, "Those dogs are crazy."

When we pulled into the courtyard of the moulin a few minutes later, the dogs were running wild and Maxine was charging at them with a push broom. One dog was muzzled. I managed to get around Maxine as she lunged at the unmuzzled dog who was barking frantically. In the chaos, Olivier came out to greet us.

We followed Olivier and Maxine inside and Henri joined them in the kitchen. Maxine was ranting about something. I hung back in the hallway outside the kitchen, looking out the French doors into the back garden. A few minutes later, Henri emerged.

"Drama, drama," he said. He then told me the unmuzzled dog had killed the family's pet rabbit that morning.

I looked in the room opposite the kitchen where the empty rabbit hutch stood. The scene of a grisly murder.

I felt a bit smug. Those dogs *are* crazy.

That evening, the four of us celebrated an agreement we had reached: Henri and I would become tenants of a small house Olivier and Maxine owned in the village, which they had rented out to tourists for several years. Self-catering holiday accommodations – known as gîtes – are popular in the rural areas of France and had provided a good income for Olivier and Maxine after they'd decided to close the moulin as a B&B several years earlier. But like the moulin, running a gîte was a lot of work. Maxine had a full-time job and Olivier, in his early 60s, was thinking about easing into retirement.

I knew they had a bigger concern as well. Olivier was due to go in for surgery in a couple of weeks. A new cluster of tumors had formed in his brain, this time at the base of his skull.

Henri and I had met with Olivier a week earlier to discuss arrangements for the move. My shipping container was due to arrive in a few weeks, in early April. The gîte was booked through May, but Olivier said I could store my belongings in the gîte's basement.

The gîte had been nicely refurbished, but the rooms were small. There would be barely enough room for my furniture let alone Henri's. When I explained to Olivier that the gîte furniture would need to be removed, he said that wouldn't be a problem. But he told us his doctors had said he'd need to rest for a month after his surgery. That worried me. On our drive home that evening, I asked Henri if he was concerned Olivier was taking on too much. Henri assured me Olivier would hire the help he needed.

Because Maxine had been out that evening, I had written her a detailed email about what we had discussed. She hadn't replied.

As the four of us sat down at the moulin, in the pall of the rabbit's untimely death, I asked her if she had received my message.

"Yes, but I didn't read it," she said dismissively, as a vape trail billowed out of her nostrils. "It was so long, so American."

I bit my tongue. I knew the dragon-lady side of Maxine, which I had seen many times as a guest at the moulin. Her foul moods and temper sometimes flared to the point that visitors criticized her in their Trip Advisor reviews. In response, she'd foolishly get into arguments with them in the comments, essentially proving their complaints to be true.

We raised our glasses to the new place Henri and I would call home. I hoped for the best. I really wanted this to be a new start for Henri and me.

Despite the conflict between Henri and me, all was amazingly peaceful in Doo-Doo Land.

Doo-Doo seemed more docile and perhaps had grown wiser with age. I wondered if he missed Praline. I often saw him napping by her grave.

Baby Girl, with her strong straight legs, was no longer little. Her young mother, now known as Maman, who had been derelict in her motherly duties when Baby Girl was young, had grown into her role. I loved watching mother and daughter play in the corral as they stood on their hind legs and danced with each other.

Henri's grandson Luc, now 9, had given Baby Girl a new name. He had decided on "Melissa," which we suspected might be the name of a girl he liked at school.

Doo-Doo and the Goat Girls all slept together in the shed without a problem. Doo-Doo had learned to climb the stairs. He shared snacks with them. No-more head-butting, like in the old days.

It seemed many lessons had been learned. Détente prevailed.

Chapter 45

Four days after the disco party, Henri seemed to be coming down with a cold. I suggested he take a Covid test. I had an extra kit that I had brought with me from the States.

I stood, masked, at the door of his room when I broke the news, as he lay in bed. The pink line on the antigen test strip had lit up like a neon light in the first minute. I read to him from my laptop the current guidance for quarantining a Covid patient at home. We only had one bathroom, which wasn't ideal. I stressed to him that he had to wear a mask when he went to the WC or the shower room.

"I will take care of you, but you need to take care of me," I told him. "If I get sick, we're both screwed."

I set up a bar stool in the hallway outside his bedroom door and brought another bar stool for him to set up beside his bed where he would take his meals. After he finished eating, he would return the tray to the stool in the hallway. I explained that, except for the tray exchanges and his trips to the bathroom, we needed to keep the door closed to his room to contain the virus.

Five hours after his Covid test, he wanted to take another one and appeared to be peeved with me when I said, "That's not how this works." I had just come home from the pharmacy with five test kits. "The pharmacist said you could test again in five days to see if you're negative. These other tests are for me. I'm supposed to test every 48 hours." I had already used one of the tests and was relieved I was negative.

Later that day, I noticed the door to his room was wide open. He was sitting in bed, reading.

"Henri, you have to keep this door closed."

He got up and, without putting on a mask, came toward me and then sat down at the foot of the bed, not even six feet from me. "Put on a mask," I said to him sternly. The look on his face said, *Make me.* As I turned away, he coughed as if to punctuate his defiance.

Infuriated, I slammed the door shut.

A little while later, I made him a hot dinner, but when I knocked on his door, he didn't answer. I opened it partway and saw that he was on the phone. "I'm talking to Paul," he said, waving me off and making a joke to him about room service.

I left the tray in the hallway and closed the door. He later informed me that his meal had been cold. No surprise. After dinner, I brought a tray with snacks – a tangerine, a banana and a bar of chocolate. Henri often gets up in the middle of the night for a piece of fruit or cookies. I opened his door to say good-night and reminded him to use the KN95 mask I had given him, when he got up in the night to go to the bathroom.

I closed his door and went to the kitchen to rinse his dishes, thinking about the spiky Covid balls that were probably crawling on my hands. I heard Henri leave his room to go the bathroom. I leaned over the kitchen counter to look down the hallway. When he emerged a few minutes later, I saw that he wasn't wearing a mask. He went into the shower room and left the door slightly ajar.

I flew down the hallway and flung open the shower-room door, hitting him broadside as he stood near the sink. He laughed.

"We just talked about wearing a mask, not even 10 minutes ago," I fumed.

He shrugged and said, *"J'ai oublié."* I forgot.

"You don't give a fuck about me," I shouted. "I'm done."

When I went to bed around 11, I knew I wouldn't get to sleep soon. My plan was to leave early the next morning. I turned on the nightstand lamp and surveyed the dirty clothes spilling out of the hamper in the corner of the room. I decided to throw in a load on the speed cycle, while I started packing. I got out a suitcase and organized my toiletries. I was very focused. Fifteen minutes later, I hung up the wet laundry in the shower room and turned on the space heater. Everything would be dry by morning. I made a checklist of essentials I might need for a week or so, and then I went to bed.

I slept soundly and woke up at 6 a.m. and took another Covid test. It was negative. I was resolved to leave. I threw in another load of wash – I realized I was running low on underwear – and finished packing. I took a shower and made coffee. It was about 8 when I was ready to go, wearing fresh undies still warm from the dryer. I noticed that the banana and tangerine were missing from the tray on the hallway barstool, taken by Henri – or a critter in the night. The thought of that made me chuckle. I put a mug of hot coffee next to the untouched chocolate bar on the tray and knocked on Henri's door.

He was still in bed, not quite awake. "*Bonjour,*" he said, slowly sitting up.

"*Bonjour,*" I replied. "I brought you coffee." He yawned. "*Bon.* I'd like some toast with butter."

"Well, you can fix that yourself. I'm leaving."

He suddenly was wide awake.

"It's not fair to keep you cooped up in your room. And it's not fair to me that you won't take precautions. So, I'm going."

When I rolled my suitcase out the front door about 20 minutes later, Henri was at the kitchen sink, unmasked. I said good-bye, but he said nothing.

Moments after I got in the car, our neighbor, Léo, pulled up alongside me in the driveway after finishing his night shift at the museum. He knew that Henri had tested positive the day before and asked how he was doing.

"He's a difficult patient and won't wear a mask, so I'm leaving."

Léo looked surprised: "Where will you go?"

"I'll stay with a friend." I said, even though I had no plan yet.

"I'll keep an eye on him."

"Thank you, Léo." I shook my head. "He's really stubborn." I let out a big sigh. "And so am I."

327

I drove to a *boulangerie* in Vernonnet, near the pharmacy where I had picked up the Covid tests the day before. Next door was a small grocery store. I hadn't had breakfast yet and was suddenly hungry.

I notice a message on my phone from Cindy, urging me to leave the apartment after I texted her about Henri's refusal to wear a mask. It was midnight her time in San Diego and I could see she was online.

We were talking on Facetime, when I noticed a white SUV – just like Henri's – had pulled into the parking lot about 50 feet from me. I looked closely at my side mirror and said to Cindy, "I don't believe this."

Henri got out of the car, not wearing a mask, and walked toward the entrance of the grocery store. He hadn't seen me when I called out, "No mask?"

He reached into his pocket and pulled out a surgical mask. As he put it on, he stood about 15 feet away, glaring at me.

I turned the phone toward him so Cindy could see him. She was shocked.

"I feel like going in there and telling everyone he tested positive for Covid yesterday," I told her.

In about 10 minutes, while I was still talking to Cindy, Henri left the store and walked back to his car via the far side of the parking lot.

As he waited at the exit to pull into traffic, I took a photo of his SUV with his license plate in plain view. I don't know why I did that, but I just wanted proof for myself that he didn't give a fuck about anybody.

I called a friend who lived nearby, in the village of Limmetz. I explained my predicament with Henri, asking her if I could spend the night. She said it wouldn't be a problem and invited me to join her for dinner as well.

Then I called Sarah, who asked me to join her for lunch. As we sat on her patio, we assessed my options.

"I'd like to go to the seaside for the weekend," I said. "I have a friend near Étretat. I could meet her for lunch. Some fresh sea air will do me good."

"What if you get sick while you're away?" she asked.

She had a good point. But I didn't want to get a place in Giverny. I could imagine the gossip that would create.

I had a relaxing evening with my friend in Limmetz and a good night's sleep. I tested negative the next morning, a Friday.

I didn't want to overstay my welcome, so I went online and booked a reasonably priced tourist flat in Vernonnet.

I spent the afternoon at Giverny's Impressionist Museum. It was the opening day for the first exhibition of the season called "Children of Impressionism."

It was a lovely collection featuring the depiction of children in Impressionist paintings, many from the greats – Monet, Renoir, Cassatt, Pissarro, Morisot. There was an enormous garden scene called *Roses et Lys* by American artist Mary Fairchild (MacMonnies) of her with her daughter at their home in Giverny where the family lived at the turn of the last century. I had first seen this painting at a Giverny Impressionist exhibit in San Diego some years ago. How wonderful to see it in Giverny, just down the road from where she painted it. Lilla Cabot Perry, an American artist from Boston, who was a friend of Monet's and also his neighbor, had a beautiful painting in the show called *At the River's Bend*.

The most stunning painting for me was by a lesser-known artist named André Brouillet. His luminous *La Petite Fille en rouge* – of a young girl in a cardinal-red dress and enormous hat, holding a running hoop – took my breath away.

I had a thrill of my own in the museum gift shop when the shop-keeper pointed to *The Secret of Marie* – both editions, in French and English – and *The Sound of His Voice* prominently on display next to two popular French authors. With both books set in Giverny, I felt so pleased and grateful that they had found a home here.

I tried not to jump up and down until I got back to the parking lot.

~~~

My energy was flagging by the time I got to the flat, a garret apartment tucked under the roof on the second floor of a large old house. I didn't have strength in my legs to carry my heavy suitcase. So I took out some items and put them in tote bags. I made seven trips – four flights up and four down for each trip – 56 flights total. I was in a heap when I finally closed the door for the evening. My throat was scratchy. I had a headache. At 5:30 the next morning, I knew. I had Covid.

I didn't leave the flat for three days. Sarah brought groceries, supplies and medicine. Paracetamol helped me take long naps – a five-hour nap the first day, a four-hour nap the next. I could barely swallow. My voice was reduced to a whisper. I felt like I had a hot burr in my throat. I longed for ice cream. Sarah added that to her shopping list.

On the third day, I started to feel like I might be rounding the bend. The apartment was comfortable and had a fully equipped kitchenette. My view of the outside world was through three skylights. I had a beautiful view of the chalky cliffs overlooking Vernonnet that caught the sun in late afternoon and looked spectacular against the cornflower-blue sky.

On the gray days, I tried not to feel the pull of melancholy. But one day, I looked up at the heavy clouds and imagined all my angel friends and family looking down on me. I spun my father's wedding ring on my finger – I had worn it ever since Kyle and Julia's wedding – and suddenly had a vision of him: I saw him crying. I fought back tears. I wouldn't let myself cry. I was in a mess and had let a man back in my life – yet again – who didn't deserve me. But I was determined this time, despite all I had done to return to Giverny to make a fresh start with Henri, to find a path of my own.

I started counting days according to my positive Covid status. The shipping container arrived on Day 4, in early April, almost three months after I woke up on that horrible January morning in Del Mar with mud oozing between my toes.

The day before the container arrived, Henri told me he had taken out renter's insurance for my belongings. But when I asked him to send me a copy of the policy, he sent an insurance coverage proposal that had expired at the end of March. He then sent me a boilerplate paragraph from the insurance company stating the house was insured against fire, flood and explosion, but there was no mention of the contents.

I emailed his insurance agent and asked her to send me a copy of the renter's policy. She didn't reply.

The day before, I had written to her in response to a strange email she had sent Henri, when he had asked for an insurance quote for my new Toyota. She wrote back saying they had no record of me in their system and that I'd have to go to driving school to prove I could handle a car.

In my email, I explained that I'd had coverage for the Lego-mobile and asked her to send me a copy of that policy, which she did. I was stunned to see that the policy was in Henri's name only, which was why the insurance company had no record of me. I had paid him the premiums for that policy.

In the U.S. that's called "fronting," when someone claims to be the primary driver in order to get a cheaper rate for a secondary driver. It often happens when parents take out a policy in their names to get a cheaper rate for a young driver in the family who's just gotten a license, when, in fact, the teenager is the primary driver. Fronting is a criminal offense with serious consequences in the U.S. Had I unknowingly been complicit in a crime because of what Henri had done? Was I uninsured during the time I had driven that car? I shuddered to think of the financial ruin I would have faced if I had been in an accident.

In a follow-up email, the agent assured me I would have been covered as an unnamed driver, but that I would have had a much higher deductible than Henri if I had ever been in an accident.

I was livid. In my conversations with Henri about why the insurance company didn't have a record of me, he played dumb.

He must have caught wind that I had been in touch with his agent. While I was still quarantining in my garret, he sent me a terse message telling me not to contact the insurance company – they weren't authorized to discuss his file with me. I sent him a terse reply, reminding him that the renter's policy he supposedly signed up for covered my belongings, not his. I told him I would get insurance elsewhere if he didn't send me the policy, with details of the coverage.

That didn't happen.

The next day, Covid Day 7, I arranged for my own insurance with Quentin, the banker. I made it clear I wanted to keep my affairs separate from Henri's and he supported me in that.

Quentin and I had a long talk by phone about what Henri had done with the Lego-mobile policy. "In France, what he did wouldn't be considered illegal – not like in the U.S.," Quentin told me. "But what he did was wrong. You were both on the title and both of you should have been on the insurance. By not putting you on the policy, he has now caused a big problem for you. You have no driving history and will have to pay a higher premium for car insurance."

Quentin drew up the policy for my belongings and sent the documents to me digitally. There was a glitch with the electronic signature function on the bank's website. I was losing my stamina and felt a headache coming on, so Quentin offered to print up the papers and drop them at the house where I was staying on his way home so that I could sign them that evening.

He emailed me as he was leaving his office at 6 p.m. I went downstairs to wait for him in my car. I watched a stream of cars zip past on the busy road outside the house. It was Good Friday, the start of a holiday weekend. When Quentin arrived with my packet of documents, I felt I had an angel in my corner.

While I was in my self-imposed quarantine, I had long Skype talks with Nancy, who had been married to a textbook narcissist. I had heard her stories from that painful time of her life. Richard was an opera singer, who had a charming, larger-than-life personality. But he had a manipulative, deceitful, dark side. His many extra-marital affairs – one in particular – ultimately ended their marriage. They settled their divorce in brutal court proceedings that left Nancy devastated. It took her a long time to recover. She moved to Germany to relaunch her own opera career and for years, never told him where she was.

As I was describing Henri's behavior to Nancy one evening, she said something that shifted all the puzzle pieces into place. "He's a narcissist, just like Richard." That made sense. Henri's ego had grown like a tumor, unchecked, for nearly 80 years.

For the next couple of days, I read about Narcissistic Personality Disorder and unlocked the mystery of Henri.

The concept of narcissism is rooted in Greek mythology. According to legend, Narcissus was an arrogant young man who spurned the advances of amorous suitors. One day, while drinking from a woodland pool, he fell in love with the handsome man he saw in the water, not realizing he was looking at his own reflection. He couldn't pull himself away and eventually died, consumed by the fire of his unrequited passion.

Over the years, the notion of vanity – excessive self-admiration and pride – worked its way into philosophy, art and literature. In the early 20th century, psychoanalysts were examining narcissism and its impact on personality and self-esteem. In 1914, Sigmund Freud published a paper about it, theorizing that a person's sense of self develops during childhood when interactions begin with the outside world – a critical period when love for self and love for others evolves. Later, psychoanalysts expanded on Freud's theories and began identifying personality disorders stemming from extreme forms of narcissism, when love for self becomes pathological.

I read that parental overindulgence during childhood often contributes to a narcissist's overblown ego. Henri once told me that when he was a boy, his parents didn't want him having lunch with his classmates at school and arranged for him to go to a local butcher shop to have a home-cooked meal prepared for him by the butcher's elderly mother. Henri had once shown me the place where the shop had been, on the winding cobbled streets behind the church in the ancient quarter of Vernon.

I asked if his brother Charles, who was just two years younger, had joined him for these hot lunches at the butcher shop.

"No, I went alone," he said.

I thought that was curious. Henri didn't have any health issues that would warrant special meals. But clearly from his childhood stories, he had been the golden child of the family and had developed a sense that he was exceptional.

As I read the lists of narcissistic traits, Henri ticked many of the boxes:

- Exhibits a grandiose sense of self-importance
- Expects to be treated as superior
- Can't handle criticism
- Tends to lash out if they feel slighted or challenged
- Lacks empathy
- Lies compulsively
- Disregards personal safety and the safety of others
- Fails to obey laws or social norms
- Tends to blame their bad behavior on others
- Feels no remorse for hurting others and no interest in apologizing unless it benefits them
- Enjoys inflicting pain on others and views it as an empowering experience

The advice when you're in a relationship with a narcissist: Be assertive, firm and consistent. Stay calm. Call out the lies. Expect a strong pushback, but hold your ground.

Mostly the articles stressed the importance of having a good support group when dealing with a narcissist. There's no easy fix. Counseling might help. But a narcissist is hard-wired. Life with one will always be difficult.

~⁔

I would have extended my stay at my little garret, but it was booked for the coming weekend. On the morning of my departure, the day before Easter, I was up at 6:30. The morning's sunrise was shrouded in fog. From the bathroom window, I could make out the four turrets of the 13th-century Chateau des Tourelles on the near side of the Seine, but I couldn't see the church of Vernon on the opposite bank.

I gathered my things and packed my suitcase. I cleaned the apartment, wiping down surfaces, handles and light switches with antiseptic wipes. I was so grateful that I'd had this space to recover from Covid, but I wanted to minimize germs I might be leaving behind.

I opened the window that looked out onto the cliff. The morning air was fresh and crisp. Birds were singing. Above the treetops, the crystals of a jet trail streaked across the sky. During the course of the week, the hillside had slowly changed from drab winter grey to a lush palette of spring greens, dotted with the lacy blossoms of wild plum trees.

I thought about the conversation I would have with Henri when I returned home – a word that no longer seemed to apply to my situation with him. I was furious with him for how he had treated me. But I was heartbroken, too. I had been so in love with him at the beginning. I thought he was a caring, generous man who would always have my back – not a man who in his own twisted torment would defiantly expose me to Covid or lie to me about things, big and small.

I remembered the day I fell in love with him. We were on our "honeymoon" trip to Malta. We had been wandering through the back streets of a village when we came upon a group of musicians in a little piazza, playing a lovely song that made you want to dance. That's exactly what happened. A group had entered the piazza ahead of us and were already dancing. Couples embraced, children twirled and laughed. Henri took me in his arms, both of us knowing we had been given an extraordinary gift.

When the song ended, everyone drifted out of the piazza. Henri and I were the last to leave. He let go of my hand for a moment and walked toward the musicians, reaching into his pocket. They nodded with appreciation as Henri put a generous tip in a violin case they had placed on the cobblestones.

That was the man I fell in love with. He will always live in my heart.

As I got ready to leave my garret hideaway that morning, I wondered if the ache of this would ever go away. Hearts heal, I told myself. Life goes on.

On the day I had arrived to start my new life with Henri, only two months earlier, he had said to me, "You are home now."

He was right about that. With or without him, I was HOME and I knew a wonderful life awaited me in my beloved Giverny.

Giverny had always had an incredible pull on me.

On one of my early visits, when I was doing research for *The Secret of Marie*, I had gone to the nearby village of Vetheuil (Joan Mitchell's home) to photograph a house where Monet had once lived. I noticed a weather vane on an old brick chimney of a neighboring house. I looked closer, not quite believing my eyes. Cut into the metal were my two initials. (I don't have a middle name.) The weather vane, which seemed to be stuck, was pointing back to Giverny.

The next day I wrote about the "RB" weather vane in my journal: "I came to Normandy this week with guidebooks, maps and GPS. But yesterday, I simply followed the *sign*. Clearly, this story has a compass of its own."

Despite a few circuitous detours along the way, I knew for certain

I was where I was meant to be. I also realized that the path that had brought me to Giverny had been well marked for a very long time.

Chapter 46

I didn't test negative until Day 14. My recovery slowed when I was back with Henri at his apartment.

In a bizarre twist, he denied he ever had Covid. "It was just a cold," he said. He seemed to have forgotten he had told me that he tested "a little bit positive" twice at the pharmacy on his Day 4 and Day 6. (When I told Nancy that, she asked if being a little bit positive was like being a little bit pregnant.) When I reminded him of his pharmacy tests, he said he didn't care whether he was still positive and had no concern that he might be infecting others. On Easter Sunday, 12 days after his first positive test, he had dinner with family. Two of them at the table – his brother Charles, in his late 70s, and his wife, in her early 80s – had never had Covid.

Henri's new mantra was "I don't care."

I finally revealed to Henri, a few days after I returned, that I knew about his lies. I knew that the car insurance policy – for which I had paid him the premiums – was in his name only, and I knew he had deceived me by pretending he didn't know why the insurance company had no record of me. I knew he hadn't taken out an insurance policy to cover my belongings on the day before the container arrived, as he had told me. He tried to accuse me of going behind his back by arranging my own insurance with Quentin. I said, "Read the text thread. I told you if you didn't send me proof of insurance, I would make my own arrangements."

Then came the big question: "Henri, are you planning to move to the house?" I asked.

Ever since we had agreed to rent the gîte, Henri seemed vague about what he planned to do with his apartment and how Facel, with his arthritic hips, was going to climb the flight of steps up to the gîte's front door.

"I'm not welcome there," he replied. "My dog isn't welcome. The housekeeper isn't welcome."

"Let's start at the bottom of that list," I said. "The housekeeper definitely is not welcome. Your dog can't go up the stairs. And you – why don't you feel welcome?"

"I can't do my laundry there."

"*You* can do your laundry anywhere, Henri. The problem is you want a woman to do it for you and that's not going to be me."

We were standing on opposite sides of the kitchen counter, where so many of our arguments had taken place. It had been a butcher's table, after all, that still carried the cuts of his blade.

I leaned toward Henri. "I know you, and I know you don't want this," I said calmly. "Don't wait until the day before the lease signing to pull out, like you did last time. Tell me now."

He stared at me for a moment and then reached over and hugged me, kissing my neck. I wasn't sure if he was overwhelmed by everything or whether he was relieved to be let off the hook.

The next day, when I told Sarah what had happened, she said, "He's relieved. You set him free. That was very big of you, Rebecca."

I had untied the rope around his wrists. I felt relief, too.

~⁓

What happened in the next few weeks was like watching a building implode in slow motion.

Maxine had asked Henri and me to come to the moulin one evening in mid-May to give her our personal details so that she could draw up a lease. She had given us a form to fill out. I listed myself as the primary tenant and left the column for the secondary tenant blank.

The night before the meeting, I had asked Henri, "What are you going to tell Maxine? Have you told them you're not going to live there?"

"I've never said those words," he said. "But that is the fact."

"Don't start playing games with me, Henri."

"I'll say that we're going to keep two separate residences, but that we're still together."

I wanted to shout, *"No! We're not still together!"* But I swallowed my words.

At our meeting at the moulin, Maxine, who sat next to me at the dining table, pointed to the blank column on the form.

"What about Henri?" she asked me. Henri sat in silence, across the table from us.

Technically, Henri should have been listed as the primary tenant – in keeping with the chauvinistic French order of things. In fact, Henri had told me that Olivier and Maxine may not approve the lease without him as the primary tenant.

I eagerly waited for Henri's reply when Maxine asked him why his name wasn't on the form.

"Rebecca will be signing the lease alone," he said.

Maxine shrugged, unfazed, and took down my information.

A cloud lifted, temporarily. I had managed, once again, to navigate the rough waters that foreigners – especially foreign women – face in France.

To my astonishment, Maxine had not yet read the "American" email I had sent her two months earlier. Again, she said, "It's too long."

"Use Google translate." I wasn't going to give her an inch on this.

"I didn't think of that," she said.

I wondered how she had run a B&B for 15 years, dealing with clients from around the world, without using translation apps.

She scanned Google's French translation of my email, dated March 10, and looked up at me, in surprise. "You don't want the furniture?"

"No, I don't have room for it. Look at what's stored in the basement."

She said something to Olivier in French. He didn't look surprised because I had told him in March that I needed to have the gîte furniture removed. They seemed to have a communication problem.

I could tell Olivier wasn't himself. He hadn't followed doctor's orders after his surgery. In fact, he had checked himself out of the Paris hospital two days following the operation, despite his doctor's objection. The next week, I saw Olivier riding around the village on a tractor. Within two weeks of the operation, after Henri and I had come down with Covid, so did Olivier and Maxine. She had been ill for a couple of days, but Olivier's recovery was much slower. His Covid headaches intensified the post-op ones he had been experiencing.

I glanced at Henri, who looked uncomfortable. I had an uneasy feeling that everything was going sideways with this "agreement."

～

On June 1, Maxine asked me to come to the moulin at nine that morning to review the lease, which I was expecting to sign that day.

She wasn't ready for me when I arrived and asked me to take a seat in the front garden. I wandered over to the basin of a fountain in the center of the driveway and took some photos of the beautiful water lilies that seemed to float on the soft clouds of the morning sky, reflected on the surface of the water.

I was intrigued by a rare black water lily Olivier had recently added to the collection and thought of Michel Bussi's bestselling novel *Nymphéas Noirs* (*Black Water Lilies*), a murder mystery set in Giverny that, in fact, takes place largely at Olivier and Maxine's moulin. I wondered if the new black water lilies in the pond were a nod to Bussi. Before Covid, tour groups used to come by the moulin to see the book's main setting. But Maxine, in her usual style, was typically hostile to those who wandered near her front gate.

After about 10 minutes, Maxine beckoned me inside. She had set up her laptop at one end of the long dining table, which was covered with folders and papers. I took a seat next to her.

She began by asking for my bank details so that she could transfer accounts to me for electricity, water and internet. It was a tedious process, as she waited on hold for customer service reps to come online. After about 20 minutes, I asked her if I could look at the lease. She seemed to have forgotten about that and rummaged through folders to find it.

"Yes, it's here," she said. "My mother gave me a copy from someone in her agency." Maxine's mother was a retired real estate agent.

It was a six-page document in French fine print. I used my Google translation app's camera feature, which allowed me to scan an entire page at a time. While I read through the document, Maxine continued with the account transfers. At one point, I had to speak with a rep who needed to confirm details with me in English. She was very nice and at the end of our conversation expressed her hope that I would enjoy my time in France. But before she could finish speaking, Maxine clicked off the call.

Finally, when Maxine had completed the transfers, she stood up, as if we were done.

"What about the lease?" I asked. I had a few issues I wanted to discuss, not the least of which was a confession Maxine had made to me a couple of months earlier that their electricity bills at the gîte were low because they'd had someone wire the meter to prevent it from recording the consumption. When I asked how they got around the meter reader, she said the electric company had to give advance notice of a visit which gave them time to pull the wire. When I told Henri about this, he seemed surprised and agreed with me that the wire needed to be removed before I moved in.

"We're not ready to sign the lease today."

"The contract you've drawn up here says June 1. That's today," I said. "You want me to pay rent from today, correct? I'm now paying utilities as of today."

"The house isn't ready," she said brusquely. "We haven't finished moving the furniture out. It's a lot of work."

"Everything needs to be out by Sunday." I opened my datebook. It was Thursday – she had four days left to clear out the house. "I have an IKEA delivery next Monday. A handyman is coming Tuesday to start assembling everything. The movers are coming next Saturday, the tenth, to bring everything up from the basement."

"I work full time and I have bigger concerns," she replied.

"You've known the timeline for two weeks," I said firmly, scrolling through my WhatsApp messages to the exchange we'd had about the dates.

I could see by her steely look of defiance that she wasn't going to let me tell her what had to be done.

I left that day without a lease. In France, a lease must be accompanied by an *état des lieux* – literally, "state of place" – which is an inventory of the contents of the house and its condition. Pages of photographs typically are attached to the lease as part of the *état des lieux*.

"When everything is moved and we clean, my mother will take the photos," Maxine said. "I don't know when that will be."

Our meeting was over.

~ɔ

On Sunday, I texted Maxine and asked for the key.

The house is not ready, she replied by text.

IKEA is coming tomorrow and I need a key to let them in. Or you can come over when they arrive and let them in, I wrote.

Then she called me. "Which rooms do we need to be clear for IKEA?"

"All of them," I replied.

"Olivier will be there this afternoon."

A short while later, Henri found me in my bedroom packing things for the move. "Olivier has asked us to come over for a drink this evening."

When we arrived, Maxine was picking greens outside the moulin's front wall. "For my kangaroo," she said, as Henri pulled his car up to the gate.

I rolled my eyes at Henri, as we rolled into the courtyard where the crazy dogs went crazy.

The four of us sat outside, at a little table by the driveway. Olivier opened an expensive bottle of champagne I had brought. Maxine clearly wasn't in a mood to celebrate as Olivier handed Henri the key. She drank a glass of champagne and then headed toward the moulin's laundry room, adjacent to the garage, saying she had work to do.

The next morning, when Henri and I walked into the house, I was stunned. The house was a mess. Dirty mattress pads and bed linens were strewn in the bedrooms. Duvets and pillows were piled in the dining room. Bags and boxes were stacked in the living room. There were pillow feathers everywhere. Henri took a broom from the kitchen and started sweeping up a pile of dirt and bits of trash that had accumulated in the middle of the living room floor.

I was furious.

I cleared the bedrooms so that the handyman could start his work the next day and made space in the living room for the IKEA boxes.

Henri left me to wait for the delivery. It had been scheduled for between 9 and noon. But in the end, they didn't arrive until 4.

In the seven hours I waited for IKEA, I had a glimpse of what my life would be like in this new place I thought would be mine.

It had a gorgeous unobstructed southern view toward the Seine, where I could see the trains pass on the far bank of the river. A field of winter wheat bordered the narrow street in front of the house and beyond that, the tower of the moulin rose above the trees that surrounded the property.

The view was both a good and bad thing. The house was totally exposed, with no tall trees of its own for shade or privacy. I was mostly concerned about privacy. I imagined binoculars peering out the top window of the moulin tower. (My writer's mind gets carried away sometimes.) The front door was nine steps up from the front yard, on a veranda where I sat for two hours that morning, watching bees take nectar from a tangle of passionflower vines that covered the veranda's railing. The vines offered no privacy. I was in plain view of everyone passing by on the main road beyond the wheat field. I certainly would be seen by anyone passing on the street below. I envisioned Henri circling the block ten times a day to see if I was home – or if another man's car might be in the driveway.

I couldn't quite imagine another man so soon. But if that day came, I wouldn't be able to keep a new gentleman a secret for very long.

That night, after dinner, I sent Maxine an email, reminding her that the bookcases and wardrobes that the handyman would be assembling the next day would need to be secured to walls. Had her mom photographed them, I asked. The plaster had cracked in several places and the wall covering was peeling. I wanted that to be documented.

At 10:50 that night, as I was settling into bed, my phone rang. I was too tired to get out of bed. The phone was charging on the dining room table. It rang about 10 times. I wondered if it might be Maxine. After the phone went quiet, I decided to check to see who had called, in case it might have been my son.

Indeed, the caller had been Maxine. I carried the phone to Henri's room, where he was reading in bed. Just then, the phone pinged with a message from her: *I talked with Olivier. We give you back the money you transfer. It won't be possible. Money that I didn't received yet.*

I read the message aloud to Henri. He was quiet for a minute. "I'm worried," he said.

The next day, he met with Maxine and Olivier, hoping to smooth things over.

I spoke with Quentin, my banker, who informed me the funds transfer I thought I had made for the security deposit and the first month's rent hadn't gone through. I had set up the beneficiary account, with their details, but I had initiated the transfer on the same day, not knowing I had to wait 48 hours to put through a first-time request. That was a fortunate mistake for me. Otherwise, if Maxine had received the funds, I would have had little hope of a refund.

While Henri was meeting with Maxine and Olivier, I had lunch with Sarah and her partner Maurice, at her place. Maurice was perplexed that she had transferred the accounts to me without a contract. "This isn't how it's done," he said.

Henri sent me a text while I was at Sarah's saying "the meeting went well."

When I saw him later that afternoon, he was vague about the details, but assured me they had pulled the wire on the meter. He said Maxine and her mother would finish the cleaning the next day and take photos.

"Henri, tomorrow is too late. The handyman needs at least three days. We won't be ready for the movers on Saturday."

"What are you saying?"

"Maxine blew it."

"Are you saying you're going to back out?"

"Back out? I've been waiting for a lease that should have been ready a week ago. She's the one who's dropped the ball here."

Henri asked if I'd like to join him and his granddaughter, who was visiting, for dinner that night. I declined and spent much of the evening on a video call with Sarah.

When Henri returned home, he plopped down on his big leather easy chair next to where I was sitting on the sofa. A task light, on a small end table between us, lit us both harshly, as if we were in an interrogation room on a TV police show.

He looked at me intently. "What have you decided?"

I took a deep breath. "I'm not going to take the house."

I could see a storm brewing in Henri's eyes, as he let out a sigh.

"Seventy-five percent of my reason is Maxine," I said resolutely. "The rest of my concerns could possibly be resolved. But there's no way I want to deal with her as my landlady."

There's always a surprise with Henri. He quietly said, "They told me today that if it had all become too complicated, they were fine with ending this."

"Why didn't you tell me that a few hours ago?" I asked.

"Because I wanted you to take the house."

"The house you said you were going to share with me – and share in the expenses? That house doesn't exist, Henri. It was a figment of your twisted imagination."

I left the room, relieved to be untangled from his manipulative scheme. He had never intended to move to that house with me. But he wanted to keep me close, within arm's reach.

～◦

Henri didn't communicate my decision to Maxine and Olivier. The next day – a Wednesday, seven days after Maxine had transferred accounts to me without a rental contract – she and her mother cleaned the house and made an inventory. But curiously, by that evening, Maxine hadn't contacted me to say the lease was ready to sign.

I had an email ready, to tell them I was bowing out. But I waited until early the next morning to send it.

I left Henri's place at 7:30 that morning to meet a friend's flight at Charles de Gaulle. I was stuck in traffic when Maxine's first ping landed: *I was warned to beware of you, I should have listened to people. Now that the house is empty and the inventory was done yesterday by my mother. You really are a strange person.*

That seemed pretty tame for Maxine. I figured she'd work up a bit more vitriol after her second cup of coffee.

By the time I got seated at a café at the arrivals area of Terminal One, an email arrived from Maxine bearing the full force of her wrath. Bottom line: She never wanted to see me again. I was totally on board with that.

I had to undo all that I'd done: I cancelled the movers and the handyman. I had to arrange for IKEA to pick up everything they had delivered. Henri posted a sign on the front gate at his apartment that flapped in the breeze, like a flag, for all to read, instructing the IKEA driver to go to the house. IKEA had confused my delivery address at the new house with my billing address at his apartment.

Delivery services, in general, were confused about where I lived because the name of the street changed just beyond Henri's mailbox, which was unmarked. In his attempt to clear things up, he had printed up a large card, which he taped to the box, with my name, his name and Leo's. When lost delivery drivers called to get directions, I'd tell them, "It's the green, ménage-à-trois mailbox by the big gate." That always got a laugh.

One day, Giverny's postman flagged me down as I was pulling out of the driveway. "What's going on with you?" he asked, pointing to the IKEA sign. "Where are you living these days?"

I needed a therapy session to answer his first question. As for the second, I kept it simple. "*Ici*. Here. I'm here for now."

Chapter 47

In the tempest of my housing debacle, a ray of sunlight shone through: Julia and Kyle called to say they were going to have a baby.

When we spoke on FaceTime, Julia looked so sweet, wrapped in a fluffy pink bathrobe as she snuggled next to Kyle on their living room sofa. She had that sleepy early-pregnancy look that I remembered so well. She thought she was about six weeks along.

They didn't want to make a big announcement yet, so I promised not to put out a blast on Facebook. I was over the moon. I was going to be a GRANDMOTHER!

After I got off the call, I went looking for Henri, who was sitting at the end of his bed, putting on his pajamas.

"I have some good news," I said.

"We could use some of that." We'd had an argument earlier in the evening. These had become daily occurrences.

"I'm going to be a grandmother!" I stood still for a moment, loving the sound of those words. But I didn't linger. I wasn't going to let his grumpy mood spoil the moment. I quickly left the room.

But as I went down the hallway, I heard him say, "That *is* wonderful news."

The next morning, I walked into the kitchen, with my cane clomping at my side. I was using it in the mornings to steady my wobbly ankles.

Henri was sitting on a barstool at the kitchen counter, having breakfast.

"Do I look like a grandmother?" I asked, waving my cane.

He smiled a little. "No, not yet."

A couple of weeks passed. I knew it was time for Julia's first doctor's appointment, so I sent them a text asking for baby news.

I got a quick reply from Kyle, asking me to delete my message. He wrote that they had been to see the doctor the day before and he couldn't detect a heartbeat.

Kyle called me later to say they would go back in a week for another ultrasound. "They can't tell if the fetus is viable," he said.

"Maybe she's not as far along as she thought," I said, trying to calm his fears. "At my first appointment, I was 10 weeks pregnant and the nurse had trouble hearing your heartbeat."

I clearly remembered that day. The nurse's name was Ruth. She was so caring and reassuring and was a brick of support all through my pregnancy.

But on the day of my first appointment, I had a few anxious moments as she slowly moved the Doppler wand over my abdomen.

The silence in the room – and in my womb – made it hard for me to breathe. I strained to hear the sound of the little being inside me and said a mother's first prayer.

I closed my eyes and saw a little boy on a swing, his curls dancing in the breeze. He threw back his head and laughed – such glee in his voice.

And then *wa-woosh, wa-woosh.* The water of my womb rippled with his laughter.

Ruth beamed, as though she had never heard the heartbeat of a new life. I cried happy tears.

At Julia's next appointment, they learned that the fetus had died at five weeks. Julia sank into a deep depression, yet had the courage to write about her trauma a few weeks later on Facebook.

What I admired most about her as she wrote about her anguish and grief was her hope that speaking out in a public way would help other women who had suffered the loss of an unborn child:

My mom died almost 4 years ago, when I was 27 & she was 52. One minute she was out jogging and the next she was barely alive. Over the next 4 days, she was in an induced coma and we didn't know if she would ever wake up. The wait was excruciating. The doctors wouldn't say it, but I knew she would most likely die. I thought I'd lost hope. But when the day came to see if she'd wake up, I sat at her bedside for hours & I knew that I was wrong. I did have hope. I think deep down you always do. The moment the neurologist told us that my mom was gone was the single worst moment of my life.

This miscarriage has brought up a lot of those feelings for me. The waiting, the agonizing, & ultimately the terrible shock. It's incredibly difficult, not just losing this pregnancy but reliving that nightmare. I know we can get through this. We will try again. But right now the pain feels all-consuming.

Through all the pain & the heart-wrenching sadness, I still feel lucky. Lucky enough to live (for now) in a state where my body and my choice come first. It's scary out there, & I'm thankful to be able to get the care I need. I know many others can't.

I'm sure people have opinions on whether posting about a miscarriage on social media is the *right* thing to do. Well… Miscarriage is real, it happens, it happened to me, & it has happened to so many others. It's not a dirty secret. It's your individual choice to share or to not share, and every choice is the *right* one. This is mine. Sending love to everyone out there who has been through the same. We can all do this.

With this, she posted her first sonogram image, which is now seared into my heart. I had *imagined* this baby. I saw a little girl with blonde curls and pink glasses (both Julia and Kyle had worn glasses when they were very young). I had nicknamed her "Beanie" because I knew she wasn't much bigger than one. During the week between Julia's appointments, I prayed Beanie would find her heartbeat. I lit candles for her. I begged my Angels on High to help her. I thought of that little boy on the swing and hoped I could bring her to life as I believed I had helped Kyle *whoosh* into the world with dear Ruth at my side.

Beneath the framed sonogram image was Julia's hand-written caption, from a Taylor Swift song: *You were bigger than the whole sky.* And next to our only glimpse of little Beanie was a lit candle.

I tried to write a comment, but the right words wouldn't come. It was getting late. I took a pillow off my bed and went to Henri's room. He was in bed and looked up from a video he was watching on his tablet.

"What is it, *chérie?*" he asked.

I couldn't speak. I lay down next to him, hugging my pillow. He kept a firm hand on my shoulder as I wept.

~

A few more weeks went by. I hadn't yet spoken to Julia. Kyle told me she had pulled away from everyone, except for him and her best friend, who lived close by.

He looked haggard. I could tell he was emotionally exhausted. He was under a lot of stress at work, dealing with the final details of a three-year construction project. I suggested he attend some of Julia's therapy sessions and schedule some individual sessions for himself. He was open to that.

It was their first brutally hard knock of married life. "You'll get through this," I told him. "It might be helpful to take out the beautiful wedding vows you wrote to each other and read them aloud again."

I wrote to Julia, trying to find the words her mother would say. I stared out the window for a long time, wanting to hear her mom's voice in my ear.

My sweet Julia,

Kyle tells me you're in a rough patch.

I sobbed after I read your Facebook post. I so admire your courage to tell the story of your loss and pain.

The comments tell a story, too. Many, many women suffer miscarriages – first-pregnancy miscarriages are not rare. My own mom had two before I was born. She went on to have my sister three years later.

The creation of life is truly a miracle. Think about everything that has to happen PERFECTLY in the early days and weeks of a pregnancy. If there's a hiccup in any of it, it's nature's way to shut things down.

I have a dear friend from my college days who, when I told her your sad news, wrote this to me: *I lost three babies in the process of getting the two children that I have. It's horrible to experience and then there's always that question, "Why me?" I have three little angels watching over me and now Julia and Kyle will have one, too. My heart is with them through this most difficult time and with you as well. Love to all.*

I love the thought of your little angel, in the arms of your mom, both of them watching over you.

I also love thinking about the children you're meant to have, eagerly waiting to be born. You and Kyle will be wonderful parents. As your Uncle Kevin said during your wedding ceremony, "These two are meant to have babies."

You need time to recover from this. But please don't let yourself curl up in a ball and sink into a prolonged depression. Step into the light. Every day. Find a patch of sunlight on the floor when you get up in the morning. Soak up sunlight on your walks. Exercise. Get those endorphins flowing. Eat good food. Rejoice in the love you and Kyle share. Open your heart to the babies who are meant to come.

I know you have suffered tremendous loss in the past four years. But as I said to you when your mom died, I know she wouldn't want you to withdraw from life and family and friends and doing what you enjoy. You will honor her by being strong and living life with the zest she did. I'm sure, as a loving mother herself, that she would want you to carry on and try again.

Lean on Kyle. He loves you dearly and will help you through this.

I love you, too, and know you can be a warrior woman.

Sending you a big hug,
Rebecca

Chapter 48

On the morning of June 21 – on a day that I had received a worrying email from Kyle about Julia's downward spiral – I received a text from Maxine, wanting an update about my housing prospects.

I told her I had an appointment the next day to see a house in Vernon. I explained the difficulty I was having getting agents to show me properties. My status as a foreigner with no French income was a huge strike against me. I offered to pay for storing my belongings at the gîte. I said I, too, had been dealing with some other problems. I told her my daughter-in-law had had a miscarriage and was having a difficult recovery. I closed by saying, *Je fais de mon mieux.* I'm doing my best.

Maxime's reply: *To let you know the price for the storage is 1000 euros per month. I ask the price to a storage place.*

Not a word of condolence. No acknowledgement that there had been a death in my family. A lost first child, a lost first grandchild.

I was dealing with a heartless, money-grubbing cretin. I told Henri, "Maxine is dead to me."

~

As the kerfuckle unfolded with Maxine and Olivier, Henri and I formed an improbable alliance. At first, he sided with them, saying I had been too demanding, which was the story Olivier was telling people.

I stood my ground. "Olivier knew back in March that I needed them to move the furniture out of the gîte," I said to Henri. "He agreed to that. If he wasn't up to the job, he could have hired someone to do it."

"It's all been too much for him," Henri said. "He has admitted to me he has been doing too much in general."

"He told us he needed to rest for a month after his surgery," I said. "But he was back to his normal routine a week later."

"I know. He can't sit still."

"Then he can't lay this on me."

"But you are too demanding," Henri countered.

"How is that? I come here to spend my life with you, and I open the wardrobe in my room to find it filled with old Covid supplies. And you make a fuss when I ask if I can remove the canned goods and stacks of toilet paper so that I can make room for my clothes. Is that too demanding of me, Henri?"

I let my anger rip. "Maxine blew me off. She didn't read my emails and texts. It was so *American* of me to write her a long message with every detail we had discussed with Olivier, every detail she needed to know. She let two months go by – *two months* – before she bothered to read that email. And then in the final days before the move, she threw a hissy fit saying it was all too much and that she had more important concerns – like picking greens for her kangaroo! They – you – cannot lay this all on me."

I was the easy scapegoat – the "demanding" American woman who wrote detailed emails and held people to account when they didn't bother to read them.

I made it clear to Henri that I would not deal directly with Maxine. From then on, he and Olivier would need to work out the removal of my things in the basement. A friend had offered storage at an empty building he owned, but eventually, I'd have to move everything again. The moving costs would be exorbitant. Henri said he'd try to reach a compromise with Olivier. I offered to pay a reasonable rate for storage – not $1,100 a month, as Maxine had demanded – until I found a place to live. And if they found a tenant in the meantime, I'd pay them a storage fee.

I was sorry to see the strain that had developed between Henri and Olivier. I knew this was a huge stress for Henri. He was the family patriarch, the peacemaker – in a way, the Godfather. He often claimed his family was the "mafia" of Giverny.

One day, I did a google search to remind myself what happened to the Corleone wives in *The Godfather*.

I was relieved to read that Vito's wife, Carmela, a devout Catholic who prayed daily for Vito's salvation, lived a long life and died of natural causes.

I thought of a photo I had taken of Henri during a visit we had made to an old church in a French village. I had captured him kneeling outside a confessional booth, peering curiously through the screen. My caption: "I'll be back in an hour, luv. I know you need some time."

Chapter 49

My college friend Marion – who had sent me the heartrending condolence note after Julia's miscarriage – came to Giverny for a visit, which really cheered me up. I hadn't seen her in nearly 10 years, so we had lots to catch up on, which was a great distraction from the daily soap opera of my Giverny life.

Marion had recently retired from her role in running a family furniture store with her husband, Stanley, in Natchitoches, Louisiana. She had been yearning to travel for years, but the store had kept her close to home.

We had known each other since we were 18. We had lived down the hall from each other in our freshman dorm at Southern Methodist University. The following year, we were suitemates with two other friends from our freshman floor, at another dorm on campus.

In those days, we knew the everyday details of each other's lives. We'd curl up on the beds – or one of us would be in a big bean bag chair my roommate, Jeannette, had made – talking about our weekend plans, our classes, a cute guy who had been at the table next to us in the cafeteria. Marion and her roommate, Vicky, were dating their future husbands, as it turned out.

We couldn't have imagined then the paths our lives would take – the children we'd have (or not) or the joys, disappointments and sorrows that would come our way. We were such innocents, not realizing what a fleeting time our college days were.

I was such a free spirit then. I didn't have a steady boyfriend and was preoccupied with my career plans. I wanted to write for a big magazine in New York and in my free time, see the world. I knew I wanted to be married and have a family someday. But I wasn't in a rush.

When Marion and I attended Vicky's wedding, in the summer of 1977, Marion had already been married for a year. She spent the weekend with me at my parents' house in Naperville, Illinois – about an hour from where Vicky was married at her parents' home north of Chicago. I can still see Marion and me – in our pajamas, lying on the twin beds in my old bedroom – talking about our lives. I had left SMU, the year after we had been suitemates, to spend a year at the University of Edinburgh, in 1974-75. I then went on to get a master's degree at Northwestern University's Medill School of Journalism the following year. My first job, with an energy newsletter company, had taken me to Washington, D.C., where I shared an apartment with a dear friend. I didn't own a car. I traveled to work by bus. I went on nice trips, but I didn't have much to show for my not-too-shabby paycheck.

Marion, on the other hand, already had a house – beautifully furnished, a perk of her work. I remember her saying to me that night, "After we get our patio furniture, we're going to start a family."

I couldn't comprehend such a well-ordered life. But as her future Christmas-card letters would reveal, creating a family proved to be excruciating for Marion. Two of the babies she lost were from triplets she was carrying. Her son was the survivor of that pregnancy. Her pregnancy with her daughter had been difficult as well.

Although Marion and I had seen each other a few times over the years, her Giverny visit was the first time we had had time together, one-on-one, since our night in 1977, talking into the wee hours after Vicky's wedding.

What amazes me about life-long friendships is how easy it is to pick up dangling threads. Sometimes there are surprises and revelations that take your breath away. I wish I had known about Marion's heartaches so that I could have been a better friend. During the years when we were raising children and running our households, we didn't have the internet or Facebook to keep in touch. Phone calls were expensive back then. It was a big deal to hop on a plane to go visit a friend. Our lives were so busy, with work, ball games and school events, summer holidays and family gatherings. I look back on that period of my life as the Black-Out Years.

But happily, I've found, that despite all that lost time, old friendships not only survive, but, in many ways, become all the more precious.

My five days with Marion were a delight. It was her dream to visit Giverny and she wasn't disappointed. I took some lovely photos of her on Monet's Japanese bridge. As we walked around the lily pond admiring the flowers, we discovered we had a common interest in gardening. Poor Stanley was back in Natchitoches watering her flower pots in an oppressive heatwave. We called him one night to see how he was holding up. I hadn't seen Stanley – or spoken to him – since college. I told him he looked much the same. He smiled and, with his soft southern drawl that I fondly recalled, he said, "Isn't it amazing how we all have failing eyesight?"

Marion had never been to France and wanted to end her visit in Paris. I planned an itinerary that I hoped would make her first experience there unforgettable.

On our first night, we got trapped at the top of the Eiffel Tower in a lightning storm for more than an hour. Our guide had cautioned us, as our group boarded an elevator at the second level, that a storm was coming. When we reached the top, Marion showed me the radar app on her phone. We didn't really need the app. All we had to do was look to the west to see a dark blue line of threatening clouds on the horizon. Paris was the bull's eye for the approaching storm.

"We're totally screwed," I said to Marion. "Let's go to the champagne bar."

When I slipped my bank card into the pay machine, I realized that a glass of Moët at the summit of the Eiffel Tower goes for $25. "What better way to ride out a storm," I said, handing Marion a glass.

We blithely posed for a photo on the open-air deck, in front of one of the Tower's lightning deflectors, with the ominous clouds in the background. In one selfie, by the champagne bar, my hair is sticking out horizontally from my head, like I'm in a wind tunnel. I sort of was, actually.

Soon, the Tower's security guards were ushering us all down the stairs to the enclosed deck below. Just as we got to the foot of the steps, it felt like we were on a rocking boat. At first, I thought it was the champagne. A big "WHOA!" rippled through those of us on the steps and in the waiting area near the elevator.

I learned the next day that winds clocked at 100 kilometers per hour (60 mph) buffeted the Tower that evening.

The elevators shut down and for an hour, I sat on a tiny wooden bench attached to a riveted steel beam that ran up to the Tower's top. I was afraid to lean back. I didn't need curlier hair.

I saw flashes of light outside the rain-streaked windows. I assumed those little lightning deflectors were doing their job. I saw one bolt crack the sky, too close for comfort.

A photo on the internet the next morning of giant bolts hitting the Tower two nights earlier made me thank my lucky stars.

When the elevators started running again, the first passengers were children – a few of whom had been reduced to tears.

Marion and I were in the first group down in another car. But when we got to Level 2, where we had boarded a few hours earlier, the elevator doors wouldn't open.

The operator, who had placed a call to Mission Control, said it had been a "test" run and we'd have to go back to the top to re-set the system. Up we went again and then back down.

"*Huis Clos*," I said, trying to inject a little French existential humor into the elevator car. No one got the joke. But I truly felt I was a character in Jean-Paul Sartre's depiction of hell as a room with no exit. On our second descent, I decided I'd had enough Eiffel Tower "fun" for a lifetime.

It all ended well. A young Australian couple in our car had just become engaged moments earlier.

"You did a good job with the special effects," I teased the groom-to-be.

Marion's big wish on her Paris visit was to buy a "really nice" handbag, which took us to the Louis Vuitton boutique at Galeries Lafayette, Paris' amazing department store with its famous stained-glass dome that took Marion's breath away.

Our delightful salesman, named Eric, seated us at a table in a quiet sales room. He gave Marion a smart phone that had 500 bags to view. But Marion knew what she was looking for and it just happened to match the silhouette of LV's premium bag, "Le Capucine." There's a price spread with this model, but Marion fell in love with the top of the range. The Capucine bag Eric showed her – which he held in his white-gloved hand – cost nearly as much as my first car.

I gasped a little as she seriously considered it. And then better judgment took hold. She scrolled through Eric's phone and asked to see a more reasonably priced bag. At this point, I realized my definition of "reasonable" was shifting in a direction opposite to Marion's.

Eric produced a gorgeous bag – in a neutral tone that will wear well in all seasons. He kept Le Capucine on the table, knowing Marion was smitten with it.

He gave her some time to think a bit and asked me if we'd like something to drink. "Water, juice…" he asked. I didn't reply *"oui"* until he said, "Champagne?"

Within a few minutes, Marion and I were sipping in the lap of luxury. The bubbly was every bit as good as the Moët we drank at the top of the Eiffel Tower shortly before lightning bolts began dancing around us.

Marion chose the "reasonable" bag, with a promise to Eric that she'd come back next year for Le Capucine. We thanked him for a wonderful ending to her visit. He said he hoped he had added a bit of "spark."

"You were the fireworks finale," I said. "We'll be back next year."

He gave us his phone number and said he'd arrange a tour of Versailles for our next visit.

I had never had so much fun shopping for a girlfriend's handbag in my life.

The best part of this story is that after our former suitemates, Vicky and Jeannette, heard about our adventures, they decided to come to Paris the next year for Marion's Le Capucine purchase and Eric's promised tour of Versailles.

Chapter 50

I had one more day in Paris after Marion left. It was the first time I'd had a travel day to myself since before Covid.

I love solo travel and when I'm traveling alone, I have a rhythm to my day. I get up early and write a Facebook post and edit photos from the day before. I have a good breakfast before I head out to my day's destination. I find a place where I can linger for lunch and write in my journal. I wander a bit in the afternoon and do some photography later in the day when the light has softened. If it's summer, I often shop for a picnic supper and go back to my B&B for a late-afternoon swim and then have my picnic by the pool. That's my idea of a perfect travel day.

On my day alone in Paris, I had a wonderful breakfast and then sank into a big sofa in the lobby of the hotel, which had a cozy Old-World feel, with comfy chairs, shelves of books, a box filled with children's games, and two polished apples adorning an end table – I thought they were fake, but they were ready to eat. I wrote the story of Marion's handbag purchase, which I emailed to Vicky and Jeannette, and then was ready to start my day.

My destination was La Samaritaine, Paris' historic department store, known for its Art Deco and Art Nouveau architecture and décor. The store, which opened in 1869, closed in 2005 because of safety concerns and reopened in 2021 after extensive renovations.

I enjoyed lunch on the top floor, under the glass roof, at a restaurant called Voyage, whose kitchen is "guided" by a Michelin chef, according to the menu. I couldn't resist the Michelin-guided

"California Roll" with crunchy shrimp, avocado and candied ginger.

Then, after a delicious ice-dream dessert, I did a little shopping. I found a pair of earrings that I know I will love for the rest of my days. They're quite unique – a mismatched pair, it would seem – but actually, they couldn't be better companions and better suited for strolls around a special lily pond I like: One earring is a pink water lily and the other, a gold-and-purple dragonfly.

I picked up a few colorful kitchen items at the Pylones shop at Gare St. Lazare, before boarding the train back to Giverny. I walked to the end of the platform, hoping to find a mostly empty car where I could prop my feet up. I went all the way to the end and was in luck. My only travel companion was a man, with wavy white hair who looked to be in his sixties, seated across the aisle from me.

We didn't speak during the trip. When we arrived in Mantes-la-Jolie, about 40 minutes from Paris, I wasn't sure how many stops there were before Vernon-Giverny. I got up at the next stop and had trouble retrieving my bag from a tight luggage space. The man saw me struggling, with my cane tucked into the side of the bag, and got up to help me.

He was going to Vernon-Giverny as well and said we had another stop to go.

We sat next to each other, on the jump seats at the end of the car, and were quickly amazed by what we had in common. He had lived in California – in Palo Alto and San Diego. He knew Pasadena well.

He had sensed my anxiety about missing the stop and saw my cane. He said something about letting go of things that aren't important and finding peace in life.

We introduced ourselves. His name was Jonathan. He was French, but spoke English well, and said he lived near Paris. He told me he came often to visit friends in Vernon and Giverny.

"I'm sure if we had more time, we'd discover we have mutual friends here," I said. But we had no time. Within minutes, we were rolling into the Vernon-Giverny station. I gave him my card, which he tucked into his pocket. He had mentioned he would be attending a photography exhibit in Vernon and would send me the details.

As the train screeched to a stop, he jumped to his feet and opened the door. He slung his backpack over his shoulder and grabbed my bag, while extending a hand to me as I gingerly stepped onto the platform. *Très gallant.*

"Who's picking you up?" he asked.

"That gentleman there." I pointed to Henri, who was on the opposite side of a high chain-link fence that ran along the edge of the platform. He was hanging onto the fence, with forefingers hooked onto the wire mesh, like he was a spectator at a ballgame.

Jonathan walked over to Henri and told him how much he had enjoyed meeting me and was amazed by how much we had in common. Henri smiled. He always marveled at the magnetic pull I had, especially when I traveled. I'd meet someone from Naperville at an art gallery in Giverny or sit next to someone on a plane who had read one of my books.

Jonathan waved at an elderly woman who was standing near Henri and walked with me as we went out onto the sidewalk. Without hesitating, Jonathan went to Henri's SUV, opened the trunk and tossed his bag inside.

Henri and I looked at each other in surprise.

"Is he coming home with us?" Henri asked.

Henri and I burst out laughing, as Jonathan realized his mistake. He slapped his forehead, laughing as he took his bag from the trunk, apologizing. The elderly woman looked flummoxed by the whole affair.

As Henri pulled away from the curb, I waved good-bye to Jonathan.

Still laughing, I looked over at Henri and said, "There wouldn't have been room for him on the ménage-à-trois mailbox."

Henri had just gotten his first glimpse – a chain-link-fence view – of my life without him.

Chapter 51

An art gallery in the village was celebrating its tenth anniversary and I had been invited to attend the *vernissage* – the opening celebration – for a month-long exhibition featuring paintings of artists who had shown their work there over the years.

The gallery, called Galerie Blanche, is named after the street where it's located – Chemin Blanche Hoschedé Monet – the same street address for Henri's apartment and the ménage-à-trois mailbox. It's a prestigious address in Giverny – the former home of Madame Baudy is opposite the gallery. Both sit on the curve where Robinson painted *The Wedding March*.

As I approached the gallery, I wistfully remembered the day I had sat out front with Nataliya and her Ukrainian friend Olena, in the fall of 2018. I have a beautiful photo of them from that day. Nataliya is wearing an apple-green floral dress that complements one of her large paintings, of an iris in full bloom, that sits next to her. It was the day the butterfly landed on her painting of Monet's lily pond that hung on the gallery's stone façade. I wished more than anything to relive that carefree day – with the movements of a butterfly taking our breath away.

I knew Nataliya had been selected to be part of the exhibition, but her painting hadn't yet arrived from Kyiv because Andriy had had a problem with the export paperwork. There was a photo of the painting in the gallery's catalog. My heart ached. It was an oil of a beautiful field of blue muscari and yellow violas – the colors of Ukraine – called *Clairière bleu-jaune (Blue-Yellow Meadow)*.

Her artist biography in the catalog beautifully captured her spirit: *Nataliya never tires of observing the ballet of shadows and lights on nature whose subtle touch reveals the secret harmony. Her floral compositions of great delicacy bear witness to this.*

I knew it was Nataliya's hope to travel to Giverny the following year. I had a good feeling about that.

I saw Marie Noëlle – Madame Red Shoes – in the crowd and went to speak with her. The gallery's owner, Stéphanie Guyot-Révérend, is her daughter-in-law. Marie Noëlle had a pastel on display in the exhibition, of a golden velvet chair that sits in her solarium, with a glimpse in the background of that magnificent stained-glass window populated with exotic plants and birds.

Stéphanie spoke for a few minutes about her "adventure" as the gallery's owner. Over the past 10 years, the gallery had opened its doors to artists, first from France, and then from around the world – England, Spain, Ukraine, Australia, the United States and China. Galerie Blanche had hosted more than 250 artists and 70 exhibitions. I so appreciated Stéphanie's effort to keep Giverny's art-colony tradition alive.

I saw an Australian artist I knew, Tanya Frazier, standing by the door to the gallery, and went over to say hello. She, too, was part the exhibition and had made a special trip to Giverny to join the celebration. Her painting – a colorful, dreamy rendering of water lilies – had already sold that evening. We made plans to meet for coffee. I hadn't seen her since 2019.

It was a hot day and the air inside the gallery was still and uncomfortably warm. The lights had been turned off, to keep things cool. I had ventured only a few steps inside and thought I'd come back another day to see the paintings when a small group of guests just inside the doorway dispersed and I saw a woman at the other end of the gallery looking at me.

I blinked hard. She was wearing a lovely, loose-fitting, white blouse over black trousers. The blouse was nearly the color of the gallery walls. She seemed like an apparition to me.

She moved slowly toward me, smiling. "Rebecca," she said.

"Can it really be you?" I choked back tears.

It was Olena.

The last time I had seen Olena was in that very room, as she translated Nataliya's story of her painting of the red poppies.

Not until we embraced did I know for sure I wasn't dreaming.

Olena shared with me the heartbreaking story of her escape from Ukraine as we had lunch the next day.

She and her 24-year-old daughter fled their home in Irpin a month after the invasion began and ended up in Poitiers, an historic university town in west-central France. Her daughter had enrolled in the university there. Olena had become a French teacher to many Ukrainians who had settled there.

Her husband and 29-year-old son had stayed behind in Kyiv. "They are patriots," Olena said proudly as she showed me photos of them on her phone.

She showed me other photos that broke my heart.

"This is my street where I lived in Irpin," she said.

A blasted apartment building, with windows blown out, towered over a huge pile of charred rubble upended in an apparent bombing. On the side of a scorched wall, a street artist had rendered the elegant form of a young girl gymnast, whose left foot was perched on top of a black hole in the side of the building. Her right arm gracefully mirrored the backward extension of her right leg. Her left hand, held high above her head, clung to a stick attached to a long ribbon that floated above and around her body, as if suspended in a breeze. To me, she embodied the beautiful youthful spirit of defiance and hope.

I took a deep breath and felt like I had inhaled a shard of glass. Olena put her arm around my shoulder and hugged me, as I started to cry.

I brushed away tears through most of our lunch together. She showed me other images of poignant artist's renderings: The silhouettes of two children on a concrete roadblock who appear to be "seesawing" on an anti-tank hedgehog. A mural of another young gymnast powerfully pushing herself into a handstand below a dangling metal beam that had been dislodged during an explosion. And then there was the much-seen image of a small boy flipping Putin onto his back – both of them in judo gis – on the whitewashed surface of a crumbling brick wall.

Olena spoke of a collection of stories she was working on about the invasion, as told by Ukrainian women who endured the attacks, fled with their children, lost their homes and everything they owned, witnessed the death of family members and friends.

I admired Olena's bravery. She had returned twice to Ukraine to see her husband and son.

"How is that possible? How do you travel?" I asked.

"By bus," she said.

"That must be very dangerous."

She nodded.

I asked how she had come to settle in Poitiers. She showed me photos on her phone of her husband who is an airplane *modéliste*. Before the invasion, he competed internationally with model planes he designed. One of the big competition venues is Poitiers, where they had made many friends over the years. I could tell as she scrolled through photos of her husband how much she missed and loved him.

When we arrived at the train station for her return trip to Poitiers, we made a plan to see each other again soon.

"Next year, we will have Nataliya with us," I told her.

We both had tears in our eyes as we waved good-bye.

The next day, Tanya and I met for coffee that turned into an early lunch that finally ended late that afternoon as the pre-dinner drinks crowd started arriving.

Tanya had been coming to Giverny for many years – since 2004, the same year as my first visit. She had taken a painting course that year with Gale Bennett, Giverny's American-artist-in-residence whose actual residence had been the Lodge.

She and I had become Facebook friends through mutual acquaintances and had finally met in 2019, when we'd spent some time together. She was hoping to get a long-term French visa that would allow her to move to Giverny. With each visit to Giverny, she had brought belongings to set up a home at some point. But after her return to Sydney in 2019, just months before Covid made travel impossible, she experienced an unexpected turn in personal and professional circumstances that rooted her again in Australia.

That day over coffee-that-turned-into-lunch, we talked a lot about the pull of Giverny we had both felt and the thousands of miles we had traveled, from opposite sides of the world, in our journeys to come here. We had both experienced some "dream shifting" as we found our place in Giverny. She no longer felt compelled to be a full-time resident. But she welcomed opportunities that would bring her back to Giverny.

The Galerie Blanche exhibition had certainly been a serendipitous opportunity for her to return. She was already planning an exhibition for the following spring at the gallery. She had stored a number of paintings in Giverny that she couldn't take back to Australia because of import restrictions on wood products – such as the wood stretchers on paintings that might be infested with insects, especially if the paintings had been stored in old buildings, which had been the case with her work.

She hadn't seen the paintings she had left behind for several years. On Tanya's last day in Giverny, Stéphanie graciously invited us to brunch at her Vernon gallery space, located in an ancient half-timbered house opposite the church. On the walls of the gallery,

Stéphanie had hung the paintings Tanya had left with her over the years.

Tanya was thrilled to see her work again, from a time when she was experimenting with Impressionistic techniques she had learned under Gale's tutelage.

What Tanya calls her breakthrough painting – a large tableau of the lily pond – was on the wall, facing her, as we had brunch served on an antique dresser, covered with a linen cloth, that served as a makeshift table.

"I want to keep that one," Tanya told Stéphanie. It was far too large for a suitcase and because of Australia's wood-import restriction, she'd need to remove the canvas from the stretcher and ship the canvas flat in a sturdy box, or possibly a crate – a big expense. A problem for another day.

A painting next to the lily-pond picture had caught my eye. It, too, was a view of the pond, but from a different vantage point, with a cluster of burgundy-colored leaves in silhouette against the rich blue hues, tinged with hints of green and rose, that she had chosen to depict the pond's surface.

I turned to Tanya and asked, "Is that one for sale?"

"You can have it as a gift," she said.

"That's very generous," I said. "What would you like for it?"

"Whatever you'd like to give me."

I had been to the bank a few days earlier and knew I had more cash than usual in my wallet. "Let me see what I have."

I took my wallet from my handbag and counted the bills. "I have 150 euros," I said, smiling.

She smiled, too. "Sold."

Just the day before, Stéphanie had hung a small painting of Tanya's at Galerie Blanche, depicting the boats the gardeners use to tend to the water lilies. Tanya told me she hoped the painting sold before her departure so that she'd have some extra cash for the trip home.

"How much do you hope it sells for?" I had asked her.

"I'd be happy with 150 euros."

When I brought home my new painting that evening, I propped it up on top of the harmonium in the living room and leaned it against the painting already on the wall – by Gale Bennett himself, whose studio had been on the other side of that wall years earlier. I knew he wouldn't mind being partly obscured. I got goosebumps as I looked at the paintings together: The master looking over the shoulder of his very talented protégé. The scenes they had painted at Monet's lily pond seemed to flow one into the other.

Tanya had done a good job of purging what she had stashed in Giverny over the years. On her last night, we had dinner at the Baudy.

"I've had a realization," she said. "I thought by bringing all my special things here, it would make this place my home. But that didn't happen."

I thought of Nataliya's realization about material things: *How fragile everything is in this world. How illusory are the material values that we create.*

In the tradition of Giverny's art-colony painters, who often left behind belongings – and paintings that paid for room and board – Tanya left me with a few of her trinkets and souvenirs that she couldn't quite squeeze into her suitcase. My favorite: A teapot she bought some years ago in North Yorkshire, England, at Swineside Teapottery, known for its unusual collectible teapots. The pot is so like us, we decided. The bottom of the pot is a steamer trunk with Orient Express stickers and the teapot lid is a suitcase (no doubt over its carry-on weight limit) that's essentially a table holding a champagne bottle, a tin of caviar, a copy of *Vogue*, tickets, a passport, and a cheetah-fur hat with a pair of gloves to keep head and hands warm.

We stopped by Galerie Blanche one last time. There on the wall was Nataliya's *Clairière bleu-jaune* that had arrived that day from Ukraine.

I looked forward to having a tea party for all my artist friends someday, in the home that's meant to be mine.

Chapter 52

We were well into summer. Maxine and Olivier had gone off on holiday, so I'd had a reprieve from her venomous texts. Henri wasn't pressuring me to leave his place, so at least I didn't have that as an added stress.

One Sunday night at dinner, Henri casually informed me that Bernadette had decided to sell Doo-Doo and the Goat Girls to a farmer who had grazing land in a nearby village. She wanted to be free to travel without the trouble and expense of arranging and paying for their care.

I was stunned. I understood the responsibility that comes with animal care – which had been hers alone. But apparently, she saw them mostly as a burden.

"When will this happen?"

"In a couple of days," he said vaguely.

I later found out that he had known this was coming for a couple of weeks, but hadn't told me.

The next morning, I woke up to find that Doo-Doo and the Goat Girls were gone. I hadn't had a chance to say good-bye.

In my last Doo-Doo Facebook post, I wrote:

I can't quite describe my feelings of loss. I have written about the animals of Doo-Doo Land for four years. Friends who come to visit me in Giverny want to meet them. A few years ago, an artist friend came to sketch Doo-Doo and Praline, the sweet goat who had been his corral mate for many years.

When I looked out the kitchen window on Monday morning, I focused on the stones in the middle of the corral that mark Praline's grave.

As many of you came to realize, my stories of Doo-Doo Land were, to a great extent, an allegorical tale. I was much like Praline, who, after suffering through her head-butting period with Doo-Doo, found an escape in the shed that became hers alone. Finally – and ironically – she left this world just a few weeks before I returned to California in 2021.

I will gather a bouquet of flowers to put on her grave today. I'm forever grateful to the animals of Doo-Doo Land, for making me smile and for giving me perspective on my life here.

LOTM says he'll get a donkey or a couple of cows to keep the corral from becoming overgrown. We'll see what that brings. But for me, Doo-Doo Land will never be the same.

I included an album of my favorite Doo-Doo Land photos that told the story I had chronicled in more than 150 installments.

After I uploaded the post, I tried to go about my day. By about four that afternoon, Doo-Doo's American followers were waking up to the sad news.

The comments reduced me to tears. I could read only a few at a time. The outpouring of empathy and gratitude was overwhelming.

One friend wrote: *I am so sorry to hear this sweet and significant chapter has ended. So many endings in the world lately...or are we just more sensitive to the changes that take place around us all the time? Every ending promises a new beginning so I wish you a wonderful new chapter for your life. Doo-Doo and Praline had much to share with you and now it's time for something new.*

From a high-school friend, who had sat next to me in a creative writing class: *I have loved these stories, as have so many others. Change can be ruthless but it can also introduce us to things we might never have noticed. You have so much to share with your armchair companions. I may never get there in person, but you have brought Giverny to me and others. Looking forward to the next chapters of life in and around this beautiful village!*

I came to dinner that night, red-eyed. Henri asked what was wrong. I railed at him for his insensitivity.

"You knew this would upset me, and your way of handling that was to let it happen without notice. YOU HAVE NO REGARD FOR ME!"

He looked at me like a father whose child has just discovered that he had thrown away her favorite doll, who was losing her stuffing. My own mother had done that to me as a child and I never forgave her.

"*Chérie*, I know where they are," he said. "I'll take you to see them."

~~~

Several days later, Maxine and Olivier returned from their holiday. Henri had seen Olivier at the *boulangerie* and told him I was waiting to hear about an application I had submitted for a house. Henri hoped a promising prospect would keep Maxine off the warpath for a week or two.

But that didn't quite work. A few days later, Henri received a call from Yuka, who had invited us to a dinner party the next evening. She had also invited Maxine and Olivier, but Maxine said she wouldn't come if I were going to be there. Incredibly, Yuka and Henri decided that I should stay home.

He informed me of this that night at dinner. "I'll be out tomorrow night," he said nonchalantly.

When he told me that I had been uninvited by Yuka but that he would still be going to the party, I felt I had been kicked in the teeth. "Has it crossed your mind to stand by me in this?" I asked him.

"I've made my decision. I'm going."

I stood up from the dining table, with half my dinner still on my plate. "Do you know how much this hurts my feelings?" My voice trembled, but I was determined not to cry.

I went outside to water my flowerbed.

Henri made himself scarce the rest of the evening.

We didn't speak the next morning as we passed in the kitchen. He was out all day. I made arrangements to meet a friend for dinner.

Henri went to Yuka's dinner party without me. When he came home, he started to tell me who had been there and what Yuka had served. He saw I wasn't interested in hearing the details of his evening, so he left the room and got ready for bed.

I went to the bathroom to wash my face and brush my teeth. As I came out into the hallway, Henri stood waiting for me, wearing only his boxer shorts, with his pot belly hanging over the elastic band of his underwear. He was grinning. I had seen that grin many times. After a row, when he knew he was in the wrong, he'd come back a while later, with a big smile, like nothing had happened. The narcissist's self-absolution. I'm sure he had learned that behavior as a child, when he'd come in from school recess after hatching mischief on the playground.

I turned away from him and went to my room, firmly shutting the door behind me.

~

The next day, I had a freak accident while I was having lunch with Sarah at her place. I was sitting in a molded plastic chair and turned to say something to her as she was coming out of the kitchen. The chair tipped sideways and I tumbled to the floor. I twisted my left leg and couldn't get to my feet for about 10 ten minutes.

Sarah asked if she should call an ambulance.

"God, no," I said, suddenly seeing myself as an old lady who couldn't get herself off the floor.

In what could have been a scene from the Jane Fonda-Lily Tomlin series *Grace & Frankie,* Sarah went out to her garden and came back with a 10-foot PVC pipe intended for a trench-in-progress at the side of her house. She looked so comical – she was wearing a denim bucket hat with a fringed rim. I burst out laughing. I had a clear picture of us as doddering old ladies.

Sarah ordered me to "grab hold" as she led the charge up a steep garden path, past arbors of blackberries and grapes, to the gate, where I had parked.

I held onto my end of the pipe, which gave me some stability, surprisingly. But what a sight we were.

I drove home, with some difficulty. I couldn't raise my left leg. I actually had to lift the leg, with both hands, to get in and out of the car.

I took a paracetamol tablet and went straight to bed. When I woke up at about 7:30 that evening, Henri was in the kitchen, starting dinner preparations. I was in a lot of pain and hobbled with my cane from my room to the kitchen doorway. He looked up at me from where he was sitting on a barstool at the counter.

"I fell today," I said. "I need you to call Sofie and ask her not to come tomorrow because I need a rest day."

As soon as he heard me say "Sofie," he flew off, raising his hand in the air, as if to say, *Not this again!*

I shouted, "Did you hear what I just said? I fell today!"

That gave him pause. "Well, that's a good reason."

"If you're not hearing everything I'm saying to you, Henri, maybe you should ask me to repeat what I've said, before you react to the one word you've heard."

He didn't ask how I fell or where I felt pain. He didn't seem interested.

I made myself a Spritz and put it on a tray with a bowl of hummus and some breadsticks. I thought he might offer to carry the tray for me. But his butt stayed on the barstool as I made two trips back and forth to the living room, still hobbling on my cane.

He set two plates on the table for dinner. But when we sat down to eat, I noticed that he had set his place with cutlery, but I had none. He had served himself a glass of wine. He had put out an empty water glass for me, but there was no water on the table.

I flinched in pain as I sat down. "Could you please get me some utensils and a bottle of water?"

He silently got up and came back with the water along with two knives and a spoon – no fork.

"Could I possibly have a fork?"

He laughed at his oversight and returned with a fork.

I held the fork in the air for a moment, ready for battle. "Was asking for this fork too *demanding* of me?"

He didn't revisit that argument. But as he sat down, he launched into an incredible denial of his hearing impairment. "I don't have a problem with other people. It's just you. You speak fast and English isn't my language."

"Apparently, you're so deaf you can't hear how ridiculous you sound."

"What is deaf?"

"Are we playing the I-don't-understand-English game now?" I shook my head. "The only language we've spoken for the past five years?"

"What does it mean – deaf?" he persisted.

"It means you can't hear," I yelled. "Which, in your case, is a big problem when you don't listen well to begin with."

A couple of weeks earlier, I needed to move my car, which I had parked outside his museum. I reluctantly handed him the keys and watched in disbelief as he drove forward – not even 10 feet – and scraped the side against the chrome bumper of a vintage MG, owned by a friend of his, that was parked next to me. When Henri got out of the car, beaming, I realized he hadn't heard me screaming at him to stop nor had he heard the car's screeching sensor alarm.

"Are you now telling me you heard the sensor alarm that day and intentionally scratched my car?" I asked.

The next day, Henri left the apartment early and didn't come home all day to see how I was doing or if I needed anything. He made a brief appearance before heading out for a dinner and concert that was being held at the *boulangerie* that evening. I had already told him to cancel

379

my reservation. I couldn't sit on a hard bench, and I figured Maxine had already had my name crossed off the guest list anyway.

I was in my usual spot on the sofa and he sat down in his favorite chair. I reached up to brush some hair from my forehead and he saw a big bruise that had formed under my arm from my fall.

He looked a bit remorseful. He asked how I had fallen, but didn't seem to care about the details. He asked if I had something in the fridge for dinner, knowing full well I hadn't been able to leave the apartment all day to go to the store.

He didn't offer to water the flowerbed before he left, which was a nightly ritual on hot days. I went out, with my cane, and took my time soaking my plants, which were outgrowing their pots.

The evening sky was beautiful. I sent up a prayer to my angels: PLEASE HELP ME FIND A PLACE TO LIVE. I so wanted to be off on my own again, in a sweet little house with *un petit jardin.*

I still couldn't believe that the dream I'd had only six months earlier, of making a new life with Henri, had gone up in smoke.

Chapter 53

A couple of weeks later, at the end of July, I drove to southern Belgium to attend a Van Gogh festival. I was glad to escape Giverny for a few days.

I had met the organizer of the festival – a friendly guy named Filip and his lovely wife Dominique, both in their 50s – in Giverny in May. That same morning, I had received the exhibition catalog for a new Van Gogh show, which was then in Amsterdam and was coming to the Orsay museum in Paris in October, about the last weeks of Van Gogh's life in Auvers-sur-Oise, France. When Filip told me about the festival, I thought what an extraordinary coincidence.

I had started to do research for my next book, which would have a story thread about Van Gogh. I was fascinated by the many controversial theories that, in recent years, had debunked long-held beliefs about Van Gogh, with plausible evidence that he hadn't committed suicide.

I knew very little about his early life and became intrigued when Filip told me that Van Gogh, in his twenties, had spent a couple of years in Belgium's Borinage coal-producing region as a preacher and ministered to the needs of the miners and their families. To better understand the miners' plight, Van Gogh descended 700 meters (about a half mile) into one of the deepest shafts of the Marcasse mining site, near the Belgian town of Colfontaine. Each year, Van Gogh lovers gathered at Marcasse in a weekend celebration, with artists, of all ages, paying homage to him.

When Filip asked if I'd like to attend, I immediately said YES.

On the night of my arrival, Filip and Dominque invited me to a wonderful dinner at their home with family and friends. I was seated across the table from an American man named Walter, in his mid-50s, who looked much younger than his years and bore an uncanny resemblance to Van Gogh, with his red hair and bushy red beard. He wore a straw hat like Van Gogh's, minus the candles. I was relieved to see that both his ears were intact. I noticed that one of Walter's paint-splattered shoes had a plastic sunflower dangling from the laces. He was staying at a house nearby where Van Gogh had once lived. Walter was a professional actor and channeled the spirit of Van Gogh as he taught painting classes for children.

The group at the table was welcoming and interested in knowing about my life in Giverny. I loved their conviviality. Most were multi-lingual. Sometimes the conversation slipped into Italian, which surprised me. Filip later told me that after World War II, Belgium offered coal to Italy in exchange for labor. Many Italian men came to the Borinage region and the Italian presence there is still strong.

I felt so much a part of them, not like in Giverny, where I might sit for a couple of hours at a lunch or dinner without anyone turning to me to ask if I was following the conversation or trying to include me.

Filip knew I was looking for a place to live in Giverny and that there had been a problem, but I hadn't told him the details.

At one point during dinner that night, he said, "Rebecca, why don't you come live here with us in the Borinage?"

The group was enthusiastic and Filip's daughter, in her late 20s, took out her phone and began scrolling through listings on a real estate website.

"What about this one?" Filip asked. "We could go see this one tomorrow. It's not far from here."

His daughter pulled up a chair next to me, so I could see the possibilities.

I was so touched by their "come join us" hospitality.

I explained that I would need to get a visa to move to Belgium. They raised their bottles of "Vincent" beer – a local brew with a sunflower and a starry-night scene on the label – to that possibility.

I instantly felt at home.

~~~

There was a fascinating conversation that evening over dinner about Van Gogh's experience in the Borinage. Many at the table knew the details of his life story and could quote from his letters to his brother Theo, who was a key family ally during Vincent's struggles with poverty and mental illness.

Walter, who sat across from me, endorsed the new theories about Van Gogh's death – that he hadn't killed himself – but instead, the fatal gunshot had been an accidental misfiring by a boy who had been in possession of a pistol when he came upon Vincent in a field above Auvers-sur-Oise.

On his deathbed, Van Gogh told police not to go looking for an assailant. He claimed to have shot himself – that it was his wish to die. But recent studies show that, based on the trajectory of the bullet, the shot could not have been self-inflicted.

"He covered up what happened to protect the boy," Walter said to me. "Van Gogh was a caring, benevolent man. When you read his letters to Theo about his experience in the Borinage, you appreciate the compassion he had for the miners and their families. He wanted to understand their plight and help them."

His compassion is apparent in a letter he wrote to Theo in 1879:

I went on a very interesting excursion not long ago; the fact is, I spent 6 hours in a mine.

In one of the oldest and most dangerous mines in the area no less, called Marcasse. This mine has a bad name because many die in it, whether going down or coming up, or by suffocation or gas exploding, or because of water in the ground, or because of old passageways caving in and so on. It's a somber place, and at first sight everything around it has something dismal and deathly about it. The workers there are usually people, emaciated and pale owing to fever, who look exhausted and haggard, weather beaten and prematurely old, the women generally sallow and withered. All around the mine are poor miners' dwellings with a couple of dead trees, completely black from the smoke, and thorn-hedges, dung-heaps and rubbish dumps, mountains of unusable coal etc.

…The villages here have something forsaken and still and extinct about them, because life goes on underground instead of above. One could be here for years, but unless one has been down in the mines one has no clear picture of what goes on here.

Going down in a mine is an unpleasant business, in a kind of basket or cage like a bucket in a well, but then a well 500-700 meters deep, so that down there, looking upward, the daylight appears to be about as big as a star in the sky.

When Walter quoted that line to me – "Looking upward, the daylight appears to be about as big as a star in the sky" – I immediately thought of Van Gogh's famous painting *The Starry Night*.

Vincent's awakening as an artist happened during his time in the Borinage. When his six-month contract as a preacher was not renewed, he moved to a nearby village where he continued preaching voluntarily. But eventually, he found himself at loose ends – forsaking a comfortable existence, even covering his face and clothes with coal soot, to experience a miner's misery – and sank into a depression.

During this period, he had drifted from his family, who regarded his evangelical mission as another of his failures. He reluctantly reached out to Theo, who had supported him financially. Theo suggested he pursue his growing interest in art.

Van Gogh turned to his surroundings in the Borinage and took inspiration from the miners, weavers and peasants he had come to know. Initially, he was self-taught in his art studies. He read books about drawing and copied works by French Barbizon painter Jean-François Millet, whom he admired.

Van Gogh destroyed most of his drawings from this early period. But the few that remain – *Coke Factory in the Borinage* (1879), *Miners in the snow* (1882), The Magros and Zannmennik houses (1879-1880), and *The diggers* (1880), which is a close copy of a Millet painting – mark Van Gogh's birth as an artist. His later works of reapers and men digging in fields, some inspired by Millet's renderings of similar scenes, harken back to Van Gogh's artistic awakening in the Borinage and are testimony to his great empathy for the human condition around him.

~

That night when I got back to my hotel in Mons, about 20 minutes from Filip's home, I found a scorching message on my phone from Maxine.

She and Olivier had sent me a registered letter earlier in the week threatening to take legal action against me because my belongings were still in the basement at the house. Just a few days before I left for Belgium, the friend who had been thinking about renting the house decided he didn't want it, which meant I'd need to find storage space in a hurry knowing that Maxine would start spewing venom at me again.

Henri had met with Maxine and Olivier to tamp things down, but hadn't succeeded. At their meeting, Henri apparently had told them I was going to be out of town.

The message that arrived on my first night in Belgium read: *Henri came to visit us and we are happy. Know it's not his furniture and he can't do anything. We don't want to get angry with him, but as far as you're concerned, it's over. We have explained everything to him and he understands we are taking legal action against you. Your furniture and boxes must be removed before July 31, so remember to return from the Netherlands before this date. He says you were thinking of doing it on August 6 or 8, but it will be too late.*

The Netherlands?

When I spoke with Henri the next morning, I asked, "Did you tell them I was in the Netherlands?"

He went quiet for a moment, then quickly recovered. "You're in Belgium."

I knew he had associated anything Van Gogh with the Netherlands, but I had clearly told him the festival was in Belgium.

We discussed how to handle the situation. It was Friday, July 28. There was no way I could have a moving crew at the house by Monday.

"How upset is she?" I asked Henri.

"You know her. She's threatening to throw your stuff into the street and have a sale."

I stifled a laugh. I imagined her setting a torch to the pile.

Henri offered to call a local moving company. I told him I'd contact the mover that had handled the container delivery. I sent Maxine a WhatsApp text that I would only communicate with her in the future by email. If she was threatening legal action against me, I wanted everything documented by email. I told her Henri and I were contacting movers and that I would send her an update.

Filip had made arrangements for me to see local sites that morning. I texted him to say I was running late. I apologized when I finally arrived at his office.

He looked concerned as he greeted me. I took a deep breath. "The owners of the house I was going to rent in Giverny are threatening to take legal action against me. I've been trying to figure out what to do."

Filip looked stunned. "What are you going to do?"

"I'll deal with it when I get back."

Both moving companies Henri and I contacted didn't have crews available until the second week of August.

When I emailed Maxine to tell her that news, she informed me she wouldn't give a moving crew access to the basement unless I paid her 4,000 euros (about $4,300).

She wrote: *We are eagerly awaiting the exact date of the move. On the other hand, don't forget to pay your debt before the movers intervene. If we have not received the transfer before, they will not access the basement. The bailiff is only waiting for our green light to intervene. Here is attached the RIB of the account on which you can make the payment.*

I sent her messages to Henri so that he was in the loop.

"This is blackmail," he said.

"I think technically it's extortion," I replied. "Regardless, my belongings are being held for ransom."

～౿

I tried not to dwell on the churning cesspool back in Giverny. On the first day of the festival, Filip introduced me to Lorent Wanson, a well-known Belgian theater producer-director-actor who envisioned transforming the Marcasse mining site into a cultural event venue.

He knew the history of Marcasse and gave me a tour, pointing out a concrete cap that covered the opening to the mine shaft where the explosion had occurred in 1953. The site was in a state of severe decay. I felt uneasy looking up into the skeletal bones of the brick buildings where pieces of tangled metal dangled overhead. Shards of glass still clung to the frames of the window panes, where creeping vines had taken hold.

Lorent said to me, "Look around us. Nature is reclaiming Marcasse."

Tufts of green sprouted from crevices where mortar had fallen away from the bricks. Improbably, a young tree was growing on the roof of one of the buildings.

Lorent pointed to a lush forest on a hill overlooking the festival site. "That's an old slag heap. Look at what has taken root there."

He wanted to take me along a muddy track to where a herd of horses grazed in a thicket of trees. But I was on my cane that day and the path looked slippery.

"Another time," I said. There had been rain a few hours earlier. The grass was slick enough. "Do you mind if I take your arm?" I asked.

"Not at all," he said, tucking my hand close to his side in the crook of his elbow.

I spent much of the day photographing the setting and the festival participants. Artists had set up their easels around the site. During the course of the afternoon, the Marcasse landscape, vases of sunflowers, and portraits of Van Gogh took form on the artists' canvases.

By the end of the day, I was inspired to put together a photo book of the event, like I had done with Henri's engine show. I photographed a tuba player, who was part of the live entertainment, as he stood in front of a mural depicting the explosion of the mine. A big burst of light that looked like a star hovered over men crying out in despair. The horn of the tuba blended in with the scene and seemed to provide its soundtrack.

In the barroom, which served as a makeshift museum, miners' helmets, picks and lanterns were on display, along with the Van Gogh-themed paintings of the day.

At one end of a long table was memorabilia from the Vincente Minnelli film *Lust for Life*, starring Kirk Douglas as Van Gogh. Minnelli had shot scenes for the movie on location at Marcasse in 1955. Photos from the filming were on exhibit. A book had been published about the production, with locals – some of them extras in the film – recounting their memories of what it was like having a Hollywood crew in their village. There's a wonderful photo in the book of Kirk Douglas standing at the door of a house that was actually a set constructed of cardboard and plywood that had been built in the street outside the entrance to the mining site.

I loved the camaraderie of the visitors, many of whom knew each other. A big group of Italians who had gathered at a table for lunch invited me to join them. I felt like I was back in Italy. The Italian-language lobe of my brain woke up and I was surprised how easy it was for me to follow their conversation. They wanted to know where

I was from in the States and how I had heard about the festival. Many of them lived at the same retirement home. They weren't much older than I. Perhaps I should consider retiring in the Borinage, I thought. This was a fun group.

At the festival the next day, I was asked to be one of four judges in a children's art exhibition that followed an afternoon art class. I loved watching the budding young artists at work. They sat at long tables that had been set up under a big tent. On the tables were samples of Van Gogh's paintings. Some of the children closely copied his work while others followed their own creative instincts. I had the impression that two of the judges were art teachers. Walter, the third judge, and I hung back a bit during the judging. I felt a bit uncomfortable ranking the pictures. They all had merit to me. Along with the other judges, I had signed 20 certificates of recognition so that each child would be acknowledged for their effort.

I was happy that the "first" prize was awarded to the youngest exhibitor – a three-year-old boy who came to the stage with his face painted as Spider Man (face painting was a popular activity that day). When they handed him his certificate and a cool toy, he was elated.

I smiled at Walter, who was sitting next to me when the boy came to the stage. Walter leaned toward me and pulled something from my hair.

"A spider," he said.

I smiled. "Spider Man."

I was sorry to see the day end. A group of us went back to Filip and Dominique's for supper. I gave them a photo I had taken of Monet's lily pond in thanks for their hospitality.

One of their friends at the table asked, "Is this where you live?"

I laughed. I pointed to Monet's pink house in the background. "That's my place."

As Filip propped the photo on top of a cabinet in the room, I looked at the scene with new eyes. It had been my dream to live in Giverny and I had been convinced that it was the place meant for me.

But I suddenly felt a shift.

Chapter 54

The day after the festival ended – on Monday, July 31 – I didn't head back to Giverny, as Maxine had demanded. Instead, I headed for Bruges, about an hour-and-a-half's drive from where I had been staying in Mons. I had never been to Bruges, but had long intended to go there. This was my chance, Maxine be damned.

As my GPS led me into the center of Bruges, I thought I was traveling through the pages of a fairy tale. Church spires towered about the crow-stepped gables of old brick rowhouses, some dating back to the 1600s. Horse-drawn carriages clattered along the cobbled streets. I drove over a stone bridge where lovely old leafy trees formed an arch over a canal.

It was love at first sight.

That evening I walked from my hotel into the main market square just a block away and stood in awe of the scene in front of me. The 270-foot Belfry tower, the city's iconic landmark from the 13th century, loomed over me, backlit by the cobalt twilight sky. The song of the carillon bells (47 of them) was punctuated by the measured rhythm of horse hooves and carriage wheels on the cobbles. The far side of the square was rimmed with a colorful row of Bruges' distinctive gabled houses that provided a backdrop for open-air restaurants crowded with diners. Bruges had nearly suffered an economic collapse during Covid. But it clearly had recovered, with tourist season in full swing.

At a nearby restaurant, away from the crowded square, I had a delicious meal of *moules frites*. On the way back to the hotel, I did some window-shopping. The handmade lace displays were gorgeous. I stood at the window of a Christmas shop and sent Nancy some photos. I loved the Christmas markets of Berlin and during my last Christmas with her, the year before I moved to Giverny, I came back to Florence with an entire suitcase full of ornaments and decorations. The caption to the Christmas-shop photos I sent her from Bruges: *Uh-oh.*

A chocolate shop was still open. How could I resist? It was a good beginning. I had no idea then how refined my palate for fine chocolate would become.

I slept well that night and woke to the sound of the Belfry's carillon. The music of Bruges is its bells.

I headed out early to explore. I had the address of two shops I had read about online that I wanted to visit: a paper shop and a tapestry shop.

I was in the market for a new journal and there was a vast selection at Alfa Papyrus. I'm particular about my journals. I don't like lined pages. I want to be free to let my pen wander on the page. I sometimes make margin notes or little sketches. I like to insert faces to convey mood and emotion. Lines get in the way.

I found a beautiful little journal with flowers made of embroidered felt on the cover. I looked longingly at the exquisite handmade papers on display – the kind for covering a book or a treasure box – but thought I'd wait for another visit. The thought of another visit made me happy.

The tapestry shop called Mille Fleurs was a step back in time. Enormous wall hangings lined the walls. They were authentic Flemish tapestries made on Jacquard looms. Some were Old World scenes of palaces and pastoral landscapes, Medieval knights on horseback, Dutch floral paintings and the canals of Bruges. I loved the ones depicting the legend of the Lady and the Unicorn – they looked like they had come from the Great halls of ancient castles. Many were the tapestry version of famous paintings by Klimt, Van Gogh, Renoir and Monet. A scene of water lilies made my heart quicken a little.

I purchased a beautiful tapestry attaché case that Klimt himself might have designed, along with some small zippered coin purses and two beautiful lace doilies. The sales ladies at the shop were friendly and helpful. I commented about all the Monet-inspired merchandise in the shop.

"We support our European artists," the saleswoman replied.

"I live in Giverny," I said.

"Really? How wonderful!"

Another woman at the counter said she had just visited Giverny. "It's such a beautiful place. You must love living there."

I smiled. "It's like living in a Monet painting." Except for the toxic cesspools, I thought.

I had only one day in Bruges. I was tempted to extend my stay another night. But I knew I had dire matters to deal with on the home front.

The trip from Bruges to Giverny is about four hours by car, across vast stretches of farmland. I missed the turn for the road I wanted to take and ended up in outer Paris rush-hour traffic, which quickly erased the pleasure of the scenic drive to that point. I took the exit from the motorway to Bonnières, which is the back way to Giverny. A narrow road leads through the sleepy village of Bennecourt, on the banks of the Seine. It was in Bennecourt that impoverished Monet threatened to throw himself into the river if the local butcher refused to accept one of his paintings as payment. As the story goes, the butcher refused.

I wended my way through the labyrinth of winding village streets that gave way to the bucolic countryside as I headed toward the next village, Limmetz. I always loved this drive, with the hill above Giverny in the distance.

But on that day, with the golden light of late afternoon casting its glow on the landscape, I felt nothing but dread.

~

Over dinner that evening, Henri reported that he'd had a meeting with Maxine and Olivier and they were willing to reduce their 4,000-euro demand to 2,500 euros. He thought I'd be pleased.

"Henri, I'm not paying them ransom to get my stuff out of their basement. How do they figure I owe them 2,500 euros?"

"Lost income."

"They canceled the deal, not me."

Henri looked wrung out. "*Chérie*, it's going to cost you a lot more if they take you to court. Maxine is sure she's going to win."

I smiled. "I'm holding the high card."

"What do you mean?"

"What if the electric company found out that they had wired the meter at the house? That's a criminal offense. Sarah says you can do jail time for that."

"You've told Sarah?"

"I've told a few people."

"Why are you bringing on more trouble? They took the wire out when they installed the new water heater."

"If they removed it when my name was on the account that makes me culpable if I don't blow the whistle. I'm here on a visa, Henri. I could get deported if I don't untangle myself from this."

"Just pay them the 2,500 euros and walk away," he said wearily.

"I will pay them 600 euros for two months' storage. That's a fair amount." While I was away, Henri had gotten a quote of 300 euros per month from a local storage facility.

"What about the rest?" he asked.

"That's family mafia business. You work that out."

Henri rubbed a hand across his forehead. As angry as I was with him for creating this mess, I was livid that his brother – 15 years younger – was an accomplice in this scheme that was putting Henri under extreme stress.

"Henri, take a breath," I said quietly. "What they're doing to *you* is criminal."

And then he suddenly found his backbone. "I won't give Olivier the money until he hands me the key to the basement."

"Maybe you should see the state of things in the basement before you hand him the money. Maxine has probably smeared horse turds on everything."

I saw a flicker of a smile.

"You're going to write them a check, aren't you?" I asked.

"Absolutely not. I want no trace of this."

At that moment, I wondered if Henri had no intention of paying the balance. Maybe this was a scheme to shake me down for whatever Maxine and Olivier thought they could get. Did they think I was a rich American with deep pockets, I wondered.

"I would think you'd want proof," I said. "What if Maxine claims you never paid her."

"Maxine wouldn't dare cross me." Henri's jaw tightened. "Call the movers tomorrow."

Feeling like I was in a scene from *Godfather: Giverny,* I said, "There's one condition. I won't call the movers until they sign an agreement saying they won't bring further claims against me – financially or otherwise. And on the day, they will give me a letter stating everything has been removed and that I never lived at the house. Quentin says I need that letter to cancel the renter's insurance."

Henri looked at me in disbelief.

I stood up from the table. "That's the deal. I won't call the movers until they sign."

To make sure of that, I sent them a lengthy "American" email that night, outlining where they stood in legal jeopardy: signing over the utilities without a lease, extorting money from me, and wiring the meter. That email would be admissible in any case they might file against me.

~⌣

Maxine and Olivier had given Henri a deadline of noon the next day to give them an answer. If we didn't agree to their terms, they said they would call the lawyer and the bailiff. I didn't understand the role of the bailiff, who, Sarah said, would simply come inspect the property to verify the claim that my belongings were in the basement.

Henri came up from his office, flustered because the agreement I had written didn't format properly and took up more than a page. His hands were shaking when he handed me the two-page document. I looked at the time. It was after 11.

"Don't let them do this to you, Henri. I sent them an email last night. They'd be really stupid to go to a lawyer."

I quickly re-formatted the document and emailed it to him. He went back downstairs to his office to print it and came back for my signature.

He returned an hour later after taking the document to Maxine and Olivier and tossed a folder next to me on the sofa. "You didn't sign it properly."

"What's the problem?"

"You're supposed to write your name clearly on the signature line. Then below, you sign like this." He raised his hand and scribbled loops and curlicues in the air.

"My handwriting is beautiful. It's perfectly legible."

"That's the problem. All the letters are connected."

I glanced around the room to see if there was a hidden camera somewhere. Surely, this was a French farce fit for television.

"So, you want me to scribble my signature like this..." I said, raising my hand in the air and imitating Henri.

"Just sign it below in another way."

"In blocks letters, like a 5-year-old?" I printed my name in capital letters. "How's that?"

I handed him the "corrected" copy and he turned toward the door.

"That's it? They signed without an argument?" I asked.

"They said they aren't worried about an investigation about the wire," he replied.

"Good. I wouldn't want them to lose any sleep."

I went to the bank that afternoon and withdrew 600 euros, in 20-euro notes. I wrapped the pile of cash in a napkin and put it on the butcher-block counter in the kitchen. Appropriate, I thought. I used a napkin because it was "dirty" money, in my eyes. I was the co-star of this new Godfather movie.

Henri came home that night, after he had made the ransom payment, with the key to the basement.

The writer-in-me was doing backflips.

～ゝ

On the day of the scheduled removal – a Saturday – the moving truck had two flat tires on the motorway en route to Giverny and had to be towed.

Olivier told Henri he wasn't surprised. I told Henri to tell Olivier that when I contact moving companies I specifically ask if their trucks have bad tires and if they say yes, I hire them.

The crew returned on Monday. But they brought a small truck, which would mean at least two trips to the storage space our friend had offered. But when we arrived with the first load, there wasn't nearly enough space. Henri began making arrangements with the driver to take the second load to a storage facility the crew had access to about 25 miles away.

"No," I said emphatically."

"What do you propose?" Henri asked testily.

"We'll do what we did last time – we'll stack it all in your living room."

For the next 10 minutes, Henri and I engaged in a battle of wills.

At first, he wouldn't budge. "It's a simple solution. They can take it to a storage facility."

"That I haven't seen. It could have a leaky roof with mice running everywhere. Absolutely not."

"We don't have room at my place."

A few weeks earlier, I had cleared out the storage space Henri had built for me above the museum hall. It would hold most of the remaining boxes. We could stack the mattresses in the living room and make room for a couple of dressers.

I leaned close to Henri. "We're in this mess because of a broken promise."

"That doesn't help us come up with a solution."

"It might help you be more accommodating."

An hour later, the second truck arrived at Henri's apartment. Henri abandoned ship, leaving me in charge. The mattresses fit snugly up against a massive bookcase in the living room. The movers lay two large dressers on their sides, blocking the TV that never seemed to work, so no loss there. The boxes fit in the storage area – just as I had predicted.

Henri came home later than usual that evening, around 8. He walked in, looking relaxed. I assumed he had smoked a pack of cigarettes since I had last seen him and had had a couple glasses of wine at the *boulangerie*.

He looked around the room and said, "I like the décor."

He went over to where the movers had pushed a little velvet arm-chair, called a "toad chair" or *fauteuil crapaud* in French, up against his big leather easy chair. The toad chair was lightweight and sized for someone with a small bottom. I was afraid to sit on it for fear the frame would splinter.

In one swift move, Henri lifted it up above the dressers where the top of my dining table formed a large shelf. The toad chair looked like an empty throne perched there, four feet above the floor.

"I think it needs a teddy bear," I said.

Henri laughed.

That was it. Henri made dinner, as usual. We had a pleasant conversation during the meal. Nothing – NOT A WORD – was said about what had happened that day.

Chapter 55

The next day I left, by train, for Bruges. It had only been two weeks since my first visit there.

But I was on a mission this time. I had lined up appointments with several real estate agents to see apartments.

At first, it seemed like a wild idea. But I could no longer see having a happy life in Giverny. I was on my own there, fending off Henri's crazy sister-in-law. Although he had been my ally – sort of – in this face-off, he wasn't truly at my side.

After I returned from the festival, I had written to Filip about what had happened. I knew he was concerned. I had thanked him again for his hospitality and, in turn, he wrote: *It was wonderful to have you here last week. I think your enthusiasm is very inspiring and communicative. But your positive attitude may probably make some people jealous because they are unhappy. That's how I interpret the attitude of the woman and some other people in Giverny.*

I read Filip's message to Henri and he nodded in agreement.

"An astute view from afar," I said.

Filip had asked me if I'd be interested in helping with an application for a grant that he and Lorent were working on, for restoring and developing the Marcasse site as a cultural-performing arts center.

The prospect of starting a new life – with nice people who were embarking on a worthwhile, interesting project – was tempting.

I stood at the kitchen window early one morning, looking out at the empty pasture where Doo-Doo and the Goat Girls had lived. Henri had promised to take me to see them. But despite my repeated requests for that to happen, he blew me off. It wasn't a priority for him. He kept saying he needed to find out from Bernadette where she had taken them. He seemed to have forgotten that he'd told me he knew where they were.

Bernadette wasn't on the scene very much anymore. It seemed she had divorced herself from her old life and Henri. He said she was still angry with him about what had happened during Covid – a three-year grudge. "I see her sometimes," he told me. "But she's away a lot and doesn't tell me where she's going."

I opened the window to listen to the birds starting to wake up in the trees on the hillside. I loved their chatter in the morning.

I started making a list of what I'd like to have in my new neighborhood in Bruges: 1) Church bells (easy). 2) Bird song and/or the clomp of horse hooves.

Filip had sent me to the real estate website he and his daughter had used to find a place for me in the Borinage, on the first night of my visit there. The site had many rental listings for Bruges. Many of the properties had twice the space and at much lower prices than in Vernon and Giverny. A spacious two-bedroom apartment rented for about 1,200 euros a month – $1,300. I had paid more than double that in Del Mar.

On the train to Bruges that day, I thought about my apartment search in Florence, in 2009. I hadn't known anyone in Florence when I arrived. I had contacted a few real estate agents in advance. But I was totally alone in my search for a new home there. Once again, I was starting from scratch.

I had made arrangements to see five apartments in Bruges. On my first day there, I posted on my private Facebook page that I was leaving Giverny because I had been caught in a "swirl of unfortunate circumstances." I didn't explain what had happened or why I was thinking about moving to Bruges. I simply wrote: *I am alone in this and would appreciate some input, so feel free to post comments as I post apartment prospects.*

The response was overwhelming. As I posted the pros and cons of each apartment, my international "Greek Chorus" weighed in with thoughtful comments, as though they were right there with me. I was hobbling on Bruges' cobblestones with my cane because of my sore and swollen ankles. Chérie, my Corolla, would be making this move with me, so finding secure parking, without a long walk for me from her parking space, was essential. I wanted an apartment on one level, preferably on the ground floor. If the apartment was on an upper floor, the building needed to have an elevator. I very much wanted a patio or terrace garden.

Two of the five apartments quickly got crossed off the list: one had an elevator that had been out of order for some time and the other (a penthouse without a terrace) had a parking option in a public garage about two blocks away. I couldn't see myself schlepping groceries or luggage from the car to the building through sleet and snow – on a cane. I was facing the reality that I needed to plan for my needs as a woman in her senior years. My Glorious Act Three, as I liked to think of it.

On my first day in Bruges, I visited the Church of Our Lady, which was near the first apartment I had visited that morning. I sat in awe of the renowned Michelangelo statue, the Madonna of Bruges, which was beautifully positioned between pink marble columns on an elevated altar. This Madonna had famously been stolen twice: Once by the French during their revolution and returned to Bruges in 1816 after Napoleon's downfall, and then during World War II by the Nazis who smuggled her out of Belgium during the Allied advance and hid her with Hitler's art stash in Austria's Altaussee salt mine where she was rescued by FDR's Monument's Men in 1945.

Feeling inspired, I began writing in my journal as Andrea Bocelli's recording of "Ave Maria" played during a midday mass. But it wasn't long before I had to lay down my pen to let the tears come.

A young woman sat down next to me and asked what I was writing.

"I'm writing about this moment," I said, wiping away tears.

She held her hand to her heart. "I feel that way, too. Are you traveling alone?"

"Yes."

"Me, too."

I understood her wanting to share this experience with someone else – a feeling I've often had in my solo travels.

I didn't ask her name, but she told me she was from Spain. She looked to be in her late 20s. She was beautiful, with long wavy brown hair, bright eyes, a warm smile and several delicate silver nose rings.

When I told her I was from California, she was surprised by how far from home I had traveled.

"I'm living in France now," I said. "But I feel I need to make a change. I'm thinking about coming here."

"Here? In Bruges?" She smiled. "It's such a beautiful place."

"It's enchanting – like a fairy tale," I said.

"Yes, like that."

We sat together for a few more minutes.

As she got up to leave, she leaned toward me and said, "I hope you find whatever makes you happy."

More tears, but happy ones.

One thing I know to be true – there are angels among us.

I spent three days in Bruges looking at apartments. I always arrived early for the appointments so that I could get a feel for the area. I liked to visit the neighborhood coffee bar where the locals gathered.

On my last day, I had lunch at a café called Books and Brunch, around the corner from the final apartment I would be seeing that afternoon. Based on the apartment's photos and description, it was my first choice: a 2-bedroom, 2-bathroom unit on the ground floor of a renovated old property, with a small garden and underground parking. All the boxes ticked.

I instantly liked Books and Brunch. The café's walls were lined with shelves of new and second-hand books, for sale and for browsing. I opened a book on the shelf next to my table and the name

"Rebecca" appeared in the middle of a page written in Dutch. I took it as a good sign.

I had butterflies as I walked to the apartment. A horse-drawn carriage passed as I took a photo of the street, with a view of the Church of Our Lady just a couple of blocks away. I liked the idea of having Michelangelo in the neighborhood.

The young Belgian woman who showed me the apartment had gone to college in San Luis Obispo, California, where she eventually got her real estate license. In the next few weeks, she was planning to take her boyfriend on a grand tour of California, Utah and the Grand Canyon.

As she was showing me around, I met Hubert, who lived in the apartment next door and was the president of the owners' association – a friendly Flemish guy who was eager to show me all the features of the property. I also met a darling young couple who were heading to San Diego for a friend's wedding the following June. I told them to be sure to visit Del Mar.

Beyond the apartment's garden wall was the private park of an estate with a home for the elderly. I wouldn't have to move far when I reach the end of my Glorious Act Three, I thought. The park's tall trees that towered over the garden wall were magnificent.

I closed my eyes and listened to the birds.

It was the perfect place in every way.

Later that afternoon, the agent sent me a form to fill out that she would submit to the owners. She said I'd have an answer the following week.

A woman at the hotel's front desk, who knew about my apartment search, was delighted I had found a place and booked a table at a Flemish restaurant next to the hotel that had been a location in the Colin Farrell film *In Bruges*.

"You must celebrate," she said. "You are now one of us. Welcome to Bruges."

Later that night, I posted on Facebook: *This story couldn't have a happier ending. I have a lump in my throat just typing that sentence. Thank you all for the good advice and support you've given me this week.*

There were times when I'd read your comments and private messages, sitting in a café or on a park bench, and I'd start to cry happy tears. I feel so fortunate to have you all in my life. Please hold one more good thought that the apartment owners (and the Belgian Embassy) will say yes to this new adventure. My love and gratitude to you all.

The friend who had advised me to keep a magic carpet for emergencies, wrote: *I am happy that you have kept your magic carpet with you!*

My reply: *Such good advice you gave me about that carpet. It's a little frayed at the edges (the lovely fringe flew off somewhere along the way). But it's still serving me well.*

The next week, the apartment owners said YES. And a few weeks after that, the Belgian Embassy gave me a green light. Not quite believing all this has transpired in the span of four weeks, I began packing my bags for Bruges.

Sarah was very sad I was leaving, but promised to come visit often. Madame Red Shoes, always up for an adventure, promised to visit, too. I knew I would miss them both terribly.

~⁓

Henri's narcissistic behavior grew worse in my final weeks with him.

He stood me up for a dinner we had booked at a restaurant one Saturday night. We rarely went out anymore, but he was interested in trying a Mexican place in Vernon that I had discovered, run by a friendly American guy from Baltimore. When Henri didn't show up at the apartment at the time we had agreed to go, I went ahead without him, thinking something had come up and he would meet me there. I called and sent several texts from the restaurant. I had a drink and an appetizer and after a half hour, without hearing from him, I became worried there might be an emergency. And then I saw those telltale WhatsApp checkmarks turn blue, showing that he had seen my messages. I called again. He didn't answer. I stayed for dinner, the only one in the restaurant dining alone. Later that night, when he tried to tell me he had forgotten about our plans and hadn't seen my texts, I said, "Henri, those blue checkmarks are trip wires for liars."

On his 80th birthday, he chose to go to a dinner organized by Maxine to which I wasn't invited. It turned out to be a much bigger affair than he had realized – it was a full-blown surprise party with many of his friends who had gathered at the hunting cabin in the woods above Giverny. When he later showed me photos of the party on his phone, I wondered if it occurred to him how excluded I felt, though, truth be told, I had declined other invites for gatherings at the cabin, cringing at the thought of the animal blood that soaked the ground there.

Henri clearly had made it known to friends that we were no longer together. My Facebook posts had announced my move to Bruges, which certainly must have been grist for the village gossip mill for a few days. Henri seemed indifferent and rarely even asked for updates as my plans evolved.

But one night, I witnessed, in shock, the unraveling of him.

Two hornets had flown into the apartment and were buzzing around the dining room chandelier. Henri had grabbed a battery-operated fly swatter, in the shape of a small racket, and took a swing as a hornet flew out from the globe of the chandelier and dove toward the table. Henri started pounding the table with the swatter, slamming it against my papers, some books of mine and a delicate piece of fabric that I had laid out to be packed.

"Please don't do that," I said as he pummeled the fabric with the racket.

He went into a frenzy, smashing the racket at least a dozen times on my things, while shouting, "You want me to stop?"

"Stop it, Henri!"

He threw down the racket and left the room.

I tried to keep my spirits up by spending time with friends. Poor Sarah had fallen in her garden and broken her ankle. When I went to see her one afternoon, I suddenly saw both of us as women turning the page to our Glorious Act Three. She greeted me at her door, sitting in a wheelchair with an oversized muslin baguette bag covering her cast to keep it clean. We needed to embroider the bag with cheerful silk-ribbon flowers, I thought. We would be ladies who grew old gracefully with stylish flair and good humor. We mustn't let ourselves down.

I was still hobbling around on my cane. My swollen legs looked like stovepipes. I had gone to the local pool a few times. Swimming was a good diuretic for me. But the pool had no steps or a ramp and I struggled to get out of the water by way of the ladder.

I felt self-conscious about the weight I had gained – nearly 15 pounds in the seven months I had been back in France.

"You need to take care of you," Henri said to me one day. "There has been such a change in you in such a short time." He put his hand several inches from his hip as if to show me how large my bottom had become.

I choked back tears.

"I'm not a doctor, but I think you have a cardio problem," he said.

If my voice hadn't been stuck in my throat at that moment, I would have said, *Yes, my cardio problem is a toxic man named Henri.*

Madame Red Shoes was a huge comfort. She and I had some wonderful outings during my last days in Giverny.

One afternoon, we paid a visit to Philippe and Véronique Perdrix, the owners of the home that had belonged to Angelina Baudy, situated on the curved street, across from Galerie Blanche, where Robinson painted *The Wedding March*. He often stayed at the white-stone house with its distinctive round window, at Madame Baudy's invitation. In an amazing revelation during our visit that day, Philippe (a direct descendent of Madame Baudy) shared with us that Robinson had photographed Marie in the back garden and that the elusive tree with the bent limb – an apricot tree – was still in place there when they moved to the property in 1983. It died several years later. He took me out to the garden to show me the place where it had stood. He and his wife didn't know the story of Marie or what became of her after Robinson left Giverny in 1892, but they solved for me The Mystery of the Tree.

As the time drew near for me to leave Giverny, I felt emotionally overwhelmed.

"I'm heartbroken," I told Madame Red Shoes.

She patted my arm. "You have been very brave. But wonderful things are coming."

As I finished packing, I gave special care to a souvenir from Bruges I had purchased: a small tapestry of Monet's lily pond, with wispy willow branches dangling above the water lilies.

I had shown it to Henri. "Not a Van Gogh?" he had asked.

"No. I want a memory of Giverny."

I thought about the early days when my romance with Henri was new. I had loved him dearly. He was charming and smart, generous, endearingly funny, well-read and well-traveled. He had brought Giverny's history to life for me. He was the "perfect package" in so many ways. But little did I know then that sometimes a monster lived under the lid.

I wondered, looking back, if he had ever really loved *me*. Or had he fallen in love with the *idea* of me – a much younger, vivacious American woman who wrote books. Had I been an ego massage for him?

I didn't have the heart, with my "cardio" problem, to ask him about that.

Life took a wonderful turn one October evening, shortly before I left for Bruges, when Kyle and Julia called to say they were pregnant again. She was 13 weeks along, due in April. They showed me the sonogram images. We loved the one with a little hand "waving" at us. All was fine.

To celebrate, Henri and I uncorked a bottle of wine I had brought back from a visit to the Loire Valley a few days earlier. It had come from a 15th-century wine cave in the village of Amboise, home to French kings and Leonardo da Vinci at the end of his life.

Before I went to bed, I posted an announcement on Facebook, along with photos of the wine-bottle label and a lovely plate of petite dessert pastries from our dinner that evening that I had arranged in the form of a child – a bite-size lemon tart for the head, a tiny square of chocolate cake for the torso, two little raspberry-tart hands and two eclairs for the legs:

So on this night, at a humble table in Giverny, we lifted a glass of a very fine French wine to a child who will be born next April to my beloved Julia & Kyle. We pulled the cork just minutes after hearing the news. To my first grandchild: I will save this bottle and give it to you on your 18th birthday, with a candle for you to blow out. We toasted you this evening and imagined you as a pastry confection. Welcome, little one! I can't wait to hold you in my arms. I want to shout from a rooftop that I'm going to be a Grammy!

The next morning, I read the post aloud to Henri, but struggled to finish it. I started to cry before I got to the end. He looked off in the distance, I suppose trying not to get caught up in the emotional undercurrent of a life that was quickly washing away around us.

On the day of my departure, Henri packed my car in a drizzling rain. I so appreciated his help with that. I could barely think straight.

As we said good-bye, we held each other tight for a moment. When I cupped his face in my hands and said, "Take care of yourself," he started to cry.

Facel followed me to the door as I was leaving. I rubbed his head as Henri looked on. "Take care of your Papa," I said to him. Facel looked at me with sad eyes, cloudy with age. He knew I was going. I knew I'd probably never see him again.

At the top of the driveway, I stopped and looked back. Unlike the day two years earlier when I had left for California, Henri was not at the door, watching me go. The man who doesn't like good-byes was true to form.

I took the high road out of the village – up the hill through the Tree Tunnel. I drove the backroads for a long stretch. I needed some time to decompress.

My heart ached. I was leaving behind a place I had loved, that I thought would be my patch of paradise for the rest of my days.

What I remember most, as I drove in the rain, was the smudge of gorgeous autumn colors along the fields by the road. I felt as though I were driving through a wet painting.

Several hours later, my GPS led me down a narrow side street in Bruges. As I stopped at the corner, I saw a reserved parking spot for a moving truck that would arrive with my precious things the next morning, across the street from my new HOME. I took a deep breath and told myself, *Be brave. Angels are near.*

EPILOGUE

During my time in Giverny, I learned the hard lessons of heartbreak: Broken hearts don't forget. They don't have to forgive. But they can let go.

When I watched my ex-husband walk out the door after our son's wedding, I felt myself let go of the anger I had held for years. In that moment, I felt grateful for the love we had shared that had brought our only child into the world.

In the grief that comes with heartbreak, I've tried to follow my advice to Julia: Open your heart and embrace what's to come. There's a world of wonderful possibilities out there. STEP INTO THE LIGHT.

Broken hearts heal. They can turn to something new and learn to love again.

I've learned that someone new – who might inspire the first chapter of a book – may be sitting next to me in an Italian piazza. Or his luggage cart may lock wheels with mine in a crowded airport. Or I might stop to admire a painting on his easel at Place du Tertre in Montmartre and minutes later, as I wait at the taxi stand, I look over my shoulder and there he is, smiling, inviting me to join him for a coffee. True stories, all.

I believe in serendipity. It opens the door to new possibilities. I've had so many chance encounters that have led to amazing experiences, friendships, love affairs.

Sometimes embracing new possibilities requires a leap of faith.

My religion is quite simple: If it's not meant to be, it won't happen. That's positive thinking with a double negative – I realize the irony in that. Believing *what's meant to be will happen*, to me, is the laissez-faire approach to life. Taking a leap, with the faith that nothing disastrous will occur, has sometimes led to incredible outcomes that have changed my life, for the better.

My new life in Bruges is testimony to that.

I have friends and family, here on earth and on High, to thank for always being near with a safety net in hand.

I especially wish to thank...

My son Kyle, who pushed my little boat off the beach, saying, "Mom, you need to do what makes you happy." And to his wife Julia, who has brought Kyle so much happiness. (They have different names in real life.)

Sarah, for her unfailing friendship that helped me through difficult times and for always being such good company. (She, too, goes by another name.)

Madame Red Shoes, for all her wisdom and good advice, often dispensed over a cup of tea in her beautiful blue-and-white-tile kitchen.

Jean-Raymond, both a wonderful chiropractor and friend who tended to the kinks in my writer's neck and was always a good listener.

Jose, the pain specialist, who (despite his thumbs of steel) soothed my injured ankles and made me laugh during my recipe-book crisis.

The present-day artists and gallery owners of Giverny who keep Monet's legacy alive.

Nataliya, Gosha, Andriy and Olena for inspiring me by their courageous example and for giving me hope that love and peace will prevail someday.

Filip and friends in the Borinage who have been so welcoming.

Henri (a pseudonym), who shared his Giverny world with me and made my life so much richer for it. And for bringing me a bouquet of lilacs from Claire Joyes' abandoned garden on the day I finished writing the first draft of this book. (He told me, with a wink, "Claire said it was okay.")

Last, but not least, Doo-Doo, Praline, Melissa and Maman, the sweet beasts of Doo-Doo Land, for making this story a poignant allegorical tale and for teaching me lessons of the heart.

AUTHOR'S NOTE

The word *enough* appears in this story 34 times.

It is a multihued word with many shades of meaning.

It can convey abundance, exasperation, a limit beyond reason, a sufficient amount, a tolerable degree or simply the warm pleasure of a full belly.

In this story, it conveys most of those things.

Henri and I couldn't get *enough* of each other in those dreamy early days of our relationship.

It was the word that ran through my mind as I stared at a little Christmas tree at four in the morning on the night of our police encounter during Covid. If it hadn't been so blustery cold that night, I would have gone outside and shouted *"ENOUGH!"* at the moon. Maybe Mimi, the neighbor's cat, would have come to comfort me.

In the end, *enough* was the word that ended a relationship that had grown toxic. When you've had *enough* heartache, you need to belt out that Barbra Streisand-Donna Summer song "ENOUGH IS ENOUGH" and move on.

Mostly, I like to think of the abundance that this word can convey – as in "there's plenty to go around." When there's *enough* joy to make you smile, *enough* love to fill your heart, *enough* light to brighten the darkness, then ENOUGH is a very good thing.

Made in the USA
Las Vegas, NV
21 December 2023

83426223R00246